Merkel Cell Carcinoma

A Multidisciplinary Approach

Molecular Medicine and Medicinal Chemistry

Book Series Editors: Professor Colin Fishwick *(School of Chemistry, University of Leeds, UK)*
Dr Paul Ko Ferrigno and Professor Terence Rabbitts FRS, FMedSci *(Leeds Institute of Molecular Medicine, St. James's Hospital, UK)*

Published:

MicroRNAs in Development and Cancer
edited by Frank J. Slack (Yale University, USA)

Forthcoming:

DNA Deamination and the Immune System: Aid in Health and Disease
edited by Sebastian Fugmann, Marilyn Diaz (National Institute of Health, USA), and Nina Papavasiliou (Rockefeller University, USA)

Fluorine in Pharmaceutical and Medicinal Chemistry: From Biophysical Aspects to Clinical Applications
edited by Véronique Gouverneur (University of Oxford, UK) and Klaus Müller (F Hoffmann-La Roche AG, Switzerland)

Molecular Exploitation of Apoptosis Pathways in Prostate Cancer
by Natasha Kyprianou (University of Kentucky, USA)

Antibody Drug Discovery
edited by Clive R. Wood (Bayer Schering Pharma, Germany)

Volume 2
Molecular Medicine and
Medicinal Chemistry

Merkel Cell Carcinoma

A Multidisciplinary Approach

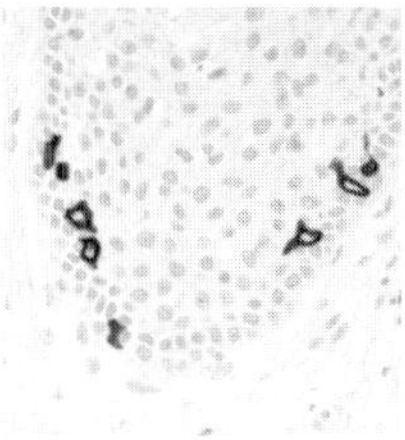

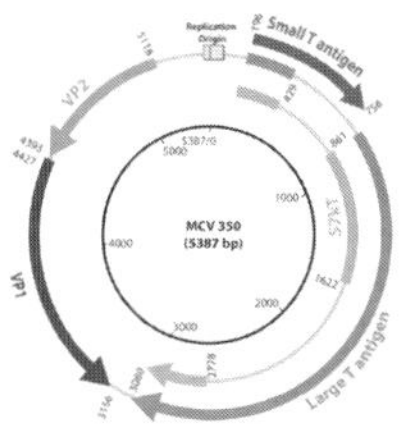

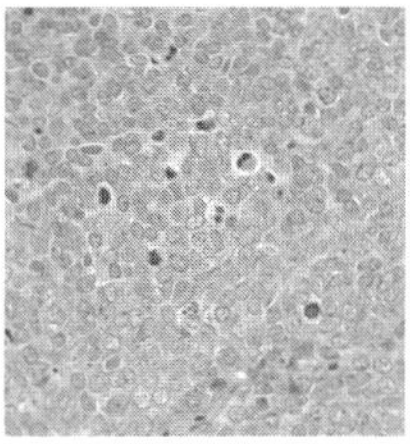

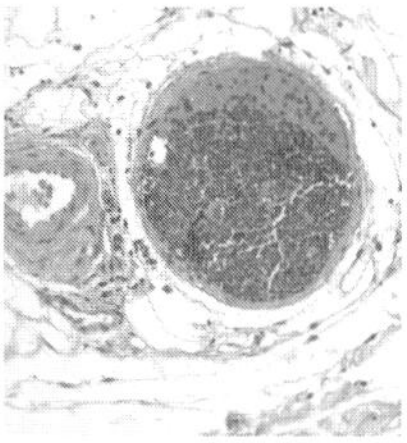

Editors

Vernon K Sondak
Jane L Messina
Jonathan S Zager
Ronald C DeConti

H Lee Moffitt Cancer Center & Research Institute,Tampa, Florida, USA

Imperial College Press

Published by

Imperial College Press
57 Shelton Street
Covent Garden
London WC2H 9HE

Distributed by

World Scientific Publishing Co. Pte. Ltd.
5 Toh Tuck Link, Singapore 596224
USA office: 27 Warren Street, Suite 401-402, Hackensack, NJ 07601
UK office: 57 Shelton Street, Covent Garden, London WC2H 9HE

British Library Cataloguing-in-Publication Data
A catalogue record for this book is available from the British Library.

Molecular Medicine and Medicinal Chemistry — Vol. 2
MERKEL CELL CARCINOMA
A Multidisciplinary Approach

ISBN-13 978-1-84816-312-6
ISBN-10 1-84816-312-6

Typeset by Stallion Press
Email: enquiries@stallionpress.com

Printed by FuIsland Offset Printing (S) Pte Ltd. Singapore

Dedication

We dedicate this book to our patients, who inspire us, and to our families, who support and sustain us. But most of all, we dedicate this book to Ronald C. DeConti, MD, who for nearly two decades has been the "go to" guy for many of the most difficult and problematic patients at Moffitt Cancer Center. His steady, insightful demeanor, his unfailing devotion to his patients and his willingness to "think outside the box" have made all of us better physicians and better people.

Vernon K. Sondak, MD
Jane L. Messina, MD
Jonathan S. Zager, MD

Tampa, Florida, USA
April 27, 2010

Contents

Contributors

Maria Agelli, MD, MS
Medical Officer
National Cancer Institute
National Institutes of Health
Department of Health and Human Services
Bethesda, Maryland, USA

Stephanie Andrews, MS, ANP-BC
Department of Cutaneous Oncology
Moffitt Cancer Center
Tampa, Florida, USA

Rosalind E. Atchison, RN, OCN
Department of Cutaneous Oncology
Moffitt Cancer Center
Tampa, Florida, USA

Melanie L. Aya-Ay, MD
Resident in Plastic and Reconstructive Surgery
University of South Florida College of Medicine
Tampa, Florida, USA

Evans C. Bailey, MD, PhD
Lecturer
Department of Dermatology
University of Michigan Medical School
Ann Arbor, Michigan, USA

Jürgen C. Becker, MD, PhD
Professor
Department of General Dermatology
Medical University of Graz
Graz, Austria

Claudia G. Berman, MD
Clinical Chief of Diagnostic Imaging
Department of Diagnostic Imaging
Moffitt Cancer Center
Professor
Department of Oncologic Sciences
University of South Florida College of Medicine
Tampa, Florida, USA

Christopher K. Bichakjian, MD
Assistant Professor
Department of Dermatology
University of Michigan Medical School
Ann Arbor, Michigan, USA

Simon Brodsky
Research Assistant
Department of Diagnostic Imaging
Moffitt Cancer Center
Tampa, Florida, USA

Basil S. Cherpelis, MD
Associate Professor
Department of Dermatology and Cutaneous Surgery
University of South Florida College of Medicine
Cutaneous Oncology Program
Moffitt Cancer Center
Tampa, Florida, USA

Limin X. Clegg, PhD, MS
Director, Biostatistics Division
Office of the Inspector General
US Department of Veterans Affairs
Washington, DC, USA

C. Wayne Cruse, MD
Professor of Surgery
Division of Plastic Surgery
Department of Surgery
University of South Florida College of Medicine
Cutaneous Oncology Program
Moffitt Cancer Center
Tampa, Florida, USA

Ronald C. DeConti, MD
Department of Cutaneous Oncology
Medical Director
Moffitt Cancer Center
Professor
Department of Oncologic Sciences
University of South Florida College of Medicine
Tampa, Florida, USA

Neil Alan Fenske, MD
Professor and Chair
Department of Dermatology and Cutaneous Surgery
University of South Florida College of Medicine
Cutaneous Oncology Program
Moffitt Cancer Center
Tampa, Florida, USA

L. Frank Glass, MD
Professor
Department of Dermatology and Cutaneous Surgery
University of South Florida College of Medicine
Cutaneous Oncology Program
Moffitt Cancer Center
Tampa, Florida, USA

Roland Houben, PhD
Department of Dermatology
Julius-Maximilians-Universität Würzburg
Würzburg, Germany

George Hruby, MBChB
Clinical Senior Lecturer
Royal Prince Alfred Hospital
The University of Sydney
Sydney, New South Wales, Australia

Charles Knapp, MD
Resident in Dermatology
University of South Florida College of Medicine
Tampa, Florida, USA

Bianca D. Lemos, MD
Resident in Dermatology
Emory University School of Medicine
Atlanta, Georgia, USA

Mary H. Lien, MD
Assistant Professor
Department of Dermatology and Cutaneous Surgery
University of South Florida College of Medicine
Cutaneous Oncology Program
Moffitt Cancer Center
Tampa, Florida, USA

Kelly M. McLean, MD
Fellow in Surgical Oncology
Moffitt Cancer Center
Tampa, Florida USA

Jane L. Messina, MD
Professor
Departments of Pathology and Cell Biology and Dermatology and Cutaneous Surgery
University of South Florida College of Medicine
Cutaneous Oncology Program
Moffitt Cancer Center
Tampa, Florida, USA

Paul Nghiem, MD, PhD
Associate Professor
Departments of Dermatology and Pathology (adjunct)
University of Washington School of Medicine
Affiliate Investigator
Fred Hutchinson Cancer Research Center
Seattle, Washington, USA

Tapan A. Padhya, MD
Director, Division of Head and Neck Oncology
Associate Professor and Vice Chairman
Department of Otolaryngology-Head and Neck Surgery
University of South Florida College of Medicine
Head and Neck Oncology Program
Moffitt Cancer Center
Tampa, Florida, USA

Angie Paniagua, RN, OCN
Department of Cutaneous Oncology
Moffitt Cancer Center
Tampa, Florida, USA

Melanie D. Prince, MD
Resident in Plastic and Reconstructive Surgery
University of South Florida College of Medicine
Tampa, Florida, USA

Christopher A. Puleo, PA-C
Department of Cutaneous Oncology
Moffitt Cancer Center
Tampa, Florida, USA

Dana E. Rollison, PhD
Associate Professor
Department of Cancer Epidemiology and Genetics
Moffitt Cancer Center
Department of Oncologic Sciences
University of South Florida College of Medicine
Department of Epidemiology and Biostatistics
University of South Florida College of Public Health
Tampa, Florida, USA

Wolfram A. Samlowski, MD
Professor and Chief
Section of Melanoma, Renal Cancer and Immunotherapy
Nevada Cancer Institute
Las Vegas, Nevada, USA

David Schrama, PhD
Assistant Professor
Department of General Dermatology
Medical University of Graz
Graz, Austria

Vernon K. Sondak, MD
Chair, Department of Cutaneous Oncology
Moffitt Cancer Center
Professor
Departments of Oncologic Sciences and Surgery
University of South Florida College of Medicine
Tampa, Florida, USA

John F. Thompson, MD
Executive Director
Melanoma Institute Australia
Professor of Melanoma and Surgical Oncology
Sydney Medical School
The University of Sydney
Sydney, New South Wales, Australia

Ashani T. Weeraratna, PhD
Head, Cancer Biology Unit
National Institute of Aging
National Institutes of Health
Baltimore, Maryland, USA

Darcelle Welker, RN, BSN, OCN
Department of Cutaneous Oncology
Moffitt Cancer Center
Tampa, Florida, USA

Sandra L. Wong, MD, MS
Assistant Professor
Department of Surgery
University of Michigan Medical School
Ann Arbor, Michigan, USA

Jonathan S. Zager, MD
Department of Cutaneous Oncology
Moffitt Cancer Center
Assistant Professor
Departments of Oncologic Sciences and Surgery
University of South Florida College of Medicine
Tampa, Florida, USA

Foreword

Ronald C. DeConti, Jonathan S. Zager, Jane L. Messina and Vernon K. Sondak

Our intention in creating this textbook is to review the clinical, etiologic and research aspects of Merkel cell carcinoma, providing clinicians, scientists and patients and their caregivers alike with a single source to find information about this rare and challenging disease. The focus is on a multidisciplinary approach firmly grounded in the latest scientific advances, in hopes of transitioning our management of Merkel cell carcinoma into the molecular era.

The initial chapters cover the epidemiology and biology of Merkel cell carcinoma, areas where some of the most rapid and unexpected advancements have taken place. Maria Agelli, MD, and Limin Clegg, PhD, provide a comprehensive review of the etiology of this disease, while Jürgen Becker, MD, PhD, David Schrama, PhD, and Roland Houben, PhD, review the burgeoning literature on its molecular biology and pathobiology. It was the epidemiologic data linking Merkel cell carcinoma to immunosuppression that led to the pioneering studies of a possible viral etiology for this tumor, a story that is related by Dana Rollison, PhD, and Jürgen Becker, MD, PhD, who summarize the multiple investigations that have demonstrated the presence of a previously undiscovered polyomavirus in the DNA of some Merkel cell carcinomas. Molecular profiling and genomic analysis is still in its infancy for Merkel cell carcinoma, but Ashani Weeraratna, PhD, provides an outstanding primer on the current value and potential future benefits of these approaches.

The pathology, clinical presentation, staging and prognostication of Merkel cell carcinoma is covered in the next set of chapters. Jane

Messina, MD, provides an outstanding overview of the pathology of localized and metastatic Merkel cell carcinoma that is as important — and as accessible — for the clinician and the researcher as for the expert dermatopathologist. Mary Lien, MD, Frank Glass, MD, and Neil Fenske, MD, describe the clinical presentation and challenging differential diagnosis for this tumor, and stress the difficulty identifying it prior to biopsy diagnosis given the myriad of other cutaneous lesions that can present in virtually the same fashion. Bianca Lemos, MD, and Paul Nghiem, MD, PhD, discuss the staging systems for Merkel cell carcinoma, and the importance of accurate staging for prognostication and for comparison of results across centers and, in this disease, across continents. Charles Knapp, MD, Jonathan Zager, MD, Jane Messina, MD and Vernon Sondak, MD, delve into the multiplicity of new prognostic markers — histologic, immunohistochemical and molecular — that may soon improve our ability to personalize care by more accurately identifying lesions at increased risk of recurrence and/or metastasis, and in the longer term by beginning to identify those tumors most likely to respond to chemotherapy or radiation.

The current standard of management for Merkel cell carcinoma is addressed by the next group of chapters. Simon Brodsky, MD, Jonathan Zager, MD, and Claudia Berman, MD, outline the most commonly used imaging modalities for Merkel cell carcinoma, including a particularly detailed and definitive discussion of radionuclide lymphoscintigraphy for identifying the sentinel node or nodes in clinically node-negative cutaneous Merkel cell carcinoma. Surgical management, including sentinel node biopsy, is then covered by Melanie Prince, MD; Wayne Cruse, MD; Vernon Sondak, MD, and Jonathan Zager, MD, who provide an overall discussion, and by Tapan Padhya, MD, Melanie Aya-ay, MD and Wayne Cruse, MD, who focus on the specific surgical aspects relevant to head and neck primary tumors. The important role of Mohs micrographic surgery for selected patients with primary Merkel cell carcinoma is nicely summarized by Basil Cherpelis, MD. Few aspects of the management of Merkel cell carcinoma have engendered more controversy than the role of radiation therapy. The chapter by George Hruby, MBChB, and John Thompson, MD, not only presents the Australian viewpoint but summarizes the key areas of the debate so that all clinicians can make more informed choices for their patients. In the next two chapters, Ronald DeConti, MD, covers the use of systemic chemotherapy for the management of established metastatic or recurrent tumors and for their prevention by adjuvant chemotherapy.

The future management of Merkel cell carcinoma, however, is likely to rely heavily on new modalities of treatment that currently are only in the earliest stages of development. Wolfram Samlowski, MD, and Jürgen Becker, MD, PhD, describe the multiple molecular targets that may have relevance to inhibitors under development, and describe the first prospective, multicenter clinical trial of a targeted therapy, the tyrosine kinase inibitor imatinib, in metastatic Merkel cell carcinoma. They highlight c-kit, survivin, VEGF and PDGF receptors, and acetylcholine receptors as exciting potential molecular targets for inhibition. Kelly McLean, MD, Ronald DeConti, MD, and Vernon Sondak, MD, discuss the potential applications of immunotherapeutic strategies to Merkel cell carcinoma, drawing heavily on efforts in other malignancies, especially small cell lung cancer and malignant melanoma.

Regardless of which, if any, new therapies emerge for Merkel cell carcinoma, one prediction for the future management of this disease is already coming true: the optimal patient care is provided by multidisciplinary teams of clinicians and researchers. Evans Bailey, MD, PhD, Sandra Wong, MD, and Christopher Bichakjian, MD, describe how they organized and conduct the successful multidisciplinary Merkel cell carcinoma clinic at the University of Michigan, Ann Arbor, Michigan, providing a model for other centers to emulate. Taking this multidisciplinary approach a step further, Christopher Puleo, PA-C, Jonathan Zager, MD, and Vernon Sondak, MD provide in Appendix I a broad set of guidelines for individualized patient management, seeking to move beyond the paradigm of "one size fits all" management algorithms to define the optimum approach for each individual patient, and at the same time identify opportunities for further research in areas where current approaches are insufficient or at least insufficiently studied. Finally, it stands to reason that if experienced clinicians are confused (or at least cannot agree) on the optimum approach, then patients and their family members and caregivers are going to be even more confused and frustrated. The final two appendices are for them. Mary Lien, MD, Darcelle

Welker RN, Stephanie Andrews, RN and Paul Nghiem, MD, address a series of “frequently asked questions” about this disease, while Rosalind Atchison, RN, Angie Paniagua, RN, and Jane Messina, MD, provide some guidance and assistance to the growing number of patients, friends and family who turn to the internet for information about this rare malignancy. If in some small way, this information assists patients and families as they battle this formidable foe, then we will have contributed something worthwhile indeed.

Acknowledgments

The authors wish to acknowledge the outstanding support and expert assistance we receive every day, but particularly in the preparation of this textbook, from Vicki Bassett, Administrative Assistant in the Moffitt Cutaneous Oncology Program.

Introduction

**Ronald C. DeConti, Jonathan S. Zager,
Jane L. Messina and Vernon K. Sondak**

So, what is the impetus for the creation of a book on a disease as rare as Merkel cell carcinoma? The answer probably lies in the fact that few diseases have led to the promulgation of so many diverse management strategies, without a consensus as to which strategy is best, as Merkel cell carcinoma has. The rarity of this disease has caused confusion from the outset, beginning with the identification of its cellular origin (the Merkel cell), our lack of understanding of the physiologic role of these cells in human skin, and the difficult nature of its pathologic diagnosis. Merkel cell carcinoma has protean manifestations, mimicking many benign and malignant skin neoplasms, and is only rarely diagnosed clinically before biopsy. Its behavior has historically been likened to both malignant melanoma and, because of its neuroendocrine features, small cell carcinoma of the lung, but as we will see neither of these tumors is an ideal template on which to base management decisions.

Our goal, as will become evident in the following chapters, is to lay the foundation for an evidence-based approach to the multidisciplinary management of Merkel cell carcinoma. We hope to provide the reader with an in depth look at the etiology, epidemiology, biology and pathology of this mysterious disease, focusing attention on recent advances in understanding its molecular origins, including evidence of a viral etiology. Despite many recent advances, most of our available information still derives largely from small, retrospective studies and individual institution data. Staging techniques have varied and staging systems have been largely derived empirically, with little or no prospective data to validate stage definitions. However, it is our intent to piece all the available information together and present a clear-cut evidence-based framework to be used as a reference in treating the patient with Merkel cell carcinoma. In the process, we hope to spark interest in ongoing research and clinical trials for this disease, and also to demonstrate that Merkel cell carcinoma is quite distinct and different from melanoma and small cell lung cancer!

It is in the arena of treatment that the most divergent opinions and practices have burgeoned. Management strategies have ranged from simple conservative or Mohs micrographic surgeries to radical resections with elective regional node dissections. The role of radiation to the primary resection bed and the regional nodal basin varies widely amongst institutions and across continents. Debate persists as to its role as an adjuvant therapy after a node dissection, its use in lieu of a node dissection, and the additive value of radiation to the primary surgical bed after a radical resection. What is evident and all can agree on is that Merkel cell carcinoma is a radiosensitive tumor, and there is a role for radiation in appropriate cases. Systemic chemotherapy, either as neoadjuvant, adjuvant or definitive treatment, also has a role to play. We hope to provide an evidence-based approach as to the potential benefits of both modalities as well as the optimal timing and integration of treatment. Certainly, a consistent philosophy espoused throughout this book is that elucidating the limitations of our knowledge will motivate organized efforts to collect meaningful outcome data that will guide future improvements in treatment.

Set against this morass of background data and clinical confusion, we have been confronted with an explosion of scientific knowledge about the basic biology and etiology of Merkel cell carcinoma, which if properly translated could lead to new clinical insights, novel prevention and treatment strategies, and improved outcomes for our patients. In this book, we have endeavored to collate what is known about the disease, and fully believe that we stand at the threshold of major improvements to our understanding and, hopefully, management of this disease.

In a very real sense, this book more literally outlines the questions that remain and the gaps in our current knowledge, rather than attempting to provide definitive answers the available evidence cannot sustain. At the same time, the directions we must go to achieve progress in this disease appear clear. Prospective evaluations of therapeutic choices based on cohorts of patients accurately diagnosed and consistent staged are clearly needed. The rarity of this tumor will necessitate improved efforts within a given institution and the cooperation of multiple institutions. We demonstrate that these efforts must include a multidisciplinary approach, with clinicians of all stripes working side-by-side with translational researchers. Hopefully, by examination of the issues raised in the chapters of this book, interested providers will develop an improved understanding of the limitations of our knowledge and, with that recognition, become more empathetic to efforts attempting to resolve that confusion by promoting and participating in the development of clinical trials which address these problems.

April 27, 2010

Chapter 1

Epidemiology and Etiology of Merkel Cell Carcinoma

Maria Agelli and Limin X. Clegg

Merkel cell carcinoma is a rare, aggressive skin cancer characterized by high incidence of local recurrences, regional nodal and distant metastases, and high mortality rate. As discussed in Chapter 6, Merkel cell carcinoma usually presents as a painless, nondescript skin lesion on the sun-exposed skin of elderly whites, who most often seek medical attention because of the lesion's rapid growth.[1] Merkel cell carcinoma presents most often as an asymptomatic, solitary, small red-purple subcutaneous nodule or indurated plaque, and usually eludes diagnosis until histopathologic examination.[2,3]

Merkel cell carcinoma has an estimated age-adjusted incidence of 3.2 per 1,000,000 person-years in the United States.[4] Its rarity, the difficult differential diagnosis with other primary and metastatic skin cancers, and the uncertainty of its origin continue to hamper studies on Merkel cell carcinoma etiology and risk factors, and on preventive and therapeutic strategies. Until very recently, what was known about Merkel cell carcinoma derived almost exclusively from case reports, a few larger case series and review articles compiling previously published case reports. Since its first report in 1972,[5] the literature has also seen a great number of articles discussing the etiopathogenesis of Merkel cell carcinoma across multiple medical and surgical disciplines.[6] However, much confusion on Merkel cell carcinoma origin and etiology still exists. The number of Merkel cell carcinoma population-based studies is very limited. Still, these studies have clarified the demographic characteristics of primary Merkel cell carcinoma, incidence and mortality trends, predictors of survival and identified potential risk factors. However, the rarity of Merkel cell carcinoma makes epidemiologic studies that could point toward the etiology Merkel cell carcinoma especially challenging.

1.1 Origin, Nomenclature and Histopathological Coding

1.1.1 *Origin*

Merkel cell carcinoma was first described by Toker in 1972 as trabecular carcinoma of the skin because of its histological appearance.[5] In their 1978 ultrastructural studies, Tang and Toker identified dense-core granules in the cytoplasm of the tumor cells. Merkel cells are the only cells in the skin known to contain this kind of granules. Therefore, it was postulated that trabecular carcinoma of the skin derived from Merkel cells.[7]

Today it is generally believed that Merkel cell carcinoma originates from Merkel cells,[8] and it is widely accepted that Merkel cells are of neuroendocrine origin.[9] However, the origin of Merkel cell carcinoma is still debated. Merkel cells were originally described by Friedrich Sigmund Merkel in 1875[10] and they were referred to as 'tastzellen' or 'touch cells.' They are localized in the basal layer of the epidermis in contact with nerve terminals and they function as mechanoreceptors.[11] Cells very similar to Merkel cells, but with no contact with nerve terminals, are also present in the epidermis. Their function is uncertain and they are considered to be part of a diffuse neuroendocrine system. These cells have also been described as Merkel cells. Some authors do not consider it likely that the origin of Merkel cell carcinoma is from Merkel cells in contact with nerve endings and functioning as mechanoreceptors. Rather, they propose that Merkel cell carcinoma may originate from those epidermal neuroendocrine cells with no contact with nerve endings.[11]

Another hypothesis is that Merkel cell carcinoma originates from pluripotent epidermal stem cells that can give rise to both neuroendocrine and epithelial cells.[12] This view is supported by the presence of squamous differentiation in certain cases of Merkel cell carcinoma and its metastases. Merkel cell carcinoma originating from a pluripotent epidermal stem cell could exhibit both squamous and neuroendocrine differentiations in the same lesion.[13]

1.1.2 *Nomenclature*

Because of the uncertainty of its origin, Merkel cell carcinoma has been reported under a variety of names since its first description by Toker as trabecular carcinoma of the skin.[5] These names include neuroendocrine carcinoma of skin, Merkel cell tumor or carcinoma, primary small cell carcinoma of the skin, APUDoma and endocrine carcinoma of the skin.[14]

The three most often-used names have been trabecular carcinoma of the skin, cutaneous neuroendocrine carcinoma and Merkel cell carcinoma, following the step-wise acquired knowledge on the cellular origin of this cancer. This has made the nomenclature for this cancer somewhat confusing and the identification of cases more difficult. The names trabecular carcinoma of the skin and cutaneous neuroendocrine carcinoma have been used because of the anatomic-histopathological (trabecular) and of the immunochemical (neuroendocrine) characteristics of this cancer.[5,7,14] The name Merkel cell carcinoma was proposed in 1980[15] and it has become prevalent over time because of the confirmed ultrastructural similarity of these neoplastic cells with Merkel cells and because it has become progressively accepted that Merkel cell carcinoma originates from Merkel cells.[8] However, many authors continue referring to Merkel cell carcinoma as cutaneous neuroendocrine carcinoma to the current date.[16–19]

1.1.3 *Histopathological coding*

The first edition of the International Classification of Diseases for Oncology (ICD-O) was published in 1976 by the World Health Organization. Before 1976, cancer registries used the Manual of Tumor Nomenclature and Coding (MOTNAC) published by the American Cancer Society to classify neoplasms. MOTNAC included codes for the morphology (histology), topography (anatomic site) and behavior of neoplasms. The morphology (trabecular) and topography (skin) codes for trabecular carcinoma of the skin were included in the MOTNAC edition used by cancer registries in 1973 through 1975.[1] The morphology code for trabecular carcinoma (8190/3) has been included in the first and following editions of the ICD-O.[20–22]

In 1986, the field trial edition[23] of the second edition of the ICD-O included morphology codes for neuroendocrine carcinoma (8246/3) and Merkel cell carcinoma (8247/3). Thus, cancer registries have been using the morphology codes for trabecular carcinoma since 1972 and for neuroendocrine carcinoma and Merkel cell carcinoma since 1986. The cancer registries participating in the Surveillance Epidemiology and End Results (SEER) program of the National Cancer Institute reported the coding of 81 cases as trabecular carcinoma of the skin, of 69 cases as neuroendocrine carcinoma of the skin, and of 884 cases as Merkel cell carcinoma between 1973 and 1999,[1] and of two cases as trabecular carcinoma of the skin, 68 cases as neuroendocrine carcinoma of the skin and 957 cases as Merkel cell carcinoma in 1992 to 2001.[24] Thus, even if the name Merkel cell carcinoma and its associated morphology code are those predominantly used to identify the cancer first described by Toker,[5] cancer registries are still reporting cases coded as neuroendocrine carcinoma of the skin and even as trabecular carcinoma of the skin. Given the rarity of this cancer, studies based on case identification through cancer registries should take into account that the same anatomic entity may still be reported under different codes (and names).

1.2 Epidemiology

Population-based data on Merkel cell carcinoma derive from analyzing the data collected by cancer registries that carry out cancer surveillance on large geographic areas.[1,4,25–30] Even the identification of a major risk factor such as immunosuppression was made possible only through the linkage of cancer registries with organ transplant and AIDS registries.[12,31–33]

The data collected by the geographic areas participating in the SEER[a] program of the National Cancer Institute[34,35] have proved invaluable to ascertain incidence trends, epidemiological characteristics and predictors of survival of primary Merkel cell carcinoma in the general population.

---

[a] http://seer.cancer.gov/

In fact, the size of the population at risk studied, corresponding to 10–14% of the United States population, is such that the number of first primary Merkel cell carcinoma incident cases is large enough to allow descriptive epidemiology and survival analysis by sex, anatomic site, stage and age at diagnosis.[b,1,4,24]

1.2.1 *Incidence trends*

1.2.1.1 *Overall incidence rates*

The SEER program started reporting on cancer in 1973 and participating cancer registries reported incident cases of trabecular carcinoma of the skin. Therefore, trends in reporting and in primary Merkel cell carcinoma age-adjusted incidence per year of diagnosis could be studied since the first description of Merkel cell carcinoma in 1972.[5] Until 1980, however, primary Merkel cell carcinoma has been reported only sporadically. The age-adjusted incidence rate of primary Merkel cell carcinoma has been steadily increasing from 1980 through 1997 (Figure 1).[1]

The incidence of malignant melanoma and of non-melanoma skin cancer (basal cell carcinoma and squamous cell carcinoma) has also been increasing over this time period. The increase in the incidence of Merkel cell carcinoma over time appears consistent with this trend. However, Merkel cell carcinoma is a very rare cancer; its clinical diagnosis is elusive and its histopathological diagnosis has been especially difficult until very recently, when a specific profile for Merkel cell carcinoma has been identified through immunohistological staining. Merkel cell carcinoma stains positive for low molecular weight cytokeratins (CAM 5.2 or AE1/AE3), neuron-specific enolase and cytokeratin-20, but not for other

[b] The SEER geographic areas included in these studies were the states of Connecticut, Iowa, New Mexico, Utah and Hawaii, the metropolitan areas of Detroit MI, San Francisco-Oakland CA, Atlanta GA, and the Puget Sound area of Seattle WA, which cover about 10% of the United States population, with the addition of the metropolitan area of Los Angeles CA, the area of San Jose-Monterey CA, and the counties of Glascock, Greene, Hancock, Jasper, Jefferson, Morgan, Putnam, Taliaferro, Warren and Washington in rural Georgia, altogether covering about 14% of the United States population.[4]

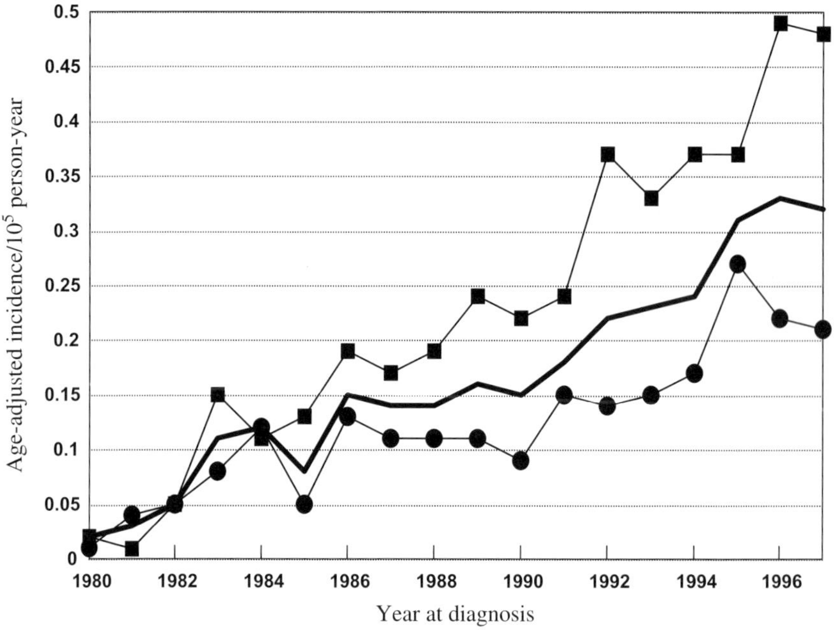

Figure 1. Age-adjusted incidence of first primary Merkel cell carcinoma by year of diagnosis (all cases —; males ▪—▪; females •—•). Modified from Agelli and Clegg (2003).[1]

markers. Furthermore, the largest proportion of primary Merkel cell carcinoma cases reported to the SEER program from 1973 to 1999 was after 1992 (73%, 758 cases out of 1034). In interpreting Merkel cell carcinoma incidence rates over time, we must keep in mind the introduction and widespread use of new diagnostic instruments, techniques and biomarkers. Electron microscopy entered major diagnostic centers in the 1980s; the staining for neuron-specific enolase started being used in 1983; ICD-O entered a morphology (histology) code associated with the name 'Merkel cell carcinoma' in 1986; and the importance of staining for cytokeratin-20 in the differential diagnosis of carcinomas was published in 1992.[36] Therefore, it is not possible at this time to distinguish how much of the increase in the incidence of primary Merkel cell carcinoma over time is an actual increase in the population and how much is instead due to improved diagnosis and increased awareness toward this very rare cancer.

The incidence of all Merkel cell carcinoma cases (primary and secondary cancers) has also been reported to have increased 8% per year from 1986 to 2001 in the population covered by the SEER program.[27] The interpretation of these results requires even more caution. In fact, improved diagnosis is especially effective in the setting of high-risk populations. Survivors of a first primary cancer are at higher risk of developing a second primary cancer, including Merkel cell carcinoma, than the general population.[37,38]

The calculated age-adjusted[c] incidence of first primary Merkel cell carcinoma for the SEER population in 1986 through 1999 was 0.24 per 100,000 person-years.[1] Since more than 70% of cases had been reported after 1992, Agelli and Clegg[4] re-calculated the age-adjusted incidence rate for primary Merkel cell carcinoma in 1992 to 2001, and it was found to be 0.32 per 100,000 person-years. These findings suggest that the incidence of primary Merkel cell carcinoma in the decade after the introduction of immunological staining for cytokeratin-20 should be considered the age-adjusted incidence of reference to ascertain whether there is a real increase of primary Merkel cell carcinoma in the general population of the United States.

1.2.2 *Incidence rates by age, race and sex*

In both males and females, incidence increases with advancing age, gradually from 50 years of age to 65 years of age, then progressively (Figure 2).

Merkel cell carcinoma is essentially a disease of older whites, who have an age-adjusted incidence of 0.36 per 100,000 person-years, more than eight times the incidence rate of blacks (0.045) and almost double the incidence of other ethnic groups (0.2).[1,24] The incidence of primary Merkel cell carcinoma is higher in males than in females in all ethnic groups, with a ratio of 2:1 in whites and blacks and a ratio of 1.5:1 in all other ethnic groups.[1,4]

---

[c] Age-adjusted to the year 2000 standard population for the United States.

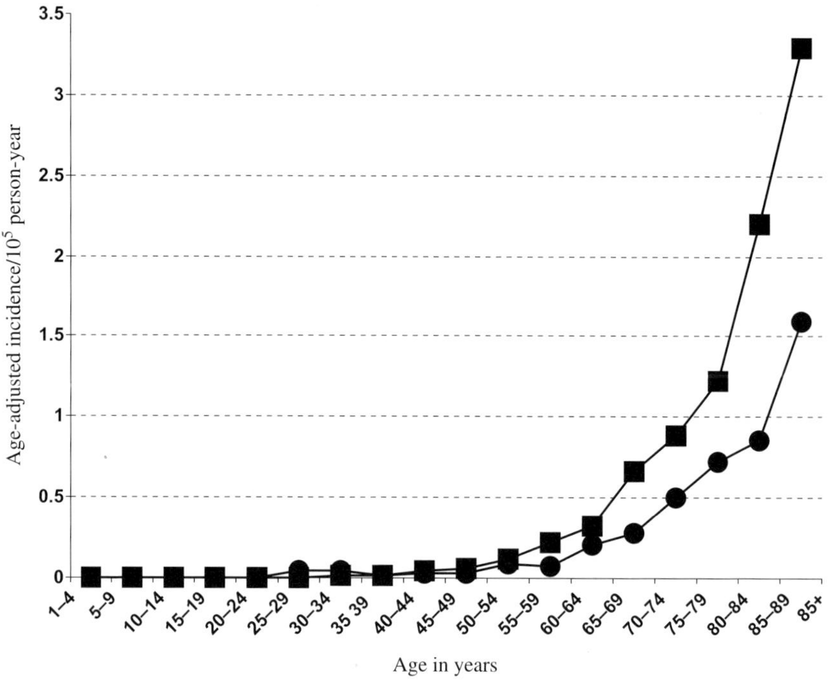

Figure 2. Age-specific incidence of first primary Merkel cell carcinoma per 100,000 person-years according to sex (males: ▪—▪; females: •—•). Reproduced with permission from Agelli and Clegg (2003).[1]

1.2.3 *Incidence rates by ultraviolet B (UVB) exposure*

Agelli and Clegg analyzed the age-adjusted incidence of first primary Merkel cell carcinoma according to ultraviolet B (UVB) radiation exposure using calculated UVB radiation indexes[28,39] for the SEER geographic areas as indicators of UVB exposure for people living in that area. The -age-adjusted incidence of whites was highest in Hawaii, the geographic location with the highest UVB radiation index. Furthermore, a statistically significant correlation ($r = 0.84$, $p = 0.005$) was present between the age-adjusted incidence of primary Merkel cell carcinoma of the head and neck in whites and the UVB radiation index of the SEER geographic

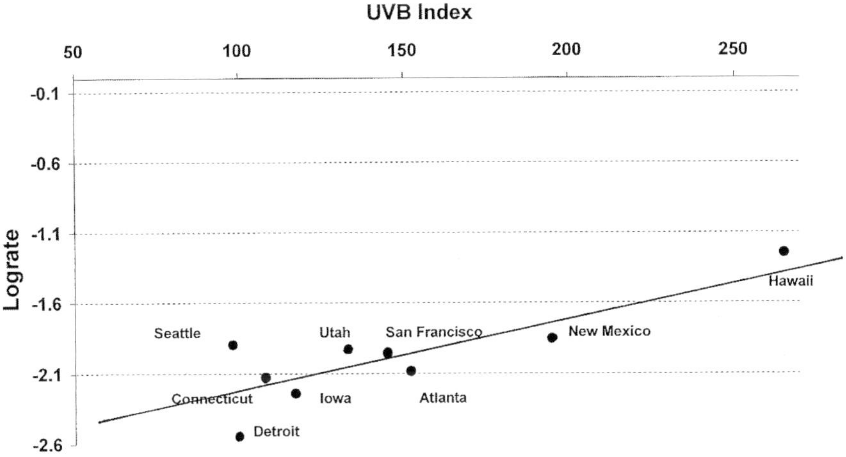

Figure 3. Linear correlation[d] of age-adjusted incidence with ultraviolet B (UVB) radiation indexes in first primary Merkel cell carcinoma of the head and neck in whites. Reproduced with permission from Agelli and Clegg (2003).[1]

areas (Figure 3). These data indicate that the major susceptibility of whites to the effects of UVB radiation may be a risk factor for Merkel cell carcinoma development in the skin areas of the body more exposed to the sun.

1.3 Characteristics of Cases

Currently, the best available information on the epidemiological characteristics of primary Merkel cell carcinoma in the general population comes from the prospective analysis of the data collected by the SEER program and is based on the 1034 cases of first primary Merkel cell carcinoma identified in 1973 to 1999[1] and on the 1027 cases identified in 1992 to 2001.[4] There are no significant differences in the epidemiological characteristics of cases identified in 1973–1999 compared with those

[d] Lograte = natural logarithm of age-adjusted incidence rates per 100,000 person-years.

identified in 1992–2001. The data obtained corroborate or complement each other.

1.3.1 *Age distribution*

In the general population, primary Merkel cell carcinoma is a disease of older whites. In fact, 94% of cases occur in whites and 76% of cases occur in people 65 years of age or older. Furthermore, almost 50% of all cases occur in people older than 75 years. Primary Merkel cell carcinoma affects males at a younger age than females (age mean: males 71 years; females 76 years, $p < 0.0001$).[1]

1.3.2 *Anatomic localization*

In both sexes, the most frequent site of primary Merkel cell carcinoma at diagnosis is the head and neck (48%), followed by the upper limb (19%), the lower limb (16%) and the trunk (11%). However, in males the anatomic site most frequently affected at diagnosis varies with age ($p < 0.0001$), with the proportion of cases on the head and neck increasing progressively from 30% in males younger than 65 years to 55% in males older than 75 years. In males younger than 65 years, the largest proportion of cases is on the trunk or limbs.[1,24]

1.3.3 *Stage at diagnosis*

The SEER program's staging system is: localized (stage I), regional lymph node involvement (stage II) and distant metastasis (stage III).[40,41] Overall, only about 50% of cases have localized disease (stage I) at diagnosis. However, there is an association between stage at diagnosis and the anatomic site of presentation. A primary site on the limbs is associated with less advanced disease compared with all other anatomic sites, while a primary on the trunk is most frequently associated with distant metastasis at the time of diagnosis. The association between anatomic site and stage at diagnosis was essentially the same in males and females.[1,4]

1.4 Relative Survival[e]

1.4.1 *Overall relative survival*

For all cases of first primary Merkel cell carcinoma, the observed five-year survival rate was 45%, but the five-year relative survival rate was 62% (Figure 4).

1.4.2 *Relative survival by stage at diagnosis*

The probability of survival decreased sharply when Merkel cell carcinoma had progressed from local to regional and metastatic disease in both

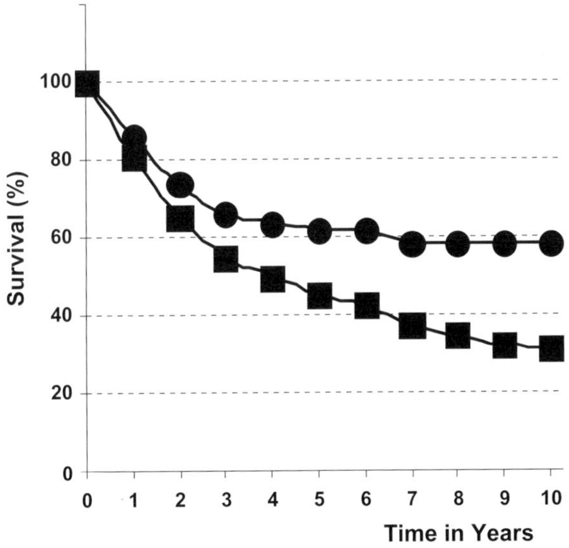

Figure 4. Observed and relative survival of first primary Merkel cell carcinoma. Observed survival = ▪—▪, relative survival = •—•. Reproduced with permission from Agelli and Clegg (2003).[1]

---

[e] The relative survival rate was calculated in lieu of the disease-specific survival rate because Merkel cell carcinoma is not indexed as a mortality code in the International Classification of Diseases. The relative survival rate is the ratio of the observed survival to the expected survival of the general population of the same age, sex and race of the patient group, and calendar year of observation.

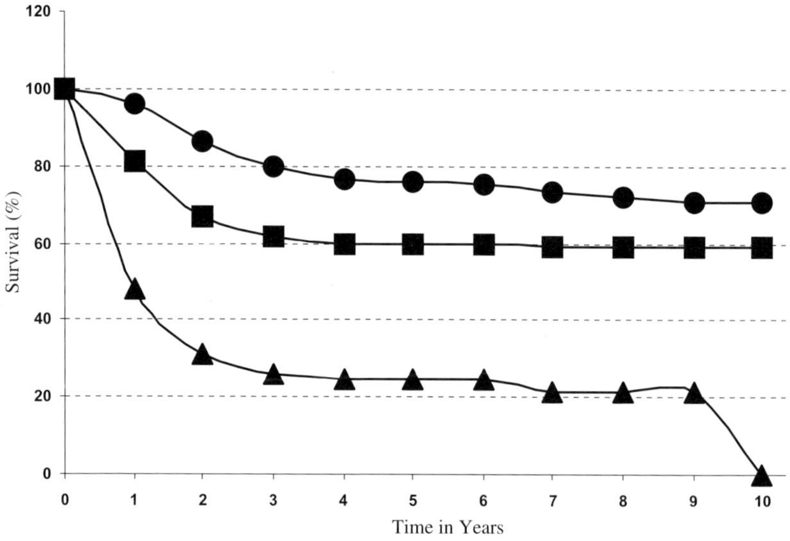

Figure 5. Merkel cell carcinoma: relative survival by stage at diagnosis. Stage I (localized) = •—•; stage II (regional) = ■—■; stage III (distant) ▲—▲. Reproduced with permission from Agelli and Clegg (2003).[1]

sexes. Overall, only 32% of patients with distant metastases at diagnosis were still alive after two years compared with 86% of patients diagnosed with localized disease. The probability of survival five years after diagnosis decreased further to 25% compared to 75% (Figure 5).

1.4.3 *Predictors of survival*

Females have a better probability of survival than males. This finding strengthened after controlling for age, stage at diagnosis and anatomic site of presentation (HR = 0.71, 95% CI = 0.59–0.87).[f,1,4] The better survival observed in females could be related to intrinsic biological differences between the two sexes.[42] However, specific modalities of treatments were not studied[1,4] and they could have been different and/or affect survival differently in males and females.

[f] HR = hazard ratio; CI = confidence interval.

1.4.3.1 *Predictors of survival by sex*

Factors associated with survival were identified through Cox proportional hazard regression analysis for males and females separately since female sex is an independent positive predictor of survival (Table 1).[1,4]

Primary site on the upper limb is associated with better survival in both sexes compared to any other anatomic site; however, statistical significance was reached only for Merkel cell carcinoma at the head and neck in males and the trunk in females.

Table 1. Hazard ratios and 95% confidence intervals for first primary Merkel cell carcinoma by age, stage, and anatomic site at time of diagnosis.

	Males		Females	
	HR	95% CI	HR	95% CI
Age in years[g]				
<65 = reference category	1.0	—	1.0	—
65–74	1.5	1.1–2.1	1.4	0.8–2.3
75+	2.3	1.7–3.1	3.3	2.2–5.1
Stage at diagnosis[h]				
Localized = reference category	1.0	—	1.0	—
Regional	1.5	1.1–2.0	1.5	1.1–2.2
Distant	3.5	2.3–5.2	4.0	2.5–6.4
Unstaged	1.9	1.3–2.6	2.1	1.4–3.0
Anatomic site[i]				
Upper limb = reference category	1.0	—	1.0	—
Head and neck	1.7	1.2–2.3	1.2	0.8–1.8
Trunk	1.3	0.9–2.1	2.8	1.7–4.6
Lower limb	1.4	0.9–2.2	1.2	0.7–1.9
Other	1.1	0.6–1.9	1.0	0.5–2.3

Source: Modified from Agelli and Clegg (2003).[1]

[g] Controlling for stage and anatomic site.

[h] Controlling for age and anatomic site.

[i] Controlling for age and stage at diagnosis.

The presence of distant metastases at time of diagnosis is a strong negative predictor of survival in both sexes, as is the case with most cancers. Other factors independently associated with worse survival are presentation on the head and neck in males and on the trunk in females, and advanced age in both sexes.

The oldest patients have a poor prognosis even if Merkel cell carcinoma is localized at diagnosis. In the elderly, the immune response may be impaired because of immunosenescence[43] and perhaps due to a chronic pro-inflammatory status, often referred to as the inflamm-aging effect.[44,45] This age-related immunodeficiency and dysregulation of the immune system cause a progressive deterioration in the ability to respond to infections and possibly to cancer, and it could explain why Merkel cell carcinoma occurs in the elderly as well as the poor survival of localized Merkel cell carcinoma in the oldest patients.

1.5 Epidemiology of Merkel Cell Carcinoma of Mucosal Anatomic Sites

About 5% of all first primary cases of Merkel cell carcinoma arise from mucosal anatomic sites.[1,4] In 1992 to 2001, the total number of cases of first primary Merkel cell carcinoma was 1027. Fifty cases (5%) were localized to mucosal anatomic sites.[1,4]

1.5.1 *Anatomic localization*

The larynx is the most frequently affected mucosal anatomic site in both sexes, as shown in Table 2.

1.5.2 *Incidence rates*

The overall age-adjusted incidence of first primary Merkel cell carcinoma at mucosal anatomic sites was 0.015 per 100,000 person-years, while the incidence of first primary Merkel cell carcinoma of the skin was 0.30 per 100,000 person-years.[4] The male to female incidence ratio was 1.3:1 (males, 0.017; females, 0.013). The age-adjusted incidence of

Table 2. Anatomic localization of first primary Merkel cell carcinoma of mucosal anatomic sites.

	Total (N = 50)		Male (N = 26)		Female (N = 24)	
	N	(%)	N	(%)	N	(%)
Mouth and tongue	7	(14.0)	4	(15.4)	3	(12.5)
Nasal cavity	12	(24.0)	6	(23.1)	6	(25.0)
Pharynx	8	(16.0)	6	(23.1)	2	(8.3)
Larynx	27	(54.0)	9	(34.6)	10	(41.7)
Genitalia	3	(6.0)	0	(0.0)	3	(12.5)
Other[j]	1	(2.0)	1	(3.8)	—	—

first primary Merkel cell carcinoma at mucosae in whites (0.016) was 1.8 times greater than in blacks (0.009) and 1.2 times greater than in other ethnic groups (0.013).[4] Thus, even if UVB radiation exposure is not a likely risk factor for Merkel cell carcinoma at mucosal anatomic sites, whites still have a higher incidence rates than all other ethnic groups.

1.5.3 *Characteristics of Merkel cell carcinoma cases at mucosal anatomic sites compared to the characteristics Merkel cell carcinoma cases at the skin*

The greatest proportion of first primary Merkel cell carcinoma cases occur in whites for either localization on the skin (94%) or on mucosae (86%), as shown in Table 3.

Cases with first primary Merkel cell carcinoma on mucosae were significantly younger than cases with first primary Merkel cell carcinoma on the skin. The mean age for cases on mucosae was 62 years while the mean age for cases on the skin was 74 years ($p < 0.0001$).[4] Males were younger than females at time of diagnosis for either first primary Merkel cell carcinoma of the skin (mean age: males 72 years; females, 76 years, $p < 0.001$) or mucosae (mean age: males, 59 years; females, 64 years,

[j] Other = overlapping mucosal anatomical sites of the head.

Table 3. Comparison of the principal characteristics in cases with first primary Merkel cell carcinoma on the skin and on mucosae.

	Skin (N = 977)		Mucosae (N = 50)	
	N	(%)	N	(%)
Sex				
Male	556	57%	26	52%
Female	421	43%	24	48%
Age groups (years)				
<65	195	20%	27	54%
≥65–74	782	80%	23	46%
Race				
White	912	93%	43	86%
Black	9	1%	3	6%
Other	56	6%	4	8%
Stage at diagnosis				
Localized	503	52%	16	32%
Regional	290	30%	23	46%
Distant	79	8%	10	20%
Unstaged	105	11%	1	2%

$p = 0.23$), but statistical significance was reached only for Merkel cell carcinoma of the skin.

1.5.4 *Survival*

Survival of individuals with primary Merkel cell carcinoma on mucosae is much worse than that of individuals with Merkel cell carcinoma on the skin (HR = 1.6, 95% CI = 1.09–2.36) even after controlling for age, sex and stage at diagnosis.

The two-year relative survival rate was 49% for first primary mucosal Merkel cell carcinoma and 76% for skin Merkel cell carcinoma (Figure 6).

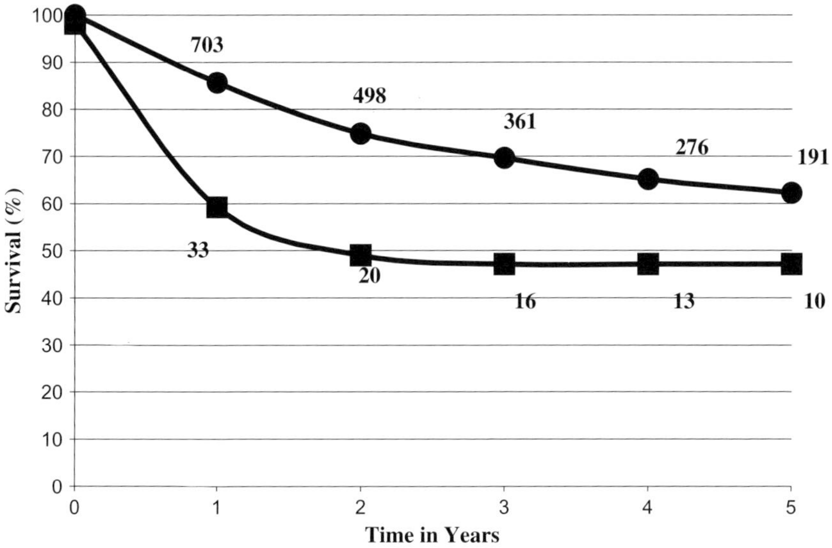

Figure 6. Relative survival of skin (N = 977, •—•) and mucosal (N = 50, ▪—▪) first primary Merkel cell carcinoma.

Primary mucosal Merkel cell carcinoma seems to be diagnosed at more advanced stages than primary skin Merkel cell carcinoma (Table 3). In addition, it is likely that localization at mucosal anatomic sites may represent a limit to more extensive and radical surgery. These two factors could explain the worse survival of primary mucosal Merkel cell carcinoma. However, cases with primary mucosal Merkel cell carcinoma were significantly younger at diagnosis than cases with primary skin Merkel cell carcinoma. There could be intrinsic factors that contribute to an earlier clinical presentation and an increased risk of death.

Published case reports describe the clinical course of mucosal Merkel cell carcinoma as aggressive, with a high risk for local recurrence and regional and distant metastasis. Fulminating courses have also been reported.[46]

Merkel cell carcinoma should be included in the differential diagnosis of head and neck mucosal lesions, especially if the tumor is submucosal.[46]

1.6 Etiology

Little is known about specific etiological factors in the pathogenesis of Merkel cell carcinoma. Recent population-based studies and the careful compilation and analysis of the many case reports published in the literature since the first description of this tumor have pointed to possible and probable risk.[1,28,31,33,37,47–50] Advanced molecular biology techniques have also allowed the identification of molecular and genetic alterations that may be in the etiologic pathway of Merkel cell carcinoma.[51] Despite this progress, the etiology of Merkel cell carcinoma remains the object of hypotheses and speculation.

1.6.1 *Skin radiation exposure*

Merkel cell carcinoma has been reported most frequently in association with exposure to ultraviolet A and B radiation, but also with exposure to ionizing radiation[52,53] and infrared radiation.[13,54,55]

Sun exposure (i.e. exposure to UVB radiation) is considered an important factor in the etiology of Merkel cell carcinoma in part because it is a recognized risk factor for malignant melanoma and other non-melanoma skin cancers.[56] However, proving that UVB radiation exposure is indeed a major risk factor for Merkel cell carcinoma has been elusive.

The concurrence of Merkel cell carcinoma with actinic keratosis, squamous cell carcinoma, basal cell carcinoma, lentigo maligna, malignant melanoma and solar elastosis has been widely reported. This association has suggested the interpretation that all these conditions share UVB radiation as a common etiological factor.[28,55–61]

Epidemiological studies have reported a probable association between Merkel cell carcinoma and sun exposure. In fact, there is a positive correlation between the incidence of Merkel cell carcinoma of the head and neck in whites and UVB radiation indexes in the geographic areas of SEER cancer surveillance.[1,4]

Recently, C $\rightarrow$ T and CC $\rightarrow$ TT mutations of the TP53 suppressor gene have been identified in Merkel cell carcinoma.[62,63] The presence of these mutations suggests that UVB radiation may be an important factor for the development of the disease.[63] In fact, these distinctive mutations are considered diagnostic of UV damage.[64,65] Studies on squamous cell carcinoma, where UVB radiation is considered the causal carcinogen, show that these mutations remain present in the progeny of the cell whose DNA had been originally damaged 50 or more years before.[65–67]

UVA radiation is a much stronger mutagen than UVB radiation.[65] The incidence of Merkel cell carcinoma in patients with psoriasis who were treated with oral methoxsalen (psoralen) and UVA photochemotherapy (PUVA) has been reported to be about 100 times higher than expected in the general population.[68,69]

Chronic exposure of the skin to thermal radiation may cause erythema *ab igne*. Case reports have described Merkel cell carcinoma arising from old burn scars and from areas of erythema *ab igne* alone or in association with squamous cell carcinoma.[13,54,55,60,70]

1.6.2 *Arsenic exposure*

The association between the consumption of arsenic-contaminated water and skin cancer has been documented since the 1960s.[71,72] Arsenic is an important environmental carcinogen that affects millions of people worldwide, especially in underdeveloped countries. Arsenic is a potent gene and chromosome mutagen that also causes mitochondrial damage.[73] Inorganic arsenicals increase the risk of skin cancer, of solid organ cancers and of cancers of the lympho-hemopoietic system. Merkel cell carcinoma has been reported in individuals with Bowen's disease and in areas of endemic chronic arsenicism.[71,74,75]

1.6.3 *Viral infection*

Very recently, a previously unknown polyomavirus has been identified in Merkel cell carcinoma tissue and named Merkel cell polyomavirus (MCV or MCPyV). This discovery brings the number of known human polyomaviruses to five (JC, BK, KI, WU and MCPyV). In the original series of tissue samples obtained from ten Merkel cell carcinoma patients, the tissues of eight patients (80%) were positive for MCPyV sequences and monoclonal viral integration[k] was observed in Merkel cell carcinoma tissue

[k] Monoclonal viral integration is a Southern blot pattern of bands indicating that the virus has integrated at different chromosomal sites before clonal expansion of the infected cell.

samples in five of ten (50%) patients.[76] Currently, MCPyV DNA sequences have been identified in 85% (n = 45), 77% (n = 30), 69% (n = 11) and 24% (n = 5) of tissue samples from Merkel cell carcinoma patients in European, American and Australian case series.[77–79] The evidence that MCPyV was integrated with the DNA of Merkel cell carcinoma cells before their clonal proliferation is a strong indication that MCPyV may be a determinant factor in Merkel cell carcinoma etiopathogenesis. However, MCPyV, even if present in a large proportion of Merkel cell carcinoma tissues, is not present in all of them. Therefore, MCPyV is not necessary for the development of Merkel cell carcinoma, in contrast to Kaposi sarcoma virus or human papilloma virus whose respective tumor does not develop in their absence. Furthermore, MCPyV DNA sequences have also been found present in tissue samples of basal cell carcinomas (13%), squamous cell carcinoma (13%) and from apparently normal skin of individuals without Merkel cell carcinoma (16%).[76,77] Therefore, the role of MCPyV in Merkel cell carcinoma etiopathogenesis remains to be clarified.

A possible role of the previously known human polyomaviruses in human carcinogenesis has been debated for years.[80] However, until the identification of the new MCPyV in Merkel cell carcinoma[76] there has been no evidence that polyomaviruses were associated with carcinogenesis in humans.[81]

Infections by polyomaviruses have been reported rarely and predominantly in patients with compromised function of the immune system.[82,83] More recently, polyomavirus infections have been studied mostly in renal transplant recipients, where polyomavirus allograft nephropathy (PVAN) has emerged since the use of potent immunosuppressive agents had become widespread in post-transplant treatment.[84,85] It is believed that the initial infection is occult and occurs before adulthood. Apparently, the virus remains latent until profound immune suppression facilitates the transition and progression from latent to active infection.[80] A similar occurrence may be postulated for MCPyV.

1.6.4 *Immunosuppression*

Many descriptive studies in the literature have been reporting the association between Merkel cell carcinoma and iatrogenic immunosuppression. Merkel cell carcinoma has been reported in almost every autoimmune disease (e.g. rheumatoid arthritis, systemic lupus erythematosus, Behçet's syndrome, Wegener's granulomatosis, autoimmune hepatitis, chronic sarcoidosis). These case reports have been increasing in frequency since the introduction of inhibitors of tumor necrosis factor (TNF) in the treatment of systemic autoimmune diseases.[86–93] Patients with systemic autoimmune diseases had been traditionally treated with drugs that cause long-term low-grade immunosuppression. The introduction of TNF-inhibitors and other potent immunosuppressant drugs in the treatment of systemic autoimmune diseases has significantly raised the degree of immunosuppression.[94] Partial regression of metastatic Merkel cell carcinoma has been reported after discontinuation of immunosuppressive therapy.[95,96]

1.6.4.1 *Organ transplantation*

Merkel cell carcinoma has been reported to occur after transplantation of the kidney, liver, heart and bone marrow; however, most reported cases are in kidney transplant patients.[97–102] The Cincinnati Tumor Registry alone identified 45 transplant patients with one or more Merkel cell carcinomas.[31,33] The mean age at time of Merkel cell carcinoma diagnosis was 53 years with 49% of patients less than 50 years old. Merkel cell carcinoma presented on average seven years after organ transplant. As in the general population, most cases were whites (80%) and males (69%). The distribution of Merkel cell carcinoma lesions was also similar to that seen in the general population with 49% of cases on the head and neck, followed by the limbs and the trunk. In nine patients (20%), Merkel cell carcinoma was present at multiple sites at time of diagnosis. Advanced disease (stages II and III) was the most frequent mode of presentation (70%). In 26 patients (57%), Merkel cell carcinoma was associated with other malignancies. In 22 patients (49%), Merkel cell carcinoma was associated with other skin cancers. Of the 45 patients diagnosed with Merkel cell carcinoma, 60% died of their disease at an average of 18 months from Merkel cell carcinoma diagnosis.

The findings on Merkel cell carcinoma in transplant recipients clearly indicate that chronic immunosuppression increases the risk of Merkel cell carcinoma. However, immunosuppression is not a risk factor specific for

Merkel cell carcinoma. In fact, transplant recipients are at higher risk for nearly any malignancy, including other skin cancers, compared with the general population. However, it appears that immunosuppression in transplant patients increases the risk of Merkel cell carcinoma more than that of other cancers. In fact, the ratio melanoma to Merkel cell carcinoma in the post-transplant population is 6:1 compared to 65:1 in the general population.[33]

1.6.4.2 *AIDS*

There are several case reports in the literature of Merkel cell carcinoma in people with the Acquired Immunodeficiency Syndrome (AIDS).[12] The study of 309,265 people with AIDS through linkage of AIDS and Cancer Registries indicates that individuals with AIDS have a relative risk of developing Merkel cell carcinoma of 13.4 compared to the general population.[32] These data have been recently confirmed.[103]

The increased risk of Merkel cell carcinoma in AIDS patients is most likely directly related to damage to the immune system caused by the human immunodeficiency virus (HIV) leaving HIV-infected patients, with or without clinically evident AIDS, susceptible to opportunistic bacterial and viral infections and to cancer development. In fact, in four of the six cases in the registries, Merkel cell carcinoma was diagnosed before the onset of clinically evident AIDS.[32] There are case reports describing remission of metastatic Merkel cell carcinoma during treatment of HIV infection.[104]

1.6.4.3 *Association with other malignancies*

Case reports and series have long been reporting the association of Merkel cell carcinoma with other cancers, mostly skin or lymphohemopoietic cancers.[48,86,105,106] However, in a population-based study that analyzed data collected by the Israel Cancer Registry, 50% of cancers associated with Merkel cell carcinoma (i.e. preceding, concurrent or following the diagnosis of Merkel cell carcinoma) were non-skin solid tumors.[37] The analysis of the SEER population showed that all other first primary cancers taken together (n = 2,048,739) had a statistical significant increased risk for developing Merkel cell carcinoma as second primary cancer (SIR* = 1.36, 95%CI = 1.19–1.55) and that 89% of Merkel cell carcinoma developed within one year from the diagnosis of the first primary cancer. Most cancers were associated with an increased risk of Merkel cell carcinoma as a second primary cancer; however, statistical significance was reached only for multiple myeloma, chronic lymphocytic leukemia, non-Hodgkin's lymphoma and malignant melanoma.[38]

In the population reporting to the Israel Tumor Registry, there was an increased risk of second primary cancers occurring during Merkel cell carcinoma follow-up (average 3.6 years). The estimated actuarial risk of developing a second primary cancer after the diagnosis of primary Merkel cell carcinoma was 2.1% for each year of follow-up.[37] In the SEER population studied by Howard *et al.*,[38] the average follow-up time for patients with primary Merkel cell carcinoma was 3.5 years. The estimated risk of developing a second primary cancer after the diagnosis of Merkel cell carcinoma was especially high during the first year of follow-up (SIR = 1.71, 95%CI = 1.21–2.33).

1.6.5 *Proposed association with squamous cell carcinoma*

It has been proposed that situations conducive to the development of squamous cell carcinomas also predispose to the development of Merkel cell carcinoma and/or the combination of the two,[56,60,63] even if the origin of the two cancers is distinct.[11,66] These proposals are based on clinical and descriptive observations and still need to be proved or disproved. The SEER program does not collect data on squamous cell carcinomas or basal cell carcinomas, and the association of Merkel cell carcinoma with squamous cell carcinoma in this population cannot be ascertained.

Squamous cell carcinoma is the tumor most commonly linked with Merkel cell carcinoma. In fact, Merkel cell carcinoma has been reported associated with squamous cell carcinoma in almost 40% of cases. The nature of the association varies. Merkel cell carcinoma has been reported to arise at the site of a previously excised squamous cell carcinoma, to be contiguous or intermingled with a squamous cell carcinoma, or to be

* SIR = Standardized incidence ratio.

surmounted by an epidermis with features of Bowen's disease or actinic keratosis.[13,37,54,55,60,105,107,108]

Squamous cell carcinoma and Merkel cell carcinoma have approximately the same age distribution. Both are diseases of the elderly, while malignant melanoma and basal cell carcinoma are more prevalent in younger individuals.[56]

Squamous cell carcinoma is caused by chronic cumulative exposure to UVB radiation, while malignant melanoma and basal cell carcinoma are associated with intense but occasional and even sporadic UVB exposure (e.g. solar burns). Merkel cell carcinoma appears also to be associated with chronic, cumulative exposure to UVB radiation.[56]

With respect to the carcinogenic effects of arsenic, it has been argued that the carcinogenic effects of arsenicals on skin may be cell-type specific since malignant melanoma does not appear to be associated with the ingestion of arsenic, while basal cell carcinoma and especially squamous cell carcinomas are.[56,109]

The behavior of squamous cell carcinoma is strongly affected by immunosuppression. The frequency of squamous cell carcinoma increases exponentially in immune-suppressed patients, especially after a transplant when it often presents at multiple sites, has an aggressive behavior and it metastasizes in 5–8% of cases.[56,63,110] The numbers and behavior of malignant melanoma do not seem to be altered by immunosuppression as much as Merkel cell carcinoma. The ratio of melanoma to Merkel cell carcinoma in the general population is 65:1 and in transplant recipients is 6:1.[28,33] Similarly, the ratio of basal cell carcinoma to squamous cell carcinoma is 4 to 1 in the general population, but in immunosuppression the frequency of basal cell carcinoma increases only by a factor of ten compared to the 65–250 times increase observed for squamous cell carcinoma.[56,63,110]

1.7 Summary

Primary Merkel cell carcinoma is an aggressive, rare cancer of elderly whites with 76% of cases occurring in people older than 65 years. It presents most often on sun-exposed areas of the skin, with 48% of cases on the head and neck. About 5% of all cases of first primary Merkel cell carcinoma present at mucosal anatomic sites at diagnosis, with most cases (54%) localized at the larynx. Primary Merkel cell carcinoma occurs more frequently in males than in females. Females have a better survival probability than males. Negative predictors for survival are advanced age at diagnosis, presentation at the head and neck in males and at the trunk in females, and presence of distant metastasis at diagnosis. Localization at a mucosal anatomic site has a very poor survival in both sexes. Patients with first primary Merkel cell carcinoma of mucosae (mean age 62 years) are significantly younger than patients with primary Merkel cell carcinoma of the skin (mean age 74 years). Merkel cell carcinoma of mucosae should be included in the differential diagnosis of head and neck mucosal lesions.

Immunosuppression increases the risk of Merkel cell carcinoma. Chronic UVB radiation exposure appears to be a major risk factor for Merkel cell carcinoma of the head and neck in older whites. A viral infection with MCPyV also appears to play a role in the etiopathogenesis of Merkel cell carcinoma. Considering the literature on Merkel cell carcinoma overall, primary Merkel cell carcinoma appears to be multifactorial in origin, as most cancers are, and likely occurring in elderly whites after a lifetime accumulation of environmental mutagenic insults when the efficiency of their immune system decreases because of immunosenescence and inflamm-aging. Each of the major potential risk factors for Merkel cell carcinoma causes directly or indirectly genetic and chromosomal abnormalities, (possible) dysregulation of mRNA stability, and can modulate gene expression. Merkel cell carcinomas are a group of genetically heterogeneous tumors,[56,63] which is consistent with a variety of different mutagenic factors acting on cell genes and chromosomes. Merkel cell carcinoma's rarity and its occurrence in old age is evidence of the resistance to carcinogenic mutation of the cells from which Merkel cell carcinoma originates.

Iatrogenic immunosuppression decreases and even abolishes the immune system defenses against cancer. Specific groups of individuals known to be immunosuppressed are at increased risk for Merkel cell carcinoma at a younger age than expected and they may be candidates for screening for Merkel cell carcinoma on the skin or mucosae. These groups of patients include people with HIV infection, the sub-population of solid organ transplant recipients and patients treated with immunosuppressant drugs because of systemic autoimmune disorders. Older whites recently diagnosed with another malignancy, especially of the lympho-hemopoietic system, are at increased risk of Merkel cell carcinoma especially in the first year of follow-up.

References

1. Agelli M., Clegg L.X. (2003). Epidemiology of primary Merkel cell carcinoma in the United States. *J Am Acad Dermatol* 49: 832–841.
2. Shipkov C.D., Dumollard J.M., Mojallal A., Seguin P. (2008). Merkel cell carcinoma vs. basal cell carcinoma: histopathologic challenges. *J Cutan Pathol* 35: 789–790.
3. Thakur S., Chalioulias K., Hayes M., While A. (2008). Bilateral primary Merkel cell carcinoma of the upper lid misdiagnosed as basal cell carcinoma. *Orbit* 27: 139–141.
4. Agelli, M., Clegg X.L., Becker J.C., Rollison D.E. (2010). The etiology and epidemiology of Merkel cell carcinoma. *Curr Prob Cancer* 34: 14–37.
5. Toker C. (1972). Trabecular carcinoma of the skin. *Arch Dermatol* 105: 107–110.
6. Haag M.L., Glass L.F., Fenske N.A. (1995). Merkel cell carcinoma. Diagnosis and treatment. *Dermatol Surg* 21: 669–683.
7. Tang C.K., Toker C. (1978). Trabecular carcinoma of the skin: an ultrastructural study. *Cancer* 42: 2311–2321.
8. Dinh V., Feun L., Elgart G., Savaraj N. (2007). Merkel cell carcinomas. *Hematol Oncol Clin North Am* 21: 527–544.
9. Szeder V., Grim M., Halata Z., Sieber-Blum M. (2003). Neural crest origin of mammalian Merkel cells. *Dev Biol* 253: 258–263.
10. Merkel F. (1875). Tastzellen and tastkoerperchen bei den hausthieren und beim menschen. *Arch Mikrosc Anat* 11: 636–652 (in German).
11. Halata Z., Grim M., Bauman K.I. (2003). Friedrich Sigmund Merkel and his "Merkel cell", morphology, development, and physiology: review and new results. *Anat Rec A Discov Mol Cell Evol Biol* 271: 225–239.
12. Youker S.R. (2003). Merkel cell carcinoma. *Adv Dermatol* 19: 185–205.

13. Hewitt J.B., Sherif A., Kerr K.M., Stankler L. (1993). Merkel cell and squamous cell carcinomas arising in erythema ab igne. *Br J Dermatol* 128: 591–592.
14. Hitchcock C.L., Kirby B.I., Laney R.G., *et al.* (1988). Neuroendocrine (Merkel cell) carcinoma of the skin: its natural history, diagnosis, and treatment. *Ann Surg* 207: 201–207.
15. Wolff-Peeters C., Marien K., Mebis J., Desmet V. (1980). A cutaneous APUDoma or Merkel cell tumor? A morphologically recognizable tumor with a biological and histological malignant aspect in contrast with its clinical behavior. *Cancer* 46: 1810–1816.
16. Dadzie O., Teixeira F. (2009). What can primary cutaneous neuroendocrine carcinomas with squamoid and neuroendocrine differentiation teach us about the origin of Merkel cells? *Int J Dermatol* 48: 91–93.
17. Lee W.J., Lee D.W., Lee M.W., *et al.* (2009). Multiple cutaneous metastases of neuroendocrine carcinoma derived from the uterine cervix. *J Eur Acad Dermatol Venereol* 4: 494–496.
18. Panelos J., Batistatou A., Paglierani M., *et al.* (2009). Expression of Notch-1 and alteration of the E-cadherin/beta-catenin cell adhesion complex are observed in primary cutaneous neuroendocrine carcinoma (Merkel cell carcinoma). *Mod Pathol* 22: 959–968.
19. Satter E.K., Derienzo D.P. (2008). Synchronous onset of multiple cutaneous neuroendocrine (Merkel cell) carcinomas localized to the scalp. *J Cutan Pathol* 35: 685–691.
20. World Health Organization (1976) *International Classification of Diseases for Oncology (ICD-O)*, First Edition, Geneva.
21. World Health Organization (1990) *International Classification of Diseases for Oncology (ICD-O)*, Second Edition, Geneva.
22. World Health Organization (2000) *International Classification of Diseases for Oncology (ICD-O)*, Third Edition, Geneva.
23. Percy C., Von Holten V. (eds.). (1986). *International Classification of Diseases for Oncology*, Field Trial Edition, National Cancer Institute, Bethesda, Maryland.
24. Agelli M. (2009). Unpublished data.
25. Brenner B., Katz A., Rakowski E., *et al.* (1996). Merkel cell carcinoma in Israel. *Isr J Med Sci* 32: 1235–1238.

26. Chuang T.Y., Su W.P., Muller S.A. (1990). Incidence of cutaneous T cell lymphoma and other rare skin cancers in a defined population. *J Am Acad Dermatol* 23: 254–256.
27. Hodgson N.C. (2005). Merkel cell carcinoma: changing incidence trends. *J Surg Oncol* 89: 1–4.
28. Miller R.W., Rabkin C.S. (1999). Merkel cell carcinoma and melanoma: etiological similarities and differences. *Cancer Epidemiol Biomarkers Prev* 8: 153–158.
29. Riou-Gotta M.O., Fournier E., Danzon A., *et al.* (2009). Rare skin cancer: a population-based cancer registry descriptive study of 151 consecutive cases diagnosed between 1980 and 2004. *Acta Oncol* 48: 605–609.
30. Vilar-Coromina N., Pérez Bueno F., Alsina Maqueda M., *et al.* (2009). Merkel cell carcinoma of the skin: population-based incidence and survival, 1995–2005. *Med Clin (Barc)* 132: 701–703 (in Spanish).
31. Buell J.F., Trofe J., Hanaway M.J., *et al.* (2002). Immunosuppression and Merkel cell cancer. *Transplant Proc* 34: 1780–1781.
32. Engels E.A., Frisch M., Goedert J.J., *et al.* (2002). Merkel cell carcinoma and HIV infection. *Lancet* 359: 497–498.
33. Penn I., First M.R. (1999). Merkel's cell carcinoma in organ recipients: report of 41 cases. *Transplantation* 68: 1717–1721.
34. Hankey B.F., Ries L.A., Edwards B.K. (1999). The Surveillance, Epidemiology, and End Results Program: a national resource. *Cancer Epidemiol Biomarkers Prev* 8: 1117–1121.
35. Ries L.G., Pollack E.S., Young J.L., Jr. (1983). Cancer patient survival: Surveillance, Epidemiology, and End Results program, 1973–1979. *J Natl Cancer Inst* 70: 693–707.
36. Moll R., Lowe A., Laufer J., Franke W.W. (1992). Cytokeratin 20 in human carcinomas. A new histodiagnostic marker detected by monoclonal antibodies. *Am J Pathol* 140: 427–447.
37. Brenner B., Sulkes A., Rakowsky E., *et al.* (2001). Second neoplasms in patients with Merkel cell carcinoma. *Cancer* 91: 1358–1362.
38. Howard R.A., Dores G.M., Curtis R.E., *et al.* (2006). Merkel cell carcinoma and multiple primary cancers. *Cancer Epidemiol Biomarkers Prev* 15: 1545–1549.
39. Scotto J., Fears T.R., Fraumeni J.F. (1996). Solar radiation. In: Schottenfeld, D.D. and Fraumeni, J.F. (eds.). *Cancer Epidemiology and Prevention*, pp. 355–372, Oxford University Press, New York.

40. Pilotti S., Rilke F., Bartoli C., Grisotti A. (1988). Clinicopathologic correlations of cutaneous neuroendocrine Merkel cell carcinoma. *J Clin Oncol* 6: 1863–1873.
41. Yiengpruksawan A., Coit D.G., Thaler H.T. *et al.* (1991) Merkel cell carcinoma. Prognosis and management. *Arch Surg* 126: 1514–1519.
42. Dwyer T., Blizzard L., Ashbolt R., *et al.* (2002). Cutaneous melanin density of Caucasians measured by spectrophotometry and risk of malignant melanoma, basal cell carcinoma, and squamous cell carcinoma of the skin. *Am J Epidemiol* 155: 614–621.
43. Aw D., Silva A.B., Palmer D.B. (2007). Immunosenescence: emerging challenges for an ageing population. *Immunology* 120: 435–446.
44. Franceschi C., Bonafè M., Valensin S., *et al.* (2000). Inflamm-aging. An evolutionary perspective on immunosenescence. *Ann N Y Acad Sci* 908: 244–254.
45. Butcher S.K., Lord J.M. (2004). Stress responses and innate immunity: aging as a contributory factor. *Aging Cell* 3: 151–160.
46. Yom S.S., Rosenthal D.I., El Naggar A.K., *et al.* (2006). Merkel cell carcinoma of the tongue and head and neck oral mucosal sites. *Oral Surg Oral Med Oral Pathol Oral Radiol Endoc* 101: 761–768.
47. Allen P.J., Zhang Z.F., Coit D.G. (1999). Surgical management of Merkel cell carcinoma. *Ann Surg* 229: 97–105.
48. Goessling W., McKee P.H., Mayer R.J. (2002). Merkel cell carcinoma. *J Clin Oncol* 20: 588–598.
49. Heath M., Jaimes N., Lemos B., *et al.* (2008). Clinical characteristics of Merkel cell carcinoma at diagnosis in 195 patients: the AEIOU features. *J Am Acad Dermatol* 58: 375–381.
50. Silva E.G., Mackay B., Goepfert H., *et al.* (1984). Endocrine carcinoma of the skin (Merkel cell carcinoma). *Pathol Annu* 19(Pt 2): 1–30.
51. Weeraratna A.T., Houben R., O'Connell M.P., Becker J.C. (2010). Lack of Wnt5A expression in Merkel cell carcinoma. *Arch Dermatol* 146: 88–89.
52. Lardy F., Gautier C., Etesse-Pichon S., *et al.* (1996). Post-radiotherapy cutaneous neuro-endocrine carcinoma. *Ann Dermatol Venereol* 123: 464–467 (in French).
53. Tuneu A, Pujol R.M., Moreno A., *et al.* (1989). Postirradiation Merkel cell carcinoma. *J Am Acad Dermatol* 20: 505–507.
54. Jones C.S., Tyring S.K., Lee P.C., Fine J.D. (1988). Development of neuroendocrine (Merkel cell) carcinoma mixed with squamous cell carcinoma in erythema *ab igne*. *Arch Dermatol* 124: 110–113.

55. Iacocca M.V., Abernethy J.L., Stefanato C.M., *et al.* (1998). Mixed Merkel cell carcinoma and squamous cell carcinoma of the skin. *J Am Acad Dermatol* 39: 882–887.
56. Boukamp P. (2005). UV-induced skin cancer: similarities — variations. *J Dtsch Dermatol Ges* 3: 493–503.
57. Andea A.A., Coit D.G., Amin B., Busam K.J. (2008). Merkel cell carcinoma: histologic features and prognosis. *Cancer* 113: 2549–2558.
58. Aydin A., Kocer N.E., Bekerecioglu M., Sari I. (2003). Cutaneous undifferentiated small (Merkel) cell carcinoma, that developed synchronously with multiple actinic keratoses, squamous cell carcinomas and basal cell carcinoma. *J Dermatol* 30: 241–244.
59. Forman S.B., Vidmar D.A., Ferringer T.C. (2008). Collision tumor composed of Merkel cell carcinoma and lentigo maligna melanoma. *J Cutan Pathol* 35: 203–206.
60. Walsh N.M. (2001). Primary neuroendocrine (Merkel cell) carcinoma of the skin: morphologic diversity and implications thereof. *Hum Pathol* 32: 680–689.
61. Whiteman D.C., Bray C.A., Siskind V., *et al.* (2008). Changes in the incidence of cutaneous melanoma in the west of Scotland and Queensland, Australia: hope for health promotion? *Eur J Cancer Prev* 17: 243–250.
62. Van Gele M., Kaghad M., Leonard J.H., *et al.* (2000). Mutation analysis of P73 and TP53 in Merkel cell carcinoma. *Br J Cancer* 82: 823–826.
63. Popp S., Waltering S., Herbst C., *et al.* (2002). UV-B-type mutations and chromosomal imbalances indicate common pathways for the development of Merkel and skin squamous cell carcinomas. *Int J Cancer* 99: 352–360.
64. Brash D.E., Rudolph J.A., Simon J.A., *et al.* (1991). A role for sunlight in skin cancer: UV-induced p53 mutations in squamous cell carcinoma. *Proc Natl Acad Sci USA* 15: 10124–10128.
65. Brash D.E. (1997). Sunlight and the onset of skin cancer. *Trends Genet* 13: 410–414.
66. Brash D.E. (2006). Roles of the transcription factor p53 in keratinocyte carcinomas. *Br J Dermatol* 154(Suppl 1): 8–10.
67. Ziegler A., Jonason A.S., Leffell D.J., *et al.* (1994). Sunburn and p53 in the onset of skin cancer. *Nature* 372: 773–776.
68. Lunder E.J., Stern R.S. (1998). Merkel-cell carcinomas in patients treated with methoxsalen and ultraviolet A radiation. *N Engl J Med* 339: 1247–1248.

69. de Gruijl F.R. (2002). Photocarcinogenesis: UVA vs. UVB radiation. *Methods Enzymol* 319: 359–366.
70. Tang C.K., Toker C., Nedwich A., Zaman A.N. (1982). Unusual cutaneous carcinoma with features of small cell (oat cell-like) and squamous cell carcinomas. A variant of malignant Merkel cell neoplasm. *Am J Dermatopathol* 4: 537–548.
71. Ho S.Y., Tsai Y.C., Lee M.C., Guo H.R. (2005). Merkel cell carcinoma in patients with long-term ingestion of arsenic. *J Occup Health* 47: 188–192.
72. Tseng W.P., Chu H.M., How S.W., *et al.* (1968). Prevalence of skin cancer in an endemic area of chronic arsenicism in Taiwan. *J Natl Cancer Inst* 40: 453–463.
73. Liu S.X., Davidson M.M., Tang X., *et al.* (2005). Mitochondrial damage mediates genotoxicity of arsenic in mammalian cells. *Cancer Res* 65: 3236–3242.
74. Huang H.P., Huang A.H., Lee J.Y. (1991). Merkel cell carcinoma: report of three cases. *J Formos Med Assoc* 90: 900–903 (in Chinese).
75. Tsuruta D., Hamada T., Mochida K., *et al.* (1998). Merkel cell carcinoma, Bowen's disease and chronic occupational arsenic poisoning. *Br J Dermatol* 139: 291–294.
76. Feng H., Shuda M., Chang Y., Moore P.S. (2008). Clonal integration of a polyomavirus in human Merkel cell carcinoma. *Science* 319: 1096–1100.
77. Becker J.C., Houben R., Ugurel S., *et al.* (2009). MC polyomavirus is frequently present in Merkel cell carcinoma of European patients. *J Invest Dermatol* 129: 248–250.
78. Garneski K.M., Warcola A.H., Feng Q., *et al.* (2009). Merkel cell polyomavirus is more frequently present in North American than Australian Merkel cell carcinoma tumors. *J Invest Dermatol* 129: 246–248.
79. Kassem A., Schöpflin A., Diaz C., *et al.* (2008). Frequent detection of Merkel cell polyomavirus in human Merkel cell carcinomas and identification of a unique deletion in the VP1 gene. *Cancer Res* 68: 5009–5013.
80. zur Hausen H. (2008). Novel human polyomaviruses — re-emergence of a well known virus family as possible human carcinogens. *Int J Cancer* 123: 247–250.
81. Poulin D.L., DeCaprio J.A. (2006). Is there a role for SV40 in human cancer? *J Clin Oncol* 24: 4356–4365.

82. Gardner S.D., Field A.M., Coleman D.V., Hulme B. (1971). New human papovavirus (B.K.) isolated from urine after renal transplantation. *Lancet* 1(7712): 1253–1257.
83. Padgett B.L., Walker D.L., ZuRhein G.M., *et al.* (1971). Cultivation of papova-like virus from human brain with progressive multifocal leucoencephalopathy. *Lancet* 1(7712): 1257–1260.
84. Acott P.D., Hirsch H.H. (2007). BK virus infection, replication, and diseases in pediatric kidney transplantation. *Pediatr Nephrol* 22: 1243–1250.
85. Bohl D.L., Brennan D.C. (2007). BK virus nephropathy and kidney transplantation. *Clin J Am Soc Nephrol* 2(Suppl 1): 36–46.
86. Cohen Y., Amir G., Polliack A. (2002). Development and rapid dissemination of Merkel-cell carcinomatosis following therapy with fludarabine and rituximab for relapsing follicular lymphoma. *Eur J Haematol* 68: 117–119.
87. Gooptu C., Woollons A., Ross J., *et al.* (1997). Merkel cell carcinoma arising after therapeutic immunosuppression. *Br J Dermatol* 137: 637–641.
88. Lentz S.R., Krewson L., Zutter M.M. (1993). Recurrent neuroendocrine (Merkel cell) carcinoma of the skin presenting as marrow failure in a man with systemic lupus erythematosus. *Med Pediatr Oncol* 21: 137–141.
89. Lillis J., Ceilley R.I., Nelson P. (2005). Merkel cell carcinoma in a patient with autoimmune hepatitis. *J Drugs Dermatol* 4: 357–359.
90. McLoone N.M., McKenna K., Edgar D., *et al.* (2005). Merkel cell carcinoma in a patient with chronic sarcoidosis. *Clin Exp Dermatol* 30: 580–582.
91. Nemoto I., Sato-Matsumura K.C., Fujita Y., *et al.* (2008). Leukaemic dissemination of Merkel cell carcinoma in a patient with systemic lupus erythematosus. *Clin Exp Dermatol* 33: 270–272.
92. Satolli F., Venturi C., Vescovi V., *et al.* (2005). Merkel-cell carcinoma in Behcet's disease. *Acta Derm Venereol* 85: 79.
93. Stone J.H., Holbrook J.T., Marriott M.A., *et al.* (2006). Solid malignancies among patients in the Wegener's Granulomatosis Etanercept Trial. *Arthritis Rheum* 54: 1608–1618.
94. Wirges M.L., Saporito F., Smith J. (2006). Rapid growth of Merkel cell carcinoma after treatment with rituximab. *J Drugs Dermatol* 5: 180–181.

95. Friedlaender M.M., Rubinger D., Rosenbaum E., *et al.* (2002). Temporary regression of Merkel cell carcinoma metastases after cessation of cyclosporine. *Transplantation* 73: 1849–1850.
96. Muirhead R., Ritchie D.M. (2007). Partial regression of Merkel cell carcinoma in response to withdrawal of azathioprine in an immunosuppression-induced case of metastatic Merkel cell carcinoma. *Clin Oncol (R Coll Radiol)* 19: 96.
97. Urbatsch A., Sams W. M., Jr., Urist M.M., Sturdivant R. (1999). Merkel cell carcinoma occurring in renal transplant patients. *J Am Acad Dermatol* 41: 289–291.
98. Gilaberte M., Pujol R.M., Sierra J., *et al.* (2000). Merkel cell carcinoma developing after bone marrow transplantation. *Dermatology* 201: 80–82.
99. Maksymiuk B., Wygoda A., Zakliczynski M., Palen P. (2002). Primary undifferentiated small cell carcinoma (Merkel cell carcinoma) in a patient after heart transplantation — case report. *Pol J Pathol* 53: 177–180.
100. Bordea C., Wojnarowska F., Millard P.R., *et al.* (2004). Skin cancers in renal-transplant recipients occur more frequently than previously recognized in a temperate climate. *Transplantation* 77: 574–579.
101. Bajetta E., Platania M., Catena L., *et al.* (2007). Merkel cell carcinoma after liver transplantation: a case report. *Tumori* 93: 323–326.
102. Bensaleh H., Perney P., Dereure O., *et al.* (2007). Merkel cell carcinoma in a liver transplant patient. *Am J Clin Dermatol* 8: 239–241.
103. Lanoy E., Dores G.M., Madeleine M.M., *et al.* (2009). Epidemiology of nonkeratinocytic skin cancers among persons with AIDS in the United States. *AIDS* 23: 385–393.
104. Burack J., Altschuler E.L. (2003). Sustained remission of metastatic Merkel cell carcinoma with treatment of HIV infection. *J R Soc Med* 96: 238–239.
105. Skelton H.G., Smith K.J., Hitchcock C.L., *et al.* (1997). Merkel cell carcinoma: analysis of clinical, histologic, and immunohistologic features of 132 cases with relation to survival. *J Am Acad Dermatol* 37: 734–739.
106. Ziprin P., Smith S., Salerno G., Rosin R.D. (2000). Two cases of Merkel cell tumour arising in patients with chronic lymphocytic leukaemia. *Br J Dermatol* 142: 525–528.
107. Cerroni L., Kerl H. (1997). Primary cutaneous neuroendocrine (Merkel cell) carcinoma in association with squamous- and basal-cell carcinoma. *Am J Dermatopathol* 19: 610–613.

108. Gomez L.G., DiMaio S., Silva E.G., Mackay B. (1983). Association between neuroendocrine (Merkel cell) carcinoma and squamous carcinoma of the skin. *Am J Surg Pathol* 7: 171–177.

109. Guo H.R., Yu H.S., Hu H., Monson R.R. (2001). Arsenic in drinking water and skin cancer: cell-type specificity. *Cancer Causes Control* 12: 909–916.

110. Euvrard S., Kanitakis J., Claudy A. (2003). Skin cancers after organ transplantation. *N Engl J Med* 348: 1681–1691.

Chapter 2

Basic Pathobiology of Merkel Cell Carcinoma

Jürgen C. Becker, David Schrama and Roland Houben

The basic biologic function of the Merkel cell, as well as the true cellular origin of the neuroendocrine carcinoma of the skin known as Merkel cell carcinoma, is a matter of dispute, as discussed in Chapter 5. Thus, it is not surprising that despite immense progress in our understanding of the pathogenesis of many cancers, little is known about the basic mechanisms underlying Merkel cell carcinoma's biology and pathogenesis. There is still a striking need for a better understanding of the molecular biology of Merkel cell carcinoma.

Douglas Hanahan and Robert A. Weinberg suggested that the vast catalogue of cancer cell genotypes is a manifestation of six essential alterations in cell physiology that collectively dictate malignant growth: evasion of apoptosis, self-sufficiency in growth signals, insensitivity to growth-inhibitory signals, limitless replicative potential, sustained angiogenesis, and tissue invasion and metastasis.[1] From an immunologist's point of view, escape from immune surveillance may be added to the list.[2] Each of these capabilities acquired during tumor development represents the successful breach of an anticancer defence mechanism. These pathways, and their potential relevance in Merkel cell carcinoma, are the subject of this chapter.

2.1 Evasion of Apoptosis

A critical step in tumorigenesis appears to be inhibition of apoptosis.[1] Apoptosis is the main form of programmed cell death in multicellular organisms, which involves a series of biochemical events leading to a characteristic cell morphology and death. The process of apoptosis is controlled by a diverse range of cell signals originating either extra- or intracellularly. These signals must be connected to the actual death pathway by way of regulatory proteins allowing an efficient initiation of this process. This is achieved by either targeting mitochondria functionality or directly transducing the signal via adapter proteins to the apoptotic caspases, a set of cystein proteases regulating and executing cell death.

In this regard, apoptotic proteins that target mitochondria affect them in different ways;[3] they may cause mitochondrial swelling through the formation of membrane pores, or they may increase the permeability of the mitochondrial membrane and cause apoptotic effectors to be released into the cytosol. Indeed, the mitochondrial apoptosis-induced channel (MAC) is an early marker of the onset of apoptosis. This ion channel is formed on the outer mitochondrial membrane in response to certain apoptotic stimuli. Members of the Bcl-2 protein family regulate apoptosis by controlling the formation of MAC: the pro-apoptotic members Bax and/or Bak form MAC, whereas the anti-apoptotic members like Bcl-2 or Bcl-xL prevent MAC formation.[3]

Over-expression of the anti-apoptotic molecule Bcl-2 was observed in three-fourths of Merkel cell carcinoma tumors in two independent studies.[4,5] The expression of Bcl-2 is a common finding in many cancers and is regarded as one of the mechanisms to avoid cell death in tumor cells. Inhibition of Bcl-2 expression *in vivo* by antisense oligonucleotides in a SCID mouse/human Merkel cell carcinoma xenograft model resulted in tumor shrinkage.[6] However, the same antisense oligonucleotides when tested in a phase II trial demonstrated only a very limited, if any, efficacy in patients with Merkel cell carcinoma.[7]

The inhibitor of apoptosis protein survivin is undetectable in most terminally differentiated human tissues. It is strongly expressed in embryonic and fetal organs and in many cancers. Interestingly, polyomaviruses, for which a causal role in Merkel cell carcinoma tumorigenesis was recently suggested,[8] are known inductors of survivin.[9] Kim and McNiff recently evaluated survivin expression in Merkel cell carcinoma.[10] All 19 cases of Merkel cell carcinoma demonstrated strong survivin staining.

Survivin protein was localized and classified into predominately nuclear or cytoplasmic compartments. However, a mixed pattern of survivin expression was also seen in three cases. Cases with a nuclear staining pattern were distinguished by an aggressive clinical course, with seven of eight patients developing metastases or dead of disease on follow-up.

2.2 Self-Sufficiency in Growth Signals

Merkel cell carcinomas grow rapidly and tumor doubling times of 5–12 days are characteristic. In aggressive subtypes, doubling can even occur within 1–5 days.[11] Cancer cells defy normal regulation of growth in a process that involves, on the one hand, lasting changes to the respective genes (genetic aberrations), and on the other hand their altered use (epigenetic aberrations). The two most important mechanisms in carcinogenesis are activation of growth-stimulating oncogenes and inactivation of tumor suppressor genes.[1] Three common molecular strategies for achieving autonomy are evident, involving alteration of (i) extracellular growth signals, (ii) transcellular transducers of those signals or (iii) intracellular circuits that translate those signals into action.

2.2.1 *Extracellular growth signals: platelet-derived growth factor receptors*

The first potential hint towards genetic alterations in growth factor receptors came from Swick *et al.*[12] They observed that three of nine (33.3%) Merkel cell carcinomas demonstrated an identical novel single heterozygous base change in exon 10 of the platelet-derived growth factor receptor-A (PDGFRA) gene leading to an amino acid substitution at codon 478. All three of those Merkel cell carcinomas expressed PDGFRA. However, it is uncertain if this change represents a true mutation or a single nucleotide polymorphism. Recently, the expression of VEGF-A, VEGF-C and PDGF-α in Merkel cell carcinoma was reported. Interestingly, all of these proteins were uniformly expressed throughout the tumors but their expression levels were rather low. There was a tendency toward higher expression in larger tumors, although the difference did not reach statistical significance.[13]

2.2.2 *Transcellular growth signal receptors/transducers*

2.2.2.1 *MAP kinase pathway*

The classical mitogen-activated protein (MAP) kinase signaling pathway plays a key role in many processes such as proliferation, suppression of apoptosis, migration and differentiation.[14] The relevance of the Raf/MEK/ERK cascade for tumorigenesis has been evident for a long time, but was underlined in 2002 with the discovery that BRAF, one of the three isoforms of Raf, is present in a mutated form in many tumor entities, particularly melanoma.[15] Thus, MAP kinase signaling, frequently activated in many epithelial cancers, is the most studied oncogenic pathway in Merkel cell carcinoma. The impact of dysregulated KIT (CD117, SCFR) as an oncogenic tyrosine kinase for autocrine stimulation of MAP kinase signaling in Merkel cell carcinoma has been addressed in several studies which have detected KIT expression in tumor samples.[13,16–18] Indeed, KIT is present in 95% of Merkel cell carcinomas, but its expression does not correlate with more aggressive behaviour.[16,17,19] Recently, Swick *et al.* determined that although eight of nine Merkel cell carcinoma tumors were positive for KIT by immunohistochemical staining, no activating mutations were present in the four exons commonly found to have mutations in this gene.[20] Similarly, the analysis of Merkel cell carcinoma samples for the presence of activating BRAF mutation did not reveal any of these.[21,22] Moreover, immunohistochemical studies revealed that despite high proliferation indices and existing expression of ERK, the ERK protein generally occurs in the non-phosphorylated form and is thus inactive.[22] The lack of ERK phosphorylation was always accompanied by a strong expression of the Raf kinase inhibitor protein (RKIP), a negative regulator of the MAPK cascade that binds to Raf and MEK and thus inhibits their interaction. These observations suggested that RKIP is responsible for turning off this signaling pathway. This assumption did not prove true since silencing of RKIP did not lead to an induction of ERK phosphorylation.[22]

The general inactivity of the 'mitogenic' cascade distinguishes Merkel cell carcinoma from many other tumors such as melanoma and raises the question if active MAP kinase signaling is perhaps even a negative selection factor for Merkel cell carcinoma cells. To test this notion, we developed UISO cells that express a Raf construct in which the natural regulatory domain is replaced by an artificial hydroxy-tamoxifen (OHT)-sensitive regulatory domain (Raf-ER) derived from the estrogen receptor.[23] OHT stimulation results in MEK and ERK activation in these cells. This activation of the MAPK pathway leads to a collapse of the cytoskeleton and subsequent apoptosis of the Merkel cell carcinoma cells. OHT-induced apoptosis could be prevented by specific MEK inhibition, indicating that apoptosis is indeed an effect mediated by the MAPK cascade.

2.2.3 *Secreted Wingless type (Wnt) ligands*

Secreted Wingless type (Wnt) ligands have been shown to activate signal transduction pathways and trigger changes in gene expression, cell behavior, adhesion and polarity.[24] The role of Wnt signaling in cancer was first suggested 20 years ago with the discovery of Wnt1 as an integration site for mouse mammary tumor virus in mouse mammary carcinoma. Over time, a wealth of evidence has implicated Wnt signaling in tumor development and progression. The Wnt pathway and its role in Merkel cell carcinoma have been evaluated by determination of nuclear accumulation of β-catenin and mutations in β-catenin and three other related genes. Liu *et al.* observed elevated β-catenin accumulation in only one out of 12 tumors and no mutations in any tumors; thus, they concluded that the Wnt pathway is not implicated in Merkel cell carcinoma.[25]

2.3 Insensitivity to Growth-Inhibitory Signals

Within a normal tissue, multiple antiproliferative signals operate to maintain cellular quiescence and tissue homeostasis. These growth-inhibitory signals are received by transmembrane cell surface receptors coupled to intracellular signaling circuits.[26] Incipient cancer cells must evade these antiproliferative signals if they are to prosper. At the molecular level, most antiproliferative signals are funneled through the retinoblastoma protein (RB) and its two relatives, RBL1 and RBL2. When in a hypophosphorylated state, RB blocks proliferation by sequestering and altering the function of E2F transcription factors that control the expression of genes

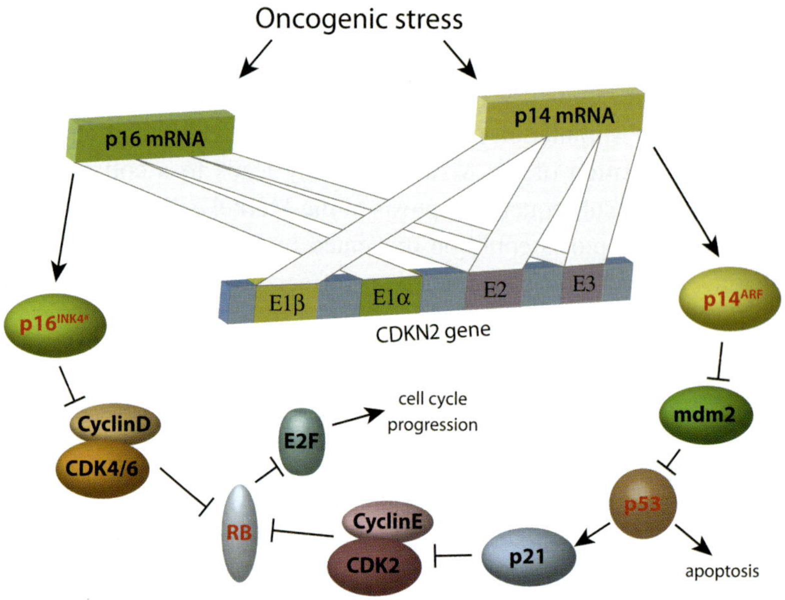

Figure 1. The control of the cell cycle progression by RB, p53 and CDK inhibitors.

essential for progression from G1 into S phase. The INK4a-ARF locus encodes two protein products, p16INK4a and p14ARF, whose respective mRNAs are generated by alternative splicing and whose expression is regulated by separate promoters (Figure 1). p16INK4a and p14ARF are integral parts of the two cell-cycle control pathways targeted most frequently during tumorigenesis, i.e. the RB and p53 pathway, respectively.[27]

The epigenetic silencing of upstream events of the RB pathway has recently been described.[28] Lassacher *et al.* observed that promoter hypermethylation of the INK4a-ARF locus is common in Merkel cell carcinoma. Their analysis revealed the presence of methylated DNA at the p14ARF promoter in eight of 19 Merkel cell carcinoma samples; in contrast, the p16INK4a promoter was only methylated in one case. This observation sheds important light on the pathogenesis of Merkel cell carcinoma because DNA methylation in promoter regions helps to regulate the gene expression. In particular, hypermethylation of CpG islands located in the promoter regions of tumor-suppressor genes such as p16INK4a, BRCA1 and hMLH is now established as an important

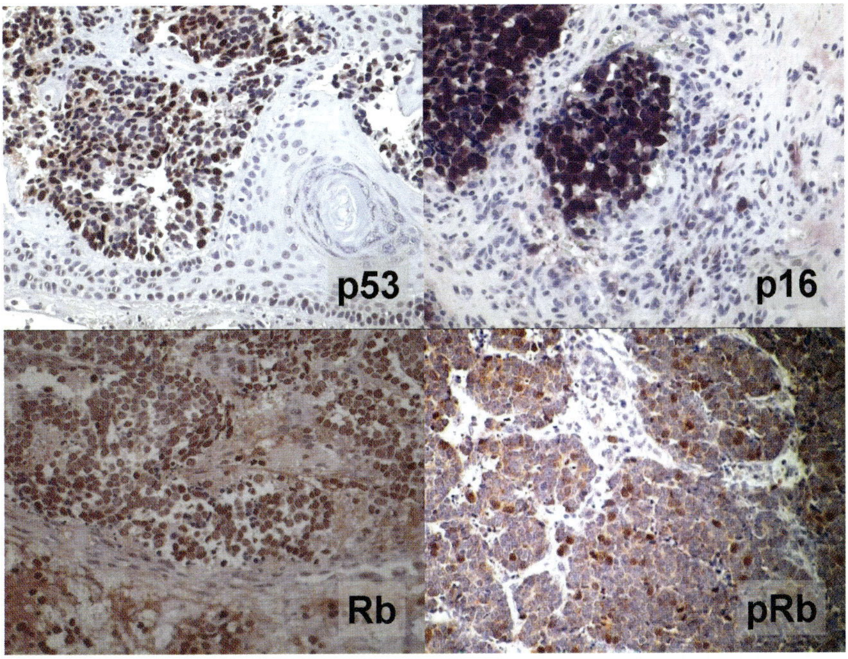

Figure 2. Detection of p53, p16INK4a, Rb and phospho-Rb in Merkel cell carcinoma tissue sections by immunohistochemistry.

mechanism of gene inactivation in cancer.[29] The high frequency of p14ARF promoter methylation compared to that of p16INK4a in Merkel cell carcinoma suggest that alterations in the p53 pathway appear to be most crucial. In accordance with this we observe high-level expression of p16INK4a in the majority of Merkel cell carcinoma tissues (Figure 2).

Mutations in p53, p14ARF promoter methylation and high levels of p16INK4a expression have been demonstrated. Data on loss of RB are contradictory and RB inactivation through viral proteins is conceivable.

A multitude of functions have been described for the tumor suppressor p53. Most importantly, as a transcription factor following DNA damage p53 regulates the expression of genes involved in the control of the cell cycle, the induction of apoptosis or senescence and DNA repair.[27] The anti-proliferative activity of p53 plays a significant role in the avoidance of tumor development, but also requires effective mechanisms to control p53 in normal proliferating cells. The most important of these mechanisms involves the control of protein stability with ubiquitination by the p53-specific ubiquitin ligase mdm2 and subsequent proteasomal degradation. Oncogenic stress results in the induction of the tumor suppressor protein p14ARF, which by binding to mdm2 inactivates it and thus prevents degradation of p53 (Figure 1).[30] In Figure 2, over-expression of p53 in Merkel cell carcinoma is depicted, which is frequently an indication of p53 being inactivated by point mutation, making it also insensitive to degradation.

p53 is the protein that is most frequently present in a mutated form in tumors. It is found altered in about 50% of human tumors, and in tumors with wild-type p53, its activation is often disturbed. p53 mutations are occasionally found in Merkel cell carcinoma. In three of 15 tumors examined, and in two of six Merkel cell carcinoma cell lines, p53 mutations were present.[31,32] On the other hand, the previously mentioned apoptosis induction associated with p53 derepression in Merkel cell carcinoma xenografts suggests that the regulation of p53 expression or stability may be disturbed in Merkel cell carcinoma.[33] For another member of the p53 family, p63, it has been shown that its expression in Merkel cell carcinoma cells correlates to a high degree with the aggressiveness of the disease.[34] p63 is a transcription factor essential for proliferation of stem cells and for stratification in epithelia, which is found to be mutated in human hereditary syndromes characterized by ectodermal dysplasia.

The proteins whose expression is induced by p53 include p21 (Figure 1). Together with p27 and the proteins of the INK4 family, p21 belongs to the inhibitors of the cyclin-dependent kinases (CDK). These CDK inhibitors, expressed upon various extra- and intracellular stimuli, can prevent the transition from the G1 to the S phase of the cell cycle.[35] By binding to cyclin/CDK complexes, these inhibitors lead to inactivation of the complexes and phosphorylation of RB does not take place. As mentioned before, in its hypo-phosphorylated state RB prevents entry into the S phase by forming an inhibiting complex with transcription factors of the E2F family and by mediating the binding of DNA-modifying enzymes.[26] After multiple phosphorylations of RB by cyclin D/CDK4/6 and cyclin E/CDK2 complexes, RB is released and degraded, the inhibition of E2F is suspended and the transcription of genes for the G1/S transition is initiated. The RB/E2F signaling pathway is of such central significance for the control of cell proliferation that it is assumed its regulation is disturbed in practically all tumors. Gene loss or inactivating mutations of RB, viral RB-inactivating oncoproteins (e.g. human papilloma virus E7), over-expression and activating mutations of CDK 4/6, amplification and over-expression of CDK2, amplification or translocation of cyclin D genes as well as inactivating mutations and loss of expression of p16INK4a and p15INK4b have been described.

For Merkel cell carcinoma, little data on the regulation of the cell cycle by RB exist and studies on a possible loss of RB are contradictory. Leonard and Hayard found LOH for the marker D13S233 (13q14.3), which is located close to the RB gene, in 18 of 24 examined Merkel cell carcinoma samples.[36] Further, in all nine Merkel cell carcinoma cell lines they analyzed, no RB could be detected in the Western blot. In contrast, Popp *et al.* reported no loss of the 13q region in ten Merkel cell carcinomas analyzed by comparative genome hybridization.[32] Our own experiments suggest that loss of RB is not a frequent occurrence in Merkel cell carcinoma (Figure 2).

The inactivity of the MAP kinase pathway, together with the report that inhibition of Ras farnesylation suppresses the growth of Merkel cell carcinoma xenografts by apoptosis induction in the naked mouse model, suggest that another Ras-dependent signaling pathway may be of special relevance in Merkel cell carcinoma.[37] The most important Ras-regulated signal pathway next to the Raf/MEK/ERK cascade involves class 1 phosphoinositide 3 kinase (PI3K) and the AKT kinase.[33] PI3K phosphorylates phosphatidylinositol 4,5-biphosphate (PIP2) to phosphatidylinositol 3,4,5-triphosphate (PIP3), an important second messenger lipid.

The antagonist of PI3K that dephosphorylates PIP3 is the phosphate and tensin homologue (PTEN), whose gene is located on chromosome 10, which is frequently inactivated in human tumors. Accumulation of PIP3 after PI3K activation leads to a translocation of AKT to the plasma membrane where it is phosphorylated by two PIP3-dependent kinases and thus becomes activated (Figure 3). AKT develops its anti-apoptotic and cell cycle-regulating effects via a series of target molecules (over 30 have already been described) such as e.g. the pro-apoptotic protein Bad, procaspase 9, forkhead transcription factors or the mammalian target of

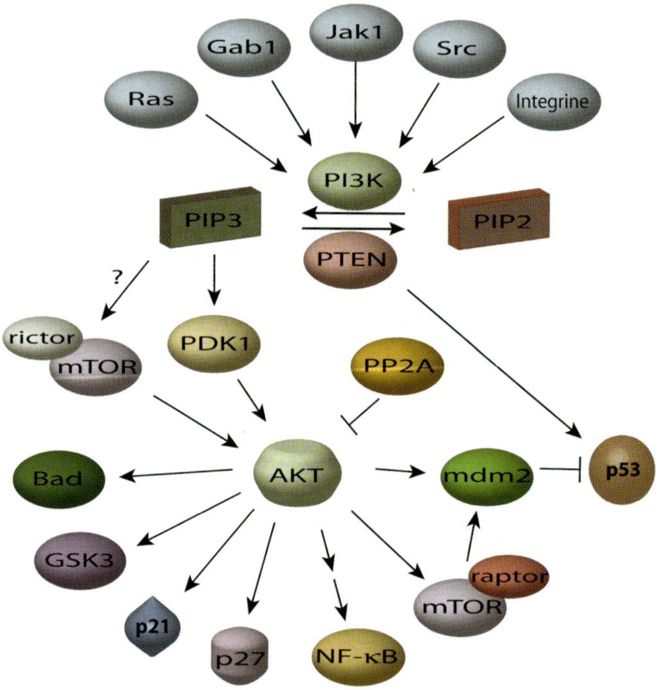

Figure 3. The PI3 kinase/AKT signal transduction pathway.

rapamycin (mTOR).[38] Surprisingly mTOR functions, on the one hand, in a rapamycin-sensitive complex with raptor as an effector of AKT; on the other hand it belongs in a rapamycin-insensitive complex with rictor to the AKT-activating kinases. Interestingly, an AKT/mTOR-regulated suppression of p53 protein expression that functions via induction of the translation of the p53-specific ubiquitin ligase mdm2 has been described. Furthermore, AKT can directly activate mdm2 and thus induce p53 protein degradation.[33] As the apoptosis induced by Ras inhibition in Merkel cell carcinoma xenografts is accompanied by p53 induction, an involvement of the PI3K/AKT signaling pathway in this process as well as in the molecular pathogenesis of Merkel cell carcinoma appears very likely.[37]

The frequent heterozygous loss of the long arm of chromosome 10 in Merkel cell carcinoma suggests that the tumor suppressor PTEN encoded there plays a relevant role.[39] However, only rarely has loss of heterozygosity (LOH) been accompanied by inactivation of the second allele by mutation or deletion, which leads the authors to conclude that additional tumor suppressors located on 10q might be 'targets' of the loss.[40] On the other hand, a recent study using Merkel cell carcinoma tissue arrays to measure the expression of various proteins (especially matrix metalloproteinases) revealed that PTEN could hardly be identified in the samples examined, which could indicate inactivation of the second allele, e.g. by epigenetic mechanisms.[41]

2.4 Limitless Replicative Potential

Mammalian cells carry an intrinsic, cell-autonomous program that limits their multiplication.[1] The early work of Hayflick demonstrated that cells in culture have a finite replicative potential which largely depends on the maintenance of the telomeres. A telomere is a region of repetitive DNA at the end of chromosomes, which protects the end of the chromosome from destruction. Telomeres are composed of TTAGGG repeats, oriented 5′-to-3′ towards the end of the chromosome, ending in an essential 3′ single-stranded G-rich overhang. Each mitosis shortens the telomere appendix on the DNA of the cell. The 'Hayflick limit' is the number of times a cell will divide before it stops due to the telomere reaching a critical length.[42] Once cells have progressed through a certain number of doublings, they stop growing — a process termed senescence. In order to avoid reaching the 'Hayflick limit,' cells that need to keep on dividing express the enzyme telomerase or use alternative lengthening of telomeres mechanisms. In Merkel cell carcinoma, telomerase activity was detected *in situ* in cryostat sections of frozen Merkel cell carcinoma biopsies and *in vitro* in cultivated Merkel cell carcinoma cells. Thus, despite their pronounced neuroendocrine differentiation and their occurrence in patients of advanced age, Merkel cell carcinomas possess telomerase activity.[43]

Senescence can also be circumvented by disabling RB and p53 tumor suppressor proteins.[44] The genetic and epigenetic aberrations in Merkel cell carcinoma impacting RB and p53 function have been described above.

The location of further genes that may be involved in tumor evolution has been inferred from experiments in which loss of constitutional heterozygosity has been detected in tumor DNA at high frequency in specific chromosomal regions. For example, cytogenetic and molecular abnormalities on the short arm of chromosome 1 have been reported in tumors such as malignant melanoma and neuroblastoma. Similar aberrations have been reported for Merkel cell carcinoma.[45] Suciu *et al.* note that cytogenetic studies have reported several chromosomal abnormalities in Merkel cell carcinomas, including trisomy of chromosomes 6 and 8.[46] Using fine needle aspiration with subsequent fluorescent *in situ* hybridization in two patients with recurrent Merkel cell carcinoma of the head and neck, the authors detected trisomy of chromosome 6 in 85% of tumor cells in one patient and trisomy 8 in 77% of cells in the other patient.

2.5 Sustained Angiogenesis

The formation of new blood vessels, a process known as angiogenesis, is important for embryonic development and wound healing as well as the development of cancer and inflammation. Indeed, angiogenesis is a microscopic feature frequently encountered in neuroendocrine tumors in various organs. Specifically, in 20–50% of Merkel cell carcinoma foci of vascular proliferation may be seen, ranging from subtle to prominent.[47] These changes include pericyte hyperplasia, pyogenic granuloma-like, hemangioendothelioma-like, epithelioid hemangioma-like, peliosis-like and follicular dendritic cell tumor-like morphologic patterns; thus, the vascular changes features are similar to those previously reported in other neuroendocrine tumors.

The 'angiogenic switch' is increasingly recognized as a rate-limiting secondary event in multistage carcinogenesis.[1] Tumors appear to activate the 'angiogenic switch' by changing the balance of angiogenesis inducers and countervailing inhibitors. One common strategy for shifting the balance involves altered gene transcription, e.g. increased expression of VEGF via activation of hypoxia induced factor-1 (HIF1). Indeed, HIF1, a transcription factor, is over-expressed in several human cancers. However, in a recent report, no activation of the HIF pathway could be demonstrated and the intensity of VEGF staining was faint in most Merkel cell carcinoma cases.[41] Nevertheless, aggressive tumors displayed significantly higher VEGF expression levels. Moreover, as already mentioned above, for Merkel cell carcinoma the expression of VEGF-A and VEGF-C has been demonstrated. There was a tendency toward higher expression in larger tumors, although the difference did not reach statistical significance.[13]

In response to various stimuli, arachidonic acid can be mobilized from phospholipids pools and converted to bioactive eicosanoids through cyclooxygenase (COX). The COX pathway generates five major prostanoids that play important roles in diverse biological processes.[48] Both prostanoids and their synthase are suspected to promote tumor progression and cancer metastasis, e.g. PGE_2 stimulates angiogenesis. COX-2 staining was reported in 77% of primary Merkel cell carcinomas (strong staining intensity 19%, moderate 23% and weak 35%). Metastases showed similar staining. Prominent mitotic activity was associated with more diffuse COX-2 immunopositivity. However, no association was found between COX-2 expression and outcome.[49.50]

2.6 Tissue Invasion and Metastasis

Invasion and metastasis are exceedingly complex processes, and their genetic and biochemical determinants remain incompletely understood.[1] Metastasis formation, which starts with dissemination of tumor cells from the primary tumor, is a complex multistep process: tumor cells detach from the primary tumor, invade surrounding tissue and basement membranes, intravasate into the lymphatic or blood circulation, and, finally, adhere and extravasate into distant organs. Degradation and remodeling of the extracellular matrix (ECM) and basement membranes by proteolytic enzymes are essential steps in these processes.[51] Different proteolytic enzyme systems, including the plasminogen activator system, aspartyl proteinases, cystein proteinases and matrix metalloproteinases (MMPs) and their tissue inhibitors (TIMPs) have been identified in tumor progression.

Individual MMPs have been identified that show increased expression and enhanced activity in tumors. However, the classic concept of increased MMP activity resulting in greater degradation of the ECM, thus facilitating tumor cell invasion and metastasis formation is currently supplemented by much wider biological function of MMPs in tumor development and progression.[51] There is increasing evidence for important roles of MMPs in interactions with non-matrix proteins including growth factors and their receptors, mediators of apoptosis and cell adhesion molecules, such as members of the integrin family and CD44.

Until recently, the expression of MMPs and their tissue inhibitors in Merkel cell carcinoma has been only occasionally explored. Analysis of 23 cases revealed a statistically significant correlation between high MMP1 and MMP3 expression levels and metastatic potential.[52] Fernandez-Figueras *et al.* reported a high expression of most MMPs in Merkel cell carcinoma, but only those of MMP7 (matrilysin) and MMP10 (stromelysin 2) were significantly related with an impaired prognosis.[41] Upregulation of both proteinases are well established predictors of poor outcome in several neoplasms including non-small cell lung carcinoma and high-grade neuroendocrine lung tumors. TIMP3 over-expression was reported by the same group to be significantly associated with an adverse outcome. Massi *et al.* also reported a TIMP3 over-expression in 91.3% of Merkel cell carcinoma cases.[52] Interestingly, TIMP3 expression is regulated by DNA hypermethylation or mutant p53-mediated transcriptional repression.

Expression of these proteases is not restricted to tumor cells but is also found in stromal and tumor infiltrating cells, indicating that the tumor microenvironment contributes to neoplasm progression. Beer *et al.* examined the role of mast cell infiltrates in 36 Merkel cell carcinomas stained with an antibody to tryptase.[53] The authors found a statistically significantly worse prognosis in patients with higher mast cell counts. The authors propose that mast cells may affect the biologic behavior of Merkel cell carcinomas by influencing angiogenesis, immunosuppression, extracellular matrix degradation and mitogenesis.

The adhesion/homing molecule CD44 has attracted much attention not only because it is expressed on many types of tumors, but also owing to its numerous functions, such as supporting cell migration and transmitting survival signals. Penneys *et al.* analyzed 25 primary, locally recurrent or metastatic Merkel cell carcinomas for expression of CD44 in order to correlate its expression with the course of disease.[54] To this end, in three of six cases in which metastasis was documented, CD44 was present. Three cutaneous lesions associated with local metastasis did not express CD44. Three primary tumors expressed CD44 but had not disseminated during the observation time. However, the number of studied lesions as well as the limited follow-up of the patients did not allow any strong conclusions.

The endothelium of blood vessels constitutes a physical barrier to cells in the circulatory system, and metastatic cells must penetrate the interendothelial junctions to invade the adjacent tissue. Addressing adhesion proteins in Merkel cell carcinoma, epithelial cadherin has recently been described as the most frequently expressed cadherin (97% of 35 investigated tumors), followed in frequency by neural cadherin (63%) and placental cadherin (43%).[55] Furthermore, expression of the neuronal cell adhesion molecule (NCAM) localized at the cell-surface membrane has been reported for the majority of Merkel cell carcinomas.

2.7 Escape from Immune Surveillance

Tumor cells themselves express many aberrant antigens that can promote eradication through immune surveillance. Thus, immune escape is a critical gateway to malignancy. Immune surveillance represents a potent, multi-armed and essential mode of cancer suppression, and immune escape is a central modifier of the clinical course of the disease.[2]

The predilection of virally induced malignancies for immunosuppressed individuals underscores the importance of a competent immune system in regulating cancer development and spread. The recent discovery of the Merkel cell polyomavirus[8] may explain the striking epidemiological association between immunosuppression and Merkel cell carcinoma (see Chapter 3). Chronically immunosuppressed individuals are more than 15 times more likely to develop Merkel cell carcinoma than age-matched controls. For example, Merkel cell carcinoma occurs much more frequently in patients with organ transplants and HIV infections (12/100,000/year) and at a significantly younger age (about 50% under 50 years of age). Similarly, other forms of T-lymphocyte immune suppression such as chronic lymphocytic leukemia are linked with Merkel cell carcinoma. Merkel cell carcinoma is also more lethal in immunosuppressed patients, with a reported disease-specific mortality of up to 56%. Interestingly, there are several case reports of Merkel cell carcinoma regression following restoration of immune function.

2.8 Future Directions

There is a striking need for a better understanding of the molecular biology of Merkel cell carcinoma. While there have been important discoveries concerning the role of apoptosis, transcellular growth factors and their pathways such as Ras/RAF/MAP kinase, inhibitors of growth such as p53 and Rb, and angiogenesis, much remains to be investigated. The gradual improvement of our comprehension of the pathogenesis of Merkel cell carcinoma will hopefully translate into an improved management of patients suffering from this highly aggressive cancer. The identification of epigenetic aberrations, particularities in signal transduction pathways and, most recently, the Merkel cell polyomavirus are exciting discoveries and will provide opportunities to explore new targeted therapies for this disease.

References

1. Hanahan D., Weinberg R.A. (2000). The hallmarks of cancer. *Cell* 100: 57–70.
2. Andersen M.H., Schrama D., Thor Straten P., Becker J.C. (2006). Cytotoxic T cells. *J Invest Dermatol* 126: 32–41.
3. Verhagen A.M., Vaux D.L. (2002). Cell death regulation by the mammalian IAP antagonist Diablo/Smac. *Apoptosis* 7: 163–166.
4. Kennedy M.M., Blessing K., King G., Kerr K.M. (1996). Expression of bcl-2 and p53 in Merkel cell carcinoma. An immunohistochemical study. *Am J Dermatopathol* 18: 273–277.
5. Feinmesser M., Halpern M., Fenig E., *et al.* (1999). Expression of the apoptosis-related oncogenes bcl-2, bax, and p53 in Merkel cell carcinoma: can they predict treatment response and clinical outcome? *Hum Pathol* 30: 1367–1372.
6. Schlagbauer-Wadl H., Klosner G., Heere-Ress E., *et al.* (2000). Bcl-2 antisense oligonucleotides (G3139) inhibit Merkel cell carcinoma growth in SCID mice. *J Invest Dermatol* 114: 725–730.
7. Shah M.H., Varker K.A., Collamore M., *et al.* G3139 (Genasense) in patients with advanced Merkel cell carcinoma. *Am J Clin Oncol* 32: 174–179.

8. Feng H., Shuda M., Chang Y., Moore P.S. (2008). Clonal integration of a polyomavirus in human Merkel cell carcinoma. *Science* 319: 1096–1100.
9. Pina-Oviedo S., Urbanska K., Radhakrishnan S., *et al.* (2007). Effects of JC virus infection on anti-apoptotic protein survivin in progressive multifocal leukoencephalopathy. *Am J Pathol* 170: 1291–1304.
10. Kim J., McNiff J.M. (2008). Nuclear expression of survivin portends a poor prognosis in Merkel cell carcinoma. *Mod Pathol* 21: 7647–7669.
11. Van Gele M., Boyle G.M., Cook A.L., *et al.* (2004). Gene-expression profiling reveals distinct expression patterns for Classic versus Variant Merkel cell phenotypes and new classifier genes to distinguish Merkel cell from small-cell lung carcinoma. *Oncogene* 23: 2732–2742.
12. Swick B.L., Ravdel L., Fitzpatrick J.E., Robinson W.A. (2008). Platelet-derived growth factor receptor alpha mutational status and immunohistochemical expression in Merkel cell carcinoma: implications for treatment with imatinib mesylate. *J Cutan Pathol* 35: 197–202.
13. Brunner M., Thurnher D., Pammer J., *et al.* (2008). Expression of VEGF-A/C, VEGF-R2, PDGF-alpha/beta, c-kit, EGFR, Her-2/Neu, Mcl-1 and Bmi-1 in Merkel cell carcinoma. *Mod Pathol* 2: 876–884.
14. Vogelstein B., Kinzler K.W. (2004). Cancer genes and the pathways they control. *Nat Med* 10: 789–799.
15. Davies H., Bignell G.R., Cox C., *et al.* (2002). Mutations of the BRAF gene in human cancer. *Nature* 417: 949–954.
16. Feinmesser M., Halpern M., Kaganovsky E., *et al.* (2004). c-kit expression in primary and metastatic Merkel cell carcinoma. *Am J Dermatopathol* 26: 458–462.
17. Strong S., Shalders K., Carr R., Snead D.R. (2004). KIT receptor (CD117) expression in Merkel cell carcinoma. *Br J Dermatol* 150: 384–385.
18. Llombart B., Monteagudo C., Lopez-Guerrero J.A., *et al.* (2005). Clinicopathological and immunohistochemical analysis of 20 cases of Merkel cell carcinoma in search of prognostic markers. *Histopathology* 46: 622–634.
19. Su L.D., Fullen D.R., Lowe L., *et al.* (2002). CD117 (KIT receptor) expression in Merkel cell carcinoma. *Am J Dermatopathol* 24: 289–293.
20. Swick B.L., Ravdel L., Fitzpatrick J.E., Robinson W.A. (2007). Merkel cell carcinoma: evaluation of KIT (CD117) expression and failure to demonstrate activating mutations in the C-KIT proto-oncogene — implications for treatment with imatinib mesylate. *J Cutan Pathol* 34: 324–329.

21. Worda M., Sreevidya C.S., Ananthaswamy H.N., *et al.* (2005). T1796A BRAF mutation is absent in Merkel cell carcinoma. *British Journal of Dermatology* 153: 229–232.
22. Houben R., Michel B., Vetter-Kauczok C.S., *et al.* (2006). Absence of classical MAP kinase pathway signalling in Merkel cell carcinoma. *J Invest Dermatol* 126: 1135–1142.
23. Houben R., Ortmann S., Schrama D., *et al.* (2007). Activation of the MAP kinase pathway induces apoptosis in the Merkel cell carcinoma cell line UISO. *J Invest Dermatol* 127: 2116–2122.
24. Chen X., Yang J., Evans P.M., Liu C. (2008). Wnt signaling: the good and the bad. *Acta Biochim Biophys Sin* (Shanghai) 40: 577–594.
25. Liu S., Daa T., Kashima K., *et al.* (2007). The Wnt-signaling pathway is not implicated in tumorigenesis of Merkel cell carcinoma. *J Cutan Pathol* 34: 22–26.
26. Chau B.N., Wang J.Y. (2003). Coordinated regulation of life and death by RB. *Nat Rev Cancer* 3: 130–138.
27. Horn H.F., Vousden K.H. (2007). Coping with stress: multiple ways to activate p53. *Oncogene* 26: 1306–1316.
28. Lassacher A., Heitzer E., Kerl H., Wolf P. (2008). p14ARF hypermethylation is common but INK4a-ARF locus or p53 mutations are rare in Merkel cell carcinoma. *J Invest Dermatol* 128: 1788–1796.
29. Becker J.C., Ugurel S., Brocker E.B., *et al.* (2006). [New therapeutic approaches for solid tumors: histone deacetylase, methyltransferase and proteasome inhibitors]. *J Dtsch Dermatol Ges* 4: 108–113.
30. Sherr C.J. (2006). Divorcing ARF and p53: an unsettled case. *Nat Rev Cancer* 6: 663–673.
31. Van Gele M., Kaghad M., Leonard J.H., *et al.* (2000). Mutation analysis of P73 and TP53 in Merkel cell carcinoma. *Br J Cancer* 82: 823–826.
32. Popp S., Waltering S., Herbst C., *et al.* (2002). UV-B-type mutations and chromosomal imbalances indicate common pathways for the development of Merkel and skin squamous cell carcinomas. *Int J Cancer* 99: 352–360.
33. Kim D., Chung J. (2002). Akt: versatile mediator of cell survival and beyond. *J Biochem Mol Biol* 35: 106–115.
34. Asioli S., Righi A., Volante M., *et al.* (2007). p63 expression as a new prognostic marker in Merkel cell carcinoma. *Cancer* 110: 640–647.

35. Ortega S., Malumbres M., Barbacid M. (2002). Cyclin D-dependent kinases, INK4 inhibitors and cancer. *Biochim Biophys Acta* 1602: 73–87.
36. Leonard J.H., Hayard N. (1997). Loss of heterozygosity of chromosome 13 in Merkel cell carcinoma. Genes Chromosomes. *Cancer* 20: 93–97.
37. Jansen B., Heere-Ress E., Schlagbauer-Wadl H., *et al.* (1999). Farnesylthiosalicylic acid inhibits the growth of human Merkel cell carcinoma in SCID mice. *J Mol Med* 77: 792–797.
38. Sarbassov D.D., Guertin D.A., Ali S.M., Sabatini D.M. (2005). Phosphorylation and regulation of Akt/PKB by the rictor-mTOR complex. *Science* 307: 1098–1101.
39. Van Gele M., Speleman F., Vandesompele J., *et al.* (1998). Characteristic pattern of chromosomal gains and losses in Merkel cell carcinoma detected by comparative genomic hybridization. *Cancer Res* 58: 1503–1508.
40. Van Gele M., Leonard J.H., Van Roy N., *et al.* (2001). Frequent allelic loss at 10q23 but low incidence of PTEN mutations in Merkel cell carcinoma. *Int J Cancer* 92: 409–413.
41. Fernandez-Figueras M.T., Puig L., Musulen E., *et al.* (2007). Expression profiles associated with aggressive behavior in Merkel cell carcinoma. *Mod Pathol* 20: 90–101.
42. Deng Y., Chan S.S., Chang S. (2008). Telomere dysfunction and tumor suppression: the senescence connection. *Nat Rev Cancer* 8: 450–458.
43. Stoppler H., Stoppler M.C., Kisiela M., *et al.* (2001). Telomerase activity of Merkel cell carcinomas and Merkel cell carcinoma-derived cell cultures. *Arch Dermatol Res* 293: 397–406.
44. Garbe J.C., Holst C.R., Bassett E., *et al.* (2007). Inactivation of p53 function in cultured human mammary epithelial cells turns the telomere-length dependent senescence barrier from agonescence into crisis. *Cell Cycle* 6: 1927–1936.
45. Leonard J.H., Cook A.L., Nancarrow D., *et al.* (2000). Deletion mapping on the short arm of chromosome 1 in Merkel cell carcinoma. *Cancer Detect Prev* 24: 620–627.
46. Suciu V., Botan E., Valent A., *et al.* (2008). The potential contribution of fluorescent in situ hybridization analysis to the cytopathological diagnosis of Merkel cell carcinoma. *Cytopathology* 19: 48–51.
47. Vazmitel M., Michal M., Shelekhova K.V., *et al.* (2008). Vascular changes in Merkel cell carcinoma based on a histopathological study of 92 cases. *Am J Dermatopathol* 30: 106–111.

48. Becker J.C., Domschke W., Pohle T. (2004). Current approaches to prevent NSAID-induced gastropathy — COX selectivity and beyond. *Br J Clin Pharmacol* 58: 587–600.
49. Joachims Z., Feinmesser R., Purim O., *et al.* (2008). Cyclooxygenase-2 expression in primary and metastatic Merkel cell carcinoma. *Appl Immunohistochem Mol Morphol* 16: 442–446.
50. Koljonen V., Lassus P., Tukiainen E., *et al.* (2005). Cyclooxygenase-2 expression in primary Merkel cell carcinoma. *J Cutan Pathol* 32: 55–58.
51. Hofmann U.B., Houben R., Brocker E.B., Becker J.C. (2005). Role of matrix metalloproteinases in melanoma cell invasion. *Biochimie* 87: 307–314.
52. Massi D., Franchi A., Ketabchi S., *et al.* (2003). Expression and prognostic significance of matrix metalloproteinases and their tissue inhibitors in primary neuroendocrine carcinoma of the skin. *Hum Pathol* 34: 80–88.
53. Beer T.W., Ng L.B., Murray K. (2008). Mast cells have prognostic value in Merkel cell carcinoma. *Am J Dermatopathol* 30: 27–30.
54. Penneys N.S., Shapiro S. (1994). CD44 expression in Merkel cell carcinoma may correlate with risk of metastasis. *J Cutan Pathol* 21: 22–26.
55. Han A.C., Soler A.P., Tang C.K., *et al.* (2000). Nuclear localization of E-cadherin expression in Merkel cell carcinoma. *Arch Pathol. Lab Med* 124: 1147–1151.

Chapter 3

Association Between Merkel Cell Polyomavirus and Merkel Cell Carcinoma

Dana E. Rollison and Jürgen C. Becker

3.1 Introduction: Viral Infections and Cancer

Viral infections have been implicated in the etiology of many types of cancer, including human papillomavirus in cervical[1] and oropharyngeal cancers,[2] hepatitis B virus in hepatocellular carcinoma,[3] Human T-cell Leukemia Virus-1 in leukemia,[4] Epstein-Barr virus in some types of lymphoma[5] and Kaposi Sarcoma Herpesvirus (KSHV) in Kaposi's sarcoma.[6] Several aspects of these established associations between viruses and cancer can inform the investigation of emerging infections as they relate to cancer. For example, detection of viral DNA in human tumor tissues at one or more copies per cell provides evidence of clonal expansion of a virally infected cell. Expression of the oncoprotein further supports an etiologic role for the virus.[7] Additionally, many cancers with infectious etiologies are more often observed in the context of immunosuppression, such as Kaposi's sarcoma, lymphomas, cervical, oropharyngeal and penile cancers in HIV-infected individuals[8] and non-melanoma skin cancers, lymphomas and cancers of the oral cavity, vulva and vagina in organ transplant recipients.[9] Evidence for a viral etiology of Merkel cell carcinoma begins with the observation that this cancer is also more common in immunocompromised individuals.

3.2 Merkel Cell Carcinoma in the Context of Immunosuppression

Merkel cell carcinoma has been documented in several types of immunosuppressed patients. For example, numerous case series have reported Merkel cell carcinoma among organ transplant recipients, as previously reviewed,[10] including one series of 41 cases reported to the Cincinnati Transplant Tumor Registry in which the mean time from transplantation to Merkel cell carcinoma diagnosis was 91 months.[11] Several case series have also indicated that Merkel cell carcinoma may be more common among individuals who have B-cell malignancies.[10] An analysis of Merkel cell carcinoma and other cancers in the National Cancer Institute's Surveillance, Epidemiology and End Results (SEER) database demonstrated statistically significantly increased risks of Merkel cell carcinoma occurring more than one year after diagnosis of other cancers, with particularly strong associations (four-fold increased risk) observed for a previous diagnosis of lymphohematopoietic cancers.[12] Additionally, HIV-infected individuals are estimated to have a 13.4-fold increased risk of developing Merkel cell carcinoma as compared to the general population.[13]

Another potential source of immunosuppression more relevant to the general population is ultraviolet (UV) radiation, and evidence from population-based cancer registries supports an association between UV radiation exposure and Merkel cell carcinoma. Based on data collected by the SEER Program from 1986–94, Merkel cell carcinoma incidence rates have increased over time,[14–16] peaking in 1996 at 0.50 per 100,000 males and 0.22 per 100,000 females. In the earliest report from SEER,[10] a statistically significant increase in Merkel cell carcinoma incidence rates was observed among geographic SEER sites with higher solar UVB indices, an association of similar magnitude to that seen with melanoma. This trend of increasing Merkel cell carcinoma incidence rates with increasing solar UVB index for the corresponding geographic SEER site was also observed in a more recent SEER report (data through 1999), but only among whites.[14]

The exact mechanism by which UV radiation may lead to increased risk of Merkel cell carcinoma is unclear, although the effect of UV radiation on the immune system is well documented. The work of Margaret

Kripke on UV-induced immunogenic skin tumors revealed profound immunologic effects of UV radiation and brought forth the discipline of 'Photoimmunology.'[17] Her group identified suppressor T lymphocytes (which are currently referred to as regulatory T cells) as pivotal for both UV-induced tumor tolerance as well as UV-induced hapten-specific tolerance.[18] Immunologic reactions commonly evolve through an intricate network of signaling and cell activation. This concept holds true for UV-induced immunosuppression, which appears to have several starting points in various photoreceptors, including DNA. For example, UV-induced DNA damage, such as cyclobutane pyrimidine dimers (CPDs), can suppress the immune response, and removal of CPDs abrogates UV-induced immunosuppression.[19]

The number of Langerhans cells and dendritic epidermal T cells decrease in the epidermis upon UV exposure, also resulting in immunosuppression.[20] However, it is presently unknown whether this cell loss is caused by cell death, loss of surface markers or migration to lymph nodes, as the results in different murine models and human systems are inconclusive. In addition to disturbed antigen presentation, UV exposure can induce immunosuppressive cytokines such as IL-10 and TNF-alpha. Cooper and colleagues observed that UVB-induced immunosuppression in humans was associated with an influx and proliferation of CD11b+ monocytes/macrophages.[21] The macrophages were found to be the main producers of Th1-suppressive IL-10, and their presence was crucial for the development of antigen-specific tolerance upon sensitization after UVB exposure. Furthermore, the isomerization of *trans*-urocanic acid to *cis*-urocanic acid and the formation of reactive oxygen species have been implicated in the development of antigen-specific tolerance.[22] Although several pathways of UV-induced immunosuppression have been described, the precise mechanism by which UV exposure may be associated with the development of Merkel cell carcinoma is unknown.

3.3 Polyomaviruses and Cancer

Given the increased risk of Merkel cell carcinoma observed with immunosuppression, Merkel cell carcinoma is a candidate cancer for a viral etiology. As such, Feng and colleagues recently investigated Merkel cell carcinoma tissues for the presence of a novel virus using digital transcriptome subtraction.[23] Their investigation resulted in the discovery of a genome encompassing 5387 base pairs of a new polyomavirus, which they named the Merkel cell polyomavirus (MCV or MCPyV).

Polyomaviruses are small (40–50 nanometers in diameter), double-stranded DNA viruses that infect multiple species, including mice, hamsters, cows, birds and primates (i.e. simian virus 40 (SV40) in rhesus macaques). As of the writing of this chapter, 14 polyomaviruses have been identified, including five that are known to infect humans — three of which were identified within the last two years: Merkel cell polyomavirus,[23] KI and WU, the latter two of which were isolated from the human respiratory tract.[24,25] Nothing is known about the natural history of these three viral infections. In contrast, JC virus (JCV) and BK virus (BKV), the other known human polyomaviruses, were discovered in 1971[26,27] and their natural history is better understood. Initial infection with JCV or BKV is asymptomatic and occurs in early childhood and adolescence, with seroprevalence ranging from 44–80% among adults.[28–30] JCV and BKV remain latent in the kidneys and can reactivate and cause disease under conditions of immunosuppression, including BKV-associated nephritis in renal transplant patients and JCV-associated progressive multifocal leukoencephalopathy (PML) in AIDS patients.

Since the discovery of the SV40 and its potential contamination of the polio vaccine in the late 1950s to early 1960s,[31] polyomaviruses have been suspected as possible causes of cancer in humans.[31,32] Polyomaviruses, including SV40, JCV and BKV, can induce tumor formation in experimentally infected animals,[33,34] where tumor development is usually preceded by the integration of the polyomavirus DNA into the host genome.[32] Polyomaviruses express genes in two phases: the early-expressed genes encoding non-structural proteins, and the late-expressed components of the viral coat and proteins that enable lysis. The early-expressed genes include the large and small T-antigens, which bind to host proteins to force the cell into S phase (the cell cycle phase when DNA is replicated) and facilitate viral replication.[35,36] T-antigen can bind to and inactivate tumor suppressor proteins p53 and pRb[29] (Figure 1), as well as interfere with other cell signaling pathways.[37–39] This viral stimulation of

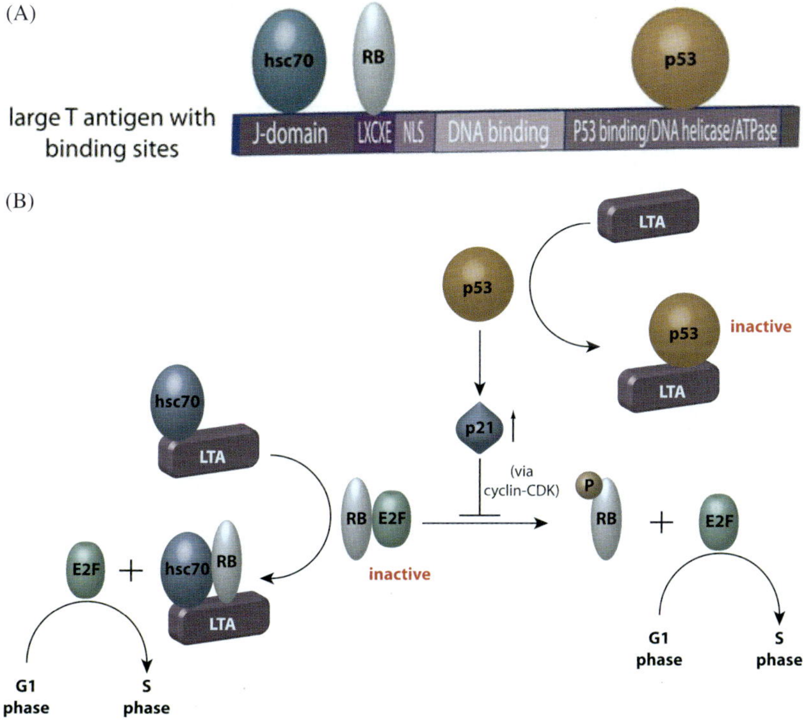

Figure 1. **(A)** The large T antigen contains binding sides for the heat shock cognate protein 70 (hsc70), retinoblastoma protein (Rb) and p53. **(B)** While p53 activity is directly inhibited by its binding to the large T antigen, the concurrent binding of hsc70 and Rb is required to disrupt the Rb/E2F complex mandatory for the G1 to S phase transition of the cell cycle.

the cell cycle is the main driving force of the oncogenic potential of polyomaviruses.[35,36]

Although JCV, BKV and SV40 can induce tumors in animal models, their role in human carcinogenesis remains controversial. DNA sequences from these three polyomaviruses have been detected in several types of human tumor tissues, including brain tumors, lymphomas and mesotheliomas,[40–48] although their integration into cellular DNA has never been demonstrated.[49] Additionally, epidemiologic case-control studies have consistently observed no positive associations between seropositivity for JCV, BKV or SV40 and cancer risk.[28,50–53] However, the transforming potential of polyomavirus T-antigen maintains these viruses as potential carcinogens.

3.4 Merkel Cell Polyomavirus

After Feng and colleagues discovered MCPyV using two cDNA libraries generated from four Merkel cell carcinoma tumor tissues, they investigated the presence of MCPyV in a separate set of ten Merkel cell carcinoma tumor tissues.[23] Of these ten tissues tested, eight (80%) contained MCPyV DNA sequences, seven of which were positive for MCPyV DNA by PCR, including four that tested positive on all three primer sets, and one that was positive only after Southern hybridization. In comparison, 8% of 59 control tissues from various body sites and 16% of control skin tissues were positive for MCPyV DNA (Table 1). The strength of the PCR signals for the Merkel cell carcinoma tissues suggested that the viral DNA was integrated in a clonal fashion (Figure 2). To test this notion, genomic DNA from Merkel cell carcinoma tumors was digested with two restriction enzymes and analyzed by Southern hybridization using a MCPyV DNA probe. The resulting banding patterns indicated a monoclonal integration of the virus in five of the eight MCPyV-positive Merkel cell carcinoma tumors, a monoclonally integrated viral concatemer in one tumor, and an indeterminate integration pattern in the remaining two tumors.[23] The distinct integration patterns between tumors imply that the virus integrated at different locations within the human genome in the different tumors. Primary and metastatic tumor tissue was available for one case with a monoclonal integration pattern, and both specimens showed an identical viral integration pattern, demonstrating that integration of MCPyV most likely preceded metastasis.[23]

Feng and colleagues sequenced the MCPyV genome and identified signature mutations in the MCPyV T-antigen sequence that appear to be specific for MCPyV-related Merkel cell carcinoma.[23,54] MCPyV large T-antigen transcripts were first described from four MCPyV-positive Merkel cell carcinoma tumor tissues. Sequencing analysis of eight additional MCPyV-positive Merkel cell carcinoma tumor tissues demonstrated that the large T-antigen gene sequence was highly conserved. However, mutations or deletions in the gene were observed in all eight tumors, resulting in premature truncation of exon 2, which encodes the large T-antigen helicase. In contrast, none of these truncating mutations were observed in four MCPyV-positive non-Merkel cell carcinoma tissues (two appendices, one bowel and one peripheral blood mononuclear cell sample). These findings suggest that truncating

Table 1. Summary of findings for Merkel cell polyomavirus (MCPyV) sequences in Merkel cell carcinoma tissues by PCR.

Study	Primers used for PCR	MCPyV in Merkel cell carcinoma tumors	MCPyV in normal tissues	MCPyV in other cancers
Feng *et al.*, 2008[23] (USA)	LT1 (1514-1953; 440 bp) forward: 5′-TACAAGCACTCCACCAAAGC-3′ reverse: 5′-TCCAATTACAGCTGGCCTCT-3′ LT3 (571-879; 309 bp) forward: 5′-TTGTCTCGCCAGCATTGTAG reverse: 5′-ATATAGGGGCCTCGTCAACC-3′ VP1 (4137-3786; 352 bp) forward: 5′-TTTGCCAGCTTACAGTGTGG-3′ reverse: 5′-TGGATCTAGGCCCTGATTTTT-3′	8 (80%) of 10 were MCPyV+ for at least one primer; 4 (40%) of 10 were MCPyV+ for all three sets primer	16% of 25 normal skin tissues	—
Garneski *et al.*, 2008[60] (North America & Australia)	Nucleotides 236-374 of the MCV350 sequence (EU375803) (139 bp) and nucleotides 1083–1181 surrounding the BamH1 restriction site (99 bp)	43% of 37	0 of 15 normal skin tissues	13% of 15 squamous cell carcinomas of the skin
Kassem *et al.*, 2008[54] (Germany)	LT1, LT3, VP1 (see Feng *et al.* above), in addition to: M1/2 (1711-1889; 179 bp) forward: 5′-GGCATGCCTGTGAATTAGGA-3′ reverse: 5′-TTGCAGTAATTTGTAAGGGGACT-3′	30 (77%) of 39 were MCPyV+ for at least one primer; 5 (13%) of 39 were MCPyV+ for all four primer sets	0 of 45 PBMC	—
Becker *et al.*, 2008[56] (Germany)	(92 bp) forward: 5′-AAACCAAAGAATAAAGCACTGA-3′ reverse: 5′-TCGCCAGCATTGTAGTCTAAAAAC-3′	75 samples were tested from 53 pts; tumors from 45 pts (85%) were MCPyV+	—	3 (13%) of 24 basal cell carcinomas of the skin

(Continued)

Table 1. (*Continued*)

Study	Primers used for PCR	MCPyV in Merkel cell carcinoma tumors	MCPyV in normal tissues	MCPyV in other cancers
Foulongne *et al.*, 2008[59] (France)	LT1, LT3, VP1 (see Feng *et al.* above)	8 (89%) of 9 were MCPyV+ for at least one primer; 1 (11%) of 9 were MCPyV+ on all three primer sets	0 of 15 biopsies of benign proliferative or inflammatory skin disease	—
Bhatia *et al.*, 2009 (USA)	Primers for quantitative PCR (97 bp) forward: 5′-GCAAAAAAACTGTCTGACGTGG-3′ reverse: 5′-CCACCAGTCAAAACTTTCCCA-3′	Tumors from 17 (74%) of 23 patients were MCPyV+	(Results from peripheral blood lymphocytes are included in the box to the right)	1 (2%) of 52 non-Merkel cell carcinoma tissues (20 breast cancers, 12 colon cancers, 20 normal peripheral blood lymphocytes)
Varga *et al.*, 2009 (Hungary)	LT1, LT3, VP1 (see Feng *et al.* above)	7 (88%) of 8 Merkel cell carcinoma tissues from 6 patients were MCPyV+ for at least one primer; 1 (13%) of 8 were MCPyV+ for all three primer sets	—	0 of 13 squamous cell carcinomas, 10 basal cell carcinomas, 3 basosquam carcinomas, and 3 melanomas
Touze *et al.*, 2009 (France)	LT1, LT3, VP1 (see Feng *et al.* above), in addition to: LT1n forward: 5′-GGCATGCCTGTGAATTAGGA-3′ reverse: 5′-TGTAAGGGGGCTTGCATAAA-3′ VP1n forward: 5′-TGCAAATCCAGAGGTTCTCC-3′ reverse: 5′-GCAGATGTGGGAGGCAATA-3′	21 (66%) of 32 were MCPyV+, including 9 (45%) of 20 FFPE tissues and 12 (100%) of 12 frozen tissues	—	0 of 9 other neuroendocrine carcinomas (5 small cell lung carcinomas, 3 intestinal carcinomas, 1 cervical carcinoma)

(*Continued*)

Table 1. (*Continued*)

Study	Primers used for PCR	MCPyV in Merkel cell carcinoma tumors	MCPyV in normal tissues	MCPyV in other cancers
Sastre-Garau *et al.*, 2009 (France)	MCPyV_ST_A and MCPyV_ST_B specific for the small T-antigen (165 bp; sequence not provided) MCPyV_LT_C and MCPyV_LT_D specific for the large T-antigen (162 bp; sequence not provided) MCPyV_VP1_A and MCPyV_VP1_B specific for VP1 gene (204 bp; sequence not provided)	10 (100%) of 10 were MCPyV+ for at least on primer; 9 (90%) of 10 were positive MCPyV+ for all three primers sets	—	0 of 1,241 tumors (32 skin, 44 cervix, 39 large bowel, 114 liver, 45 uveal tract, 172 ovary, 687 breast, 104 bone and soft tissue, 4 other)
Duncavage *et al.*, 2009 (USA)	LT1, LT3 (see Feng *et al.* above) MCVPS1 (109 bp) forward: 5′-TCAGCGTCCCAGGCTTCAGA -3′ reverse: 5′-TGGTGGTCTCCTCTCTGCTACTG-3′	41 tissues from 29 patients were tested: 9 (22%) were MCPyV+ for LT1; 17 (41%) were MCPyV+ for LT3; 32 (78%) were MCPyV+ for MCVPS1, including 22 (76%) of 29 unique patients	—	—
Wetzels *et al.*, 2009 (the Netherlands)	Modified LT3 (250 bp) forward: 5′-ATCTGCACCTTTTCTAGACTCC-3′ reverse: 5′-ATATAGGGGCCTCGTCAACC-3′	4 (40%) of 10 were MCPyV+	—	0 of 10 small cell lung cancers were MCPyV+

(*Continued*)

Table 1. *(Continued)*

Study	Primers used for PCR	MCPyV in Merkel cell carcinoma tumors	MCPyV in normal tissues	MCPyV in other cancers
Helmbold *et al.*, 2009 (Germany)	(195 bp) forward: 5′-CTTGGGAAAGTTTTGACTGGTGGCAA-3′ reverse: 5′-GGGCCTCGTCAACCTAGATGGGAAAG-3′	90 (92%) of 98 Merkel cell carcinoma tissues from 91 patients were MCPyV+	3 (17%) of 18 normal skin samples were MCPyV+; 1 (4%) of 26 blood samples were MCPyV+	—
Sihto *et al.*, 2009 (Finland)	LT1, LT3, VP1 (see Feng *et al.* above) Primers for quantitative PCR: LT3 (74 bp) forward: 5′-GCATCTGCACCTTTTCTAGACTC -3′ reverse: 5′-TTTTGCCTTATAGACTTTTCCATATCT -3′	54 (50%) of 114 were MCPyV+ LT3; 12 (11%) were MCPyV+ for VP1; 32 (30%) were MCPyV+ for LT1; 91 (80%) of 114 were MCPyV+ by qPCR	—	—

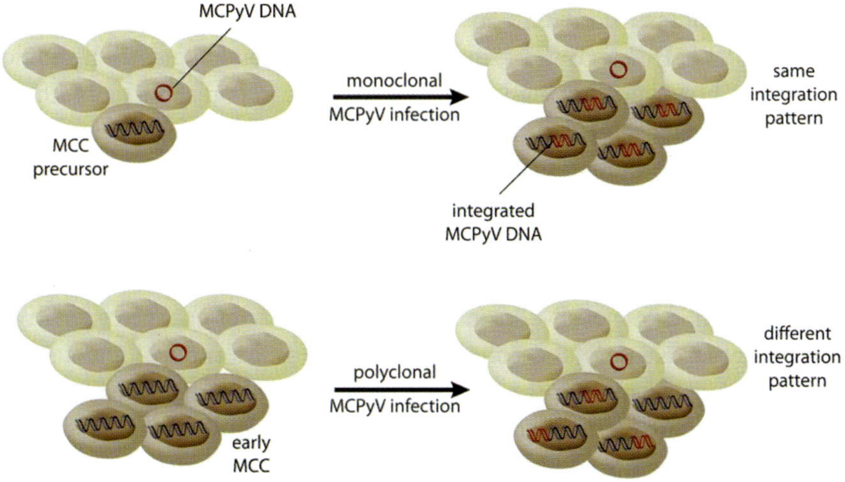

Figure 2. Clonal versus polyclonal viral integration.

mutations in the large T-antigen gene may be used to characterize tumorigenic MCPyV infections. The T-antigen locus contains many of the features common to oncogenic polyomaviruses, including an LxCxE motif that may directly bind phosphorylated Rb protein.[23] In all published Merkel cell carcinoma-related MCPyV genome sequences, premature stop codons are predicted within the second exon of the large T-antigen.[23,55] The predicted truncated proteins potentially preserve some of the cell cycle progression activities of the amino terminus of large T but prevent cell-lethal genomic instability related to the replicative functions of the carboxyl terminus.[35,36] If the large T-antigen were intact, replication initiated at an integrated origin would lead to genomic instability and cell death. Indeed, in permissive cells transformed by SV40, the large T-antigen is often mutated such that the viral replication functions are inactive but cell cycle progression functions are preserved.

3.5 Merkel Cell Polyomavirus in Merkel Cell Carcinoma Tissues

The findings of MCPyV in Merkel cell carcinoma by Feng and colleagues have since been replicated by twelve independent groups (Table 1),[54,56–67] including studies from Germany, France, Hungary and Finland that used the same LT1, LT3 and VP1 primer sets described by Feng *et al.* It should be noted, however, that only in some of these reports did the authors assess whether or not the MCPyV DNA harbored a truncating mutation as described by Shuda *et al.*[55] or whether the MCPyV DNA was indeed integrated into the host DNA. Varga and colleagues observed MCPyV DNA sequences in eight of nine paraffin-embedded Merkel cell carcinoma tissues from Hungary, including one that tested positive for all three primers, while none of 29 other skin tumors tested were positive for MCPyV.[66] Kassem and colleagues[54] tested 39 Merkel cell carcinoma formalin-fixed tissues for the presence of MCPyV sequences in a German patient population. Thirty (77%) of the Merkel cell carcinoma tissues were positive for MCPyV DNA, with only five (13%) tissues testing positive using all four primer sets. As described by the authors, formalin fixation may fragment DNA, which, in turn, may result in different rates of amplification across primer sets that vary in length (i.e. number of base pairs). In contrast to the Merkel cell carcinoma tissues, none of 45 whole blood samples from healthy blood donors tested positive for MCPyV. Foulongne and colleagues investigated MCPyV sequences in nine Merkel cell carcinoma tissues from patients in France,[59] including six formalin-fixed and three fresh tissues. Eight (89%) of the nine Merkel cell carcinoma tissues were positive for MCPyV DNA, although only one tested positive using all three primer sets. Fifteen fresh biopsies of benign proliferative or inflammatory skin diseases were investigated as controls, none of which were positive for MCPyV DNA. A second group from France described MCPyV DNA in 45% of formalin-fixed Merkel cell carcinoma tissues and 100% of 12 fresh tissues, further highlighting the impact tissue preparation may have on PCR results.[65] Zero of nine neuroendocrine carcinomas of the lung, intestine and cervix tested positive for MCPyV DNA.

Other groups have observed similar prevalence of MCPyV DNA in Merkel cell carcinoma tissues utilizing different PCR primers than those described by Feng and colleagues. A third French group detected MCPyV DNA in 100% of ten fresh-frozen Merkel cell carcinoma tissues, including nine that were positive for all three primer sets used, which were specific for sequences corresponding to the small T-antigen, large

T-antigen and VP1 genes and ranging in length from 162 to 204 base pairs.[63] In contrast, none of 1,241 other tumors of the skin, cervix, large bowel, liver, uveal tract, ovary, breast, bone or soft tissue were MCPyV positive. Duncavage and colleagues used LT1 and LT3 primers in addition to MCVPS1, which produces an amplicon 109 base pairs in length.[58] Of 41 paraffin-embedded Merkel cell carcinoma tissues tested from 29 patients, 22% and 41% were positive for LT1 and LT3, respectively, while 78% were positive for MCVPS1. A Dutch group utilized a modified LT3 primer set, corresponding to an amplicon 109 base pairs in length, and observed MCPyV DNA sequences in 40% of 10 paraffin-embedded Merkel cell carcinoma tissues.[67] In contrast, none of ten fresh-frozen small cell lung cancer tissues were positive using the same modified LT3 primer set. Helmbold and colleagues observed MCPyV DNA in 92% of 98 paraffin-embedded Merkel cell carcinoma tissues, using a primer set that produces an amplicon 195 base pairs in length.[61] Of the 18 normal skin samples and 26 blood samples used as controls, 17% and 4% were MCPyV positive, respectively.

Quantitative PCR may be more sensitive for the detection of MCPyV DNA and facilitates the comparison of MCPyV viral load across patient groups. For example, of 114 paraffin-embedded Merkel cell carcinoma tissues obtained from Finnish patients from 1979–2004, Sihto and colleagues observed MCPyV DNA in 50%, 11% and 32% using LT3, VP1 and LT1, respectively.[64] However, 80% of the 114 tissues were positive on quantitative PCR utilizing a modified LT3 primer that produced an amplicon 74 base pairs in length. Becker and colleagues investigated the presence of MCPyV in 75 formalin-fixed tumor tissues obtained from 53 Merkel cell carcinoma patients in Germany using real-time PCR techniques. MCPyV DNA sequences were detected in tumors from 45 of the 53 patients (85%). Among the eight patients for whom paired samples of primary tumor and metastatic tissue were available, MCPyV findings were concordant between primary and metastatic tissues, with MCPyV present in both samples for six patients and in neither sample for two patients. MCPyV sequences were present in a slightly greater proportion of patients with metastatic disease (88%) as compared to patients without metastatic disease (80%), although this difference was not statistically significant. By comparison, only three of 24 basal cell carcinoma tissues

(13%) were positive for MCPyV sequences with viral copy numbers four logs lower than Merkel cell carcinoma tissues. Bhatia and colleagues detected MCPyV DNA in Merkel cell carcinoma tumor tissues from 17 of 23 patients (74%), with viral loads ranging from zero to 1.2 viral copies.[57] Among these samples, higher MCPyV viral load was significantly associated with pRb, TdT and CD44 expression.

Garneski and colleagues investigated the presence of MCPyV DNA in 16 and 21 formalin-fixed Merkel cell carcinoma tissues from patients in North America and Australia, respectively.[60] Using real-time PCR with primers sets designed to amplify regions of the MCPyV genome corresponding to the small and large T-antigens, MCPyV DNA was detected in 43% of the total 37 Merkel cell carcinoma tissues. Viral load varied fourfold among the MCPyV positive Merkel cell carcinoma tissues. In contrast, MCPyV DNA was present in two of 15 squamous cell carcinoma tissues (13%) and zero of 15 normal skin tissues obtained from individuals in North America who were matched to the Merkel cell carcinoma cases on age and sex. In two individuals for whom pairs of primary tumor and nodal tissues were available, both tissues tested positive for MCPyV. No differences in overall survival were observed between MCPyV positive and negative Merkel cell carcinoma patients.

When samples from North America and Australia were considered separately, the prevalence of MCPyV DNA in Merkel cell carcinoma tissues was greater for those samples obtained from North America as compared to Australia (69% versus 24%, $p = 0.009$).[60] Although the Australian samples collected in the 1990s were older than the North American samples collected after 2000, DNA degradation was ruled out as an explanation for the MCPyV prevalence difference across continents, due to the demonstration of high-quality DNA obtained from both sets of samples. The authors suggest that the lower MCPyV prevalence observed in the Australian samples may be due to the higher level of sun exposure, although the biological underpinnings of an inverse association between sun exposure and MCPyV-associated Merkel cell carcinoma are unclear, especially given that increased sun exposure may induce immunosuppression, potentially increasing susceptibility to a virally-induced cancer. In addition, sun exposure patterns vary greatly across North America; thus, the degree of sun exposure experienced by the North American patients is unclear. Furthermore, our own unpublished data in cooperation with Richard Scolyer could not demonstrate a significant difference in the prevalence of MCPyV DNA in Merkel cell carcinoma between Australian and European samples, with both ranging around 80%.

3.6 Merkel Cell Polyomavirus and Merkel Cell Carcinoma Survival

Accumulating evidence suggests that patients with MCPyV-positive Merkel cell carcinoma may experience better survival compared to patients with MCPyV-negative tumors. For example, among the 23 Merkel cell carcinoma patients in the study by Bhatia *et al.*, those with ≥ 0.06 viral copies per cell experienced higher median survival as compared to those patients with ≤ 0.0035 viral copies per cell (86 months versus 20 months, $p = 0.015$).[57] Similarly, among 114 Finnish Merkel cell carcinoma patients described by Sihto and colleagues, the observed five-year survival was 45% for patients with MCPyV-positive Merkel cell carcinoma, as compared to 13% for MCPyV-negative Merkel cell carcinoma patients ($p < 0.001$).[64] Even after adjusting for sex and the presence of nodal metastases, the presence of MCPyV DNA was significantly associated with improved survival (hazard ratio 0.42, 95% confidence interval 0.25 – 0.71).

3.7 MCPyV in Other Cancers

MCPyV has been examined in the context of other cancers. For example, as described in Table 1, several studies included tumor tissues from other cancer sites as controls for the Merkel cell carcinoma tumor tissues. MCPyV was either absent or present at very low prevalence among these tissues. In addition, other cancer types have been the primary focus of several additional studies. Ridd *et al.* did not detect MCPyV DNA in 85 squamous cell carcinomas from organ transplant recipients.[68] In contrast, Kassem *et al.* investigated MCPyV DNA in basal and squamous cell carcinomas from both immunocompetent and immunocompromised individuals and observed higher proportions of MCPyV-positive tissues among immunocompromised patients, including 52% and 72% of squamous and basal cell carcinomas among immunosuppressed patients, respectively, versus 25% and 38% among immunocompetent patients.[69] Dworkin and colleagues observed a similar prevalence of MCPyV DNA in SCC tissues from immunocompentent individuals, reporting viral DNA in 26 of 177 squamous cell carcinoma tissues from 58 individuals, representing a prevalence of 15% of tissues and 45% of individuals.[70] MCPyV was also detected in 17% of adjacent normal tissues. A single study of polyomaviruses in melanomas did not detect MCPyV sequences in any of 37 melanoma tissues.[71]

Previous descriptive epidemiology studies have described an association between the incidence of MCPyV and lymphomas.[10,72] Shuda and colleagues investigated lymphoid tissues for the presence of MCPyV; five of 161 B-cell lymphomas (3%) and one of 104 T-cell lymphomas (1%) were MCPyV positive, whereas 31 healthy lymphoid tissues were MCPyV negative.[73] Helmbold and colleagues investigated MCPyV DNA sequences in small cell lung cancer, which like Merkel cell carcinoma is a neuroendocrine tumor. MCPyV DNA sequences were detected in seven of 18 small cell lung cancer tumors tested (39%), but not in any of 18 normal blood samples.[74] Bluemn *et al.* detected no MCPyV T-antigen RNA in 28 prostate cancer tissues, a cancer with a strong inflammatory component that has been previously hypothesized to be associated with a viral infection.[75] Again, not all reports assessed the integration of the MCPyV DNA into the host genome nor the presence of truncating mutations in the T-antigen coding region.

Little is known about the natural history of MCPyV infection, including the anatomic site of initial infection, presence of a latent phase, and mode of transmission. Several studies have begun to investigate the presence of MCPyV in normal tissues in order to answer some of these questions. For example, Dworkin *et al.* detected MCPyV DNA in the mouthwash sample of a single patient with squamous cell carcinoma, and subsequently investigated 11 additional mouthwash samples from individuals with non-oral, non-skin cancers but did not find MCPyV DNA in any of the samples.[70] Similarly, MCPyV is rarely found in normal lymphoid tissues.[73] A study of lymphoid tissues obtained at autopsy reported MCPyV DNA in only one of 42 AIDS patients and none of 55 immunocompetent patients.[76]

Other polyomaviruses, including JCV,[77] KI and WU[78], can be detected in the respiratory tract, and several groups have investigated the presence of MCPyV in these tissues. Goh *et al.* detected MCPyV DNA in 4% of 607 nasopharyngeal aspirates obtained from individuals with respiratory tract infections, including <1% of aspirates from children younger than 15 years and 9% of aspirates from individuals 15 years and older.[79] These findings are consistent with a second study that detected MCPyV DNA in 1% of 526 nasopharyngeal aspirates obtained from patients with respiratory infections, most of whom were children.[80] Similarly, Kantola *et al.* detected MCPyV DNA in 4% of 229 tonsil tissues obtained from tonsillectomy patients, 2% of 106 nasal swabs and zero of 75 fecal samples obtained from 51 children with leukemia, and 2% of 140 nasopharyngeal aspirates obtained from wheezing children.[81]

The prevalences of MCPyV DNA sequences described above for the respiratory tract are considerably lower than the prevalence of MCPyV antibodies recently described in two different populations using similar virus-like particle-based ELISA assays.[62,82] For example, among 166 healthy blood donors from the United States, IgG antibodies against the MCV339 VP1 and VP2 proteins were observed in 107 (64%).[82] Interestingly, the anti-VP1 antibody titers were significantly higher in patients with MCPyV positive Merkel cell carcinoma as compared to patients with MCPyV negative tumors or controls. In a separate study of 1501 healthy adult blood donors, the prevalence of IgG antibodies against MCPyV 339 VP1 was 46%, with age-specific seroprevalences ranging from 1–5, 5–10 and 10–15 years 43% among those 21–49 years of age to 61% among those older than 70 years.[62] Data from a separate pediatric population indicate that initial exposure to MCPyV occurs at very young ages, with seroprevalences of 20%, 30% and 40% for children aged 1–5, 5–10 and 10–15 years, respectively.[62]

3.8 Conclusion and Future Directions

In summary, the increased risk of Merkel cell carcinoma in immunosuppressed patients, the presence of MCPyV DNA in Merkel cell carcinoma tissues and its clonal pattern of integration support a role for MCPyV in Merkel cell carcinoma carcinogenesis. However, the existing tumor studies are not sufficient to establish causality. Future tumor studies should incorporate multiple primers from the previously published papers in order to facilitate comparison. In addition, both formalin-fixed and fresh-frozen Merkel cell carcinoma tissues should be tested using the same set of primers to investigate the effects of tissue preservation on viral DNA. Characterizing these differences in primer selection and tissue preparation will assist in the interpretation of differences in MCPyV prevalence across studies. Additional markers of infection should also be investigated in MCPyV patients, including expression of the T-antigen in Merkel cell carcinoma tissues and corresponding antibody responses.[83] To this end, markers of Merkel cell carcinoma infection are needed, including antibodies to both MCPyV capsid and the T-antigen. Clinical characteristics of MCPyV-positive versus MCPyV-negative Merkel cell carcinomas need to be further characterized, including stage at diagnosis and overall survival.

In parallel, molecular biology laboratories should continue to elucidate the mechanism(s) by which MCPyV can induce carcinogenesis. The effects of the proposed oncoproteins, the large and small T-antigens, need to be evaluated. Similarly, the effects of silencing of the gene products in MCPyV-positive Merkel cell carcinoma cell lines by si/shRNA and their over-expression in NIH3T3 cells should be studied. These experiments will only be possible when Merkel cell carcinoma cell lines, particularly MCPyV-positive lines, become readily available.

Finally, epidemiologic approaches are also needed to establish causality, including case-control studies that compare prevalence of MCPyV infection in Merkel cell carcinoma cases versus controls and can provide a measure of association between the two. Comparisons of MCPyV prevalence across geographic regions may provide insight into cofactors that work in conjunction with MCPyV to cause disease, such as sun exposure and other factors that may affect the immune system. Studies of the natural history of MCPyV in immunocompromised patients without Merkel cell carcinoma are also needed in order to characterize high-risk populations for future prevention strategies.

Although additional evidence is needed to characterize the role of MCPyV infection in Merkel cell carcinoma etiology and prognosis, MCPyV may be a promising target for future Merkel cell carcinoma treatment and prevention strategies. For example, antiviral therapies may provide a new avenue for Merkel cell carcinoma treatment. Furthermore, if a vaccine could be developed against MCPyV, then primary prevention of Merkel cell carcinoma may be possible through vaccination of high-risk populations.

References

1. Steben M., Duarte-Franco E. (2007). Human papillomavirus infection: epidemiology and pathophysiology. *Gynecol Oncol* 107: S2–S5.
2. Gillison M.L. (2004). Human papillomavirus-associated head and neck cancer is a distinct epidemiologic, clinical, and molecular entity. *Semin Oncol* 31: 744–754, 2004.
3. Kremsdorf D., Soussan P., Paterlini-Brechot P., Brechot C. (2006). Hepatitis B virus-related hepatocellular carcinoma: paradigms for viral-related human carcinogenesis. *Oncogene* 25: 3823–3833.
4. Matsuoka M., Jeang K.T. (2007). Human T-cell leukaemia virus type 1 (HTLV-1) infectivity and cellular transformation. *Nat Rev Cancer* 7: 270–280.
5. Kutok J.L., Wang F. (2006). Spectrum of Epstein-Barr virus-associated diseases. *Annu Rev Pathol* 1: 375–404.
6. Chang Y., Cesarman E., Pessin M.S., *et al.* (1994). Identification of herpesvirus-like DNA sequences in AIDS-associated Kaposi's sarcoma. *Science* 266: 1865–1869.
7. Pagano J.S., Blaser M., Buendia M.A., *et al.* (2004). Infectious agents and cancer: criteria for a causal relation. *Semin Cancer Biol* 14: 453–471.
8. Engels E.A., Biggar R.J., Hall H.I., *et al.* (2008). Cancer risk in people infected with human immunodeficiency virus in the United States. *Int J Cancer* 123: 187–194.
9. Adami J., Gabel H., Lindelof B., *et al.* (2003). Cancer risk following organ transplantation: a nationwide cohort study in Sweden. *Br J Cancer* 89: 1221–1227.
10. Miller R.W., Rabkin C.S. (1999). Merkel cell carcinoma and melanoma: etiological similarities and differences. *Cancer Epidemiol Biomarkers Prev* 8: 153–158.
11. Penn I., First M.R. (1999). Merkel's cell carcinoma in organ recipients: report of 41 cases. *Transplantation* 68: 1717–1721.

12. Howard R.A., Dores G.M., Curtis R.E., *et al.* (2006). Merkel cell carcinoma and multiple primary cancers. *Cancer Epidemiol Biomarkers Prev* 15: 1545–1549.
13. Engels E.A., Frisch M., Goedert J.J., *et al.* (2002). Merkel cell carcinoma and HIV infection. *Lancet* 359: 497–498.
14. Agelli M., Clegg L.X. (2003). Epidemiology of primary Merkel cell carcinoma in the United States. *J Am Acad Dermatol* 49: 832–841.
15. Hodgson N.C. (2005). Merkel cell carcinoma: changing incidence trends. *J Surg Oncol* 89: 1–4.
16. Vortmeyer A.O., Merino M.J., Boni R., *et al.* (1998). Genetic changes associated with primary Merkel cell carcinoma. *Am J Clin Pathol* 109: 565–570.
17. Kripke M.L., Fisher M.S. (1976). Immunologic parameters of ultraviolet carcinogenesis. *J Natl Cancer Inst* 57: 211–215.
18. Greene M.I., Sy M.S., Kripke M., Benacerraf B. (1979). Impairment of antigen-presenting cell function by ultraviolet radiation. *Proc Natl Acad Sci USA* 76: 6591–6595.
19. Miyauchi-Hashimoto H., Tanaka K., Horio T. (1996). Enhanced inflammation and immunosuppression by ultraviolet radiation in xeroderma pigmentosum group A (XPA) model mice. *J Invest Dermatol* 107: 343–348.
20. Kolgen W., Both H., van Weelden H., *et al.* (2002). Epidermal Langerhans cell depletion after artificial ultraviolet B irradiation of human skin in vivo: apoptosis versus migration. *J Invest Dermatol* 118: 812–817.
21. Cooper K.D., Oberhelman L., Hamilton T.A., *et al.* (1992). UV exposure reduces immunization rates and promotes tolerance to epicutaneous antigens in humans: relationship to dose, CD1a-DR+ epidermal macrophage induction, and Langerhans cell depletion. *Proc Natl Acad Sci USA* 89: 8497–8501.
22. Ullrich S.E., Nghiem D.X., Khaskina P. (2007). Suppression of an established immune response by UVA — a critical role for mast cells. *Photochem Photobiol* 83: 1095–1100.
23. Feng H., Shuda M., Chang Y., Moore P.S. (2008). Clonal integration of a polyomavirus in human Merkel cell carcinoma. *Science* 319: 1096–1100.
24. Allander T., Andreasson K., Gupta S., *et al.* (2007). Identification of a third human polyomavirus. *J Virol* 81: 4130–4136.

25. Gaynor A.M., Nissen M.D., Whiley D.M., *et al.* (2007). Identification of a novel polyomavirus from patients with acute respiratory tract infections. *PLoS Pathog* 3: e64.
26. Padgett B.L., Walker D.L., ZuRhein G.M., *et al.* (1971). Cultivation of papova-like virus from human brain with progressive multifocal leucoencephalopathy. *Lancet* 1: 1257–1260.
27. Gardner S.D., Field A.M., Coleman D.V., Hulme B. (1971). New human papovavirus (B.K.) isolated from urine after renal transplantation. *Lancet* 1(7712): 1253–1257.
28. Rollison D.E., Engels E.A., Halsey N.A., *et al.* (2006). Prediagnostic circulating antibodies to JC and BK human polyomaviruses and risk of non-Hodgkin lymphoma. *Cancer Epidemiol Biomarkers Prev* 15: 543–550.
29. Shah K. (1996). Polyomaviruses. In: Fields B., Knipe D., Howley P. (eds.) *Field's Virology*, pp. 2027–2043, Lippincott-Raven, Philadelphia.
30. Carter J.J., Madeleine M.M., Wipf G.C., *et al.* (2003). Lack of serologic evidence for prevalent simian virus 40 infection in humans. *J Natl Cancer Inst* 95: 1522–1530.
31. Shah K.V. (2007). SV40 and human cancer: a review of recent data. *Int J Cancer* 120: 215–223.
32. zur Hausen H. (2008). Novel human polyomaviruses — re-emergence of a well known virus family as possible human carcinogens. *Int J Cancer* 123: 247–250.
33. Major E.O., Mourrain P., Cummins C. (1984). JC virus-induced owl monkey glioblastoma cells in culture: biological properties associated with the viral early gene product. *Virology* 136: 359–367.
34. Shah K.V., Daniel R.W., Strandberg J.D. (1975). Sarcoma in a hamster inoculated with BK virus, a human papovavirus. *J Natl Cancer Inst* 54: 945–950.
35. Caracciolo V., Reiss K., Khalili K., *et al.* (2006). Role of the interaction between large T antigen and Rb family members in the oncogenicity of JC virus. *Oncogene* 25: 5294–5301.
36. Moens U., Van G.M., Johannessen M. (2007). Oncogenic potentials of the human polyomavirus regulatory proteins. *Cell Mol Life Sci* 64: 1656–1678.
37. Gan D.D., Khalili K. (2004). Interaction between JCV large T-antigen and beta-catenin. *Oncogene* 23: 483–490.

38. Reiss K., Khalili K., Giordano A., Trojanek J. (2006). JC virus large T-antigen and IGF-I signaling system merge to affect DNA repair and genomic integrity. *J Cell Physiol* 206: 295–300.
39. Trojanek J., Croul S., Ho T., *et al.* (2006). T-antigen of the human polyomavirus JC attenuates faithful DNA repair by forcing nuclear interaction between IRS-1 and Rad51. *J Cell Physiol* 206: 35–46.
40. Bergsagel D.J., Finegold M.J., Butel J.S., *et al.* (1992). DNA sequences similar to those of simian virus 40 in ependymomas and choroid plexus tumors of childhood. *N Engl J Med* 326: 988–993.
41. Caldarelli-Stefano R., Boldorini R., Monga G., *et al.* (2000). JC virus in human glial-derived tumors. *Hum Pathol* 31: 394–395.
42. Carbone M., Pass H.I., Rizzo P., *et al.* (1994). Simian virus 40-like DNA sequences in human pleural mesothelioma. *Oncogene* 9: 1781–1790.
43. Corallini A., Pagnan M., Viadana P., *et al.* (1987). Association of BK virus with human brain tumors and tumors of pancreatic islets. *Int J Cancer* 39: 60–67.
44. Del Valle L., Gordon J., Assimakopoulou M., *et al.* (2001). Detection of JC virus DNA sequences and expression of the viral regulatory protein T-antigen in tumors of the central nervous system. *Cancer Res* 61: 4287–4293.
45. Dorries K., Loeber G., Meixensberger J. (1987). Association of polyomaviruses JC, SV40, and BK with human brain tumors. *Virology* 160: 268–270.
46. Shivapurkar N., Wiethege T., Wistuba I.I., *et al.* (1999). Presence of simian virus 40 sequences in malignant mesotheliomas and mesothelial cell proliferations. *J Cell Biochem* 76: 181–188.
47. Vilchez R.A., Butel J.S. (2003). SV40 in human brain cancers and non-Hodgkin's lymphoma. *Oncogene* 22: 5164–5172.
48. Weggen S., Bayer T.A., von Deimling A., *et al.* (2000). Low frequency of SV40, JC and BK polyomavirus sequences in human medulloblastomas, meningiomas and ependymomas. *Brain Pathol* 10: 85–92.
49. Viscid R.P., Shah K.V. (2008). Cancer. A skin cancer virus? *Science* 319: 1049–1050.
50. Engels E.A., Viscidi R.P., Galloway D.A., *et al.* (2004). Case-control study of simian virus 40 and non-Hodgkin lymphoma in the United States. *J Natl Cancer Inst* 96: 1368–1374.

51. Engels E.A., Rollison D.E., Hartge P., *et al.* (2005). Antibodies to JC and BK viruses among persons with non-Hodgkin lymphoma. *Int J Cancer* 117: 1013–1019.
52. Rollison D.E., Helzlsouer K.J., Alberg A.J., *et al.* (2003). Serum antibodies to JC virus, BK virus, simian virus 40, and the risk of incident adult astrocytic brain tumors. *Cancer Epidemiol Biomarkers Prev* 12: 460–463.
53. Rollison D.E., Helzlsouer K.J., Halsey N.A., *et al.* (2005). Markers of past infection with simian virus 40 (SV40) and risk of incident non-Hodgkin lymphoma in a Maryland cohort. *Cancer Epidemiol Biomarkers Prev* 14: 1448–1452.
54. Shuda M., Feng H., Kwun H.J., *et al.* (2008). T antigen mutations are a human tumor-specific signature for Merkel cell polyomavirus. *Proc Natl Acad Sci USA* 105: 16272–16277.
55. Kassem A., Schopflin A., Diaz C., *et al.* (2008). Frequent detection of Merkel cell polyomavirus in human Merkel cell carcinomas and identification of a unique deletion in the VP1 gene. *Cancer Res* 68: 5009–5013.
56. Becker J.C., Houben R., Ugurel S., *et al.* (2008). MC polyomavirus is frequently present in Merkel cell carcinoma of European patients. *J Invest Dermatol* 129: 248–250.
57. Bhatia K., Goedert J.J., Modali R., *et al.* (2009). Merkel cell carcinoma subgroups by Merkel cell polyomavirus DNA relative abundance and oncogene expression. *Int J Cancer* [Epub ahead of print].
58. Duncavage E.J., Zehnbauer B.A., Pfeifer J.D. (2009). Prevalence of Merkel cell polyomavirus in Merkel cell carcinoma. *Mod Pathol* 22: 516–521.
59. Foulongne V., Kluger N., Dereure O., *et al.* (2008). Merkel cell polyomavirus and Merkel cell carcinoma, France. *Emerg Infect Dis* 14: 1491–1493.
60. Garneski K.M., Warcola A.H., Feng Q., *et al.* (2008). Merkel cell polyomavirus is more frequently present in North American than Australian Merkel cell carcinoma tumors. *J Invest Dermatol* 129: 246–248.
61. Helmbold P., Lahtz C., Enk A., *et al.* (2009). Frequent occurrence of RASSF1A promoter hypermethylation and Merkel cell polyomavirus in Merkel cell carcinoma. *Mol Carcinog* 48: 903–909.
62. Kean J.M., Rao S., Wang M., Garcea R.L. (2009). Seroepidemiology of human polyomaviruses *PLoS Pathog* 5: e1000363.

63. Sastre-Garau X., Peter M., Avril M.F., *et al.* (2009). Merkel cell carcinoma of the skin: pathological and molecular evidence for a causative role of MCPyV in oncogenesis. *J Pathol* 218: 48–56.
64. Sihto H., Kukko H., Koljonen V., *et al.* (2009). Clinical factors associated with Merkel cell polyomavirus infection in Merkel cell carcinoma. *J Natl Cancer Inst* 101: 938–945.
65. Touze A., Gaitan J., Maruani A., *et al.* (2009). Merkel cell polyomavirus strains in patients with Merkel cell carcinoma. *Emerg Infect Dis* 15: 960–962.
66. Varga E., Kiss M., Szabo K., Kemeny L. (2009). Detection of Merkel cell polyomavirus DNA in Merkel cell carcinomas. *Br J Dermatol* 161: 930–932.
67. Wetzels C.T., Hoefnagel J.G., Bakkers J.M., *et al.* (2009). Ultrastructural proof of polyomavirus in Merkel cell carcinoma tumour cells and its absence in small cell carcinoma of the lung. *PLoS One* 4: e4958.
68. Ridd K., Yu S., Bastian B.C. (2009). The presence of polyomavirus in non-melanoma skin cancer in organ transplant recipients is rare. *J Invest Dermatol* 129: 250–252.
69. Kassem A., Technau K., Kurz A.K., *et al.* (2009). Merkel cell polyomavirus sequences are frequently detected in nonmelanoma skin cancer of immunosuppressed patients. *Int J Cancer* 125: 356–361.
70. Dworkin A.M., Tseng S.Y., Allain D.C., *et al.* (2009). Merkel cell polyomavirus in cutaneous squamous cell carcinoma of immunocompetent individuals. *J Invest Dermatol* 129: 2868–2874.
71. Giraud G., Ramqvist T., Ragnarsson-Olding B., Dalianis T. (2008). DNA from BK virus and JC virus and from KI, WU, and MC polyomaviruses as well as from simian virus 40 is not detected in non-UV-light-associated primary malignant melanomas of mucous membranes. *J Clin Microbiol* 46: 3595–3598.
72. Brenner B., Sulkes A., Rakowsky E., *et al.* (2001). Second neoplasms in patients with Merkel cell carcinoma. *Cancer* 91: 1358–1362.
73. Shuda M., Arora R., Kwun H.J., *et al.* (2009). Human Merkel cell polyomavirus infection I. MCPyV T antigen expression in Merkel cell carcinoma, lymphoid tissues and lymphoid tumors. *Int J Cancer* 125: 1243–1249.
74. Helmbold P., Lahtz C., Herpel E., *et al.* (2009). Frequent hypermethylation of RASSF1A tumour suppressor gene promoter and presence of Merkel cell polyomavirus in small cell lung cancer. *Eur J Cancer* 45: 2207–2211.

75. Bluemn E.G., Paulson K.G., Higgins E.E., *et al.* (2009). Merkel cell polyomavirus is not detected in prostate cancers, surrounding stroma, or benign prostate controls. *J Clin Virol* 44: 164–166.
76. Sharp C.P., Norja P., Anthony I., *et al.* (2009). Reactivation and mutation of newly discovered WU, KI, and Merkel cell carcinoma polyomaviruses in immunosuppressed individuals. *J Infect Dis* 199: 398–404.
77. Monaco M.C., Jensen P.N., Hou J., *et al.* (1998). Detection of JC virus DNA in human tonsil tissue: evidence for site of initial viral infection. *J Virol* 72: 9918–9923.
78. Ren L., Gonzalez R., Xie Z., *et al.* (2008). WU and KI polyomavirus present in the respiratory tract of children, but not in immunocompetent adults. *J Clin Virol* 43: 330–333.
79. Goh S., Lindau C., Tiveljung-Lindell A., Allander T. (2009). Merkel cell polyomavirus in respiratory tract secretions. *Emerg Infect Dis* 15: 489–491.
80. Bialasiewicz S., Lambert S.B., Whiley D.M., *et al.* (2009). Merkel cell polyomavirus DNA in respiratory specimens from children and adults. *Emerg Infect Dis* 15: 492–494.
81. Kantola K., Sadeghi M., Lahtinen A., *et al.* (2009). Merkel cell polyomavirus DNA in tumor-free tonsillar tissues and upper respiratory tract samples: Implications for respiratory transmission and latency. *J Clin Virol* 5: 292–295.
82. Tolstov Y.L., Pastrana D.V., Feng H., *et al.* (2009). Human Merkel cell polyomavirus infection II. MCPyV is a common human infection that can be detected by conformational capsid epitope immunoassays. *Int J Cancer* 125: 1250–1256.
83. Shah K.V., Rollison D.E. (2001). Investigation of the SV40 — human cancer association: look for the full signature of the virus. *Dis Markers* 17: 159–161.

Chapter 4

Discovering Merkel Cell Carcinoma Through Gene Expression Profiling

Ashani T. Weeraratna

4.1 Introduction

Gene expression profiling techniques such as microarray analysis and the serial analysis of gene expression (SAGE) have emerged from being novel and expensive techniques to relatively common analysis tools in many laboratory settings. These tools have helped us to understand the molecular events associated with various biological processes, from cell development to tumor progression. This is particularly useful when trying to define the global changes that underlie the spread of unusual and highly aggressive cancers such as Merkel cell carcinoma. Merkel cells are low-sensitivity pressure receptors of neuroendocrine origin.[1] These cells are positioned below the epidermis and mostly within follicular epithelium, and once malignant have access to both hematogenous and lymphatic routes of spread, making for highly aggressive tumors.[2] Their position and function also implies that they exist in a unique and dependent interaction with both their microenvironment and the external environment. By understanding the molecular basis of what goes awry with these cells as they become malignant, we may better understand the biology of their interactions with their environment, and vice versa.

4.2 New Findings in Merkel Cell Carcinoma Using Genomic Approaches

Sequencing on a large scale has become accessible through the development of sequencing machines capable of handling large volumes of sequence information, with relatively short turnaround. Even so, sequencing large volumes of DNA is a laborious and inefficient process, and techniques such as the serial analysis of gene expression (SAGE) and microarray analysis were developed in an effort to analyze the transcriptome of cells more efficiently. SAGE relies upon the concatemerization and subsequent sequencing of small segments of cDNA (10–17 base pairs). This is based on the principle that if the human genome is estimated to contain 33,000–35,000 genes, then the variety provided by the 4^{10} or 4^{16} possible combinations of these 10–16 base pair sequences should be sufficient to identify all expected transcripts from the human genome.[3]

Until recently, SAGE held the advantage over microarray technology by being able to identify previously undiscovered transcripts. This became less of an advantage once the human genome was sequenced, as this allowed for the design oligomers corresponding to all known genes and expressed sequence tags (ESTs). Most modern arrays contain over 44,000 genes, corresponding to all known transcripts and many ESTs in the human genome. Microarray platforms are no longer limited to identifying transcript changes, they are also used to analyze changes in copy number (comparative genomic hybridization (CGH) arrays)[4] and for high throughput analyses of single nucleotide polymorphisms.[5] In cancer research, arrays have gone beyond simple gene discovery experiments. They have been used as a tool to confirm the biological effects of genes initially discovered as important in a disease by its profiling,[6] and have been used to assess therapeutic response in patients undergoing chemotherapy.[7] They can focus on the specific subsets of genes within a disease state, and what conditions can effect changes in these 'gene signatures.'[8,9] They have been used to study the interactions of tumor cells with their environments.[10–12] All of these types of studies highlight the versatility and utility of microarray analysis as a tool to study the biology of disease. Although microarray studies may show some discrepancies in data from one study to the next, they are a particularly useful tool in studying cancer pathobiology, and may become a vital part of the move toward individualized molecular therapy.[13] Below we discuss the use of microarray platforms in Merkel cell carcinoma research.

4.2.1 *Comparative genomic hybridization*

Only a handful of studies exist that have assessed the genetic changes associated with Merkel cell carcinoma. One of the earliest CGH studies identified chromosomal changes at 1, 6, 18q and 20.[14] Other studies have added 10q23, 8q21, 3q, 5p and loss of 4p15-pter to this list.[15–18] A more recent study analyzed a larger sample of tumors and found that chromosomal gains in Merkel cell carcinoma outnumbered chromosomal losses by more than two-fold.[15] These gains included chromosomes 6, 1 and 5 as previously reported, and the losses were most commonly found on chromosomes 13 and 4. Interestingly there appears to be no correlation between any one chromosomal gain/loss and the clinical course of these cancers. Not surprisingly, however, the more metastatic tumors tend to have larger numbers of DNA alterations (3 to 1 as reported in this study), perhaps due to genetic instability in these tumors. Mutations in common cancer-related genes such as PTEN, RAS, P53, etc., tend to be rare in Merkel cell carcinoma,[18–20] although some recent evidence links mutations in P53 in Merkel cell carcinoma to UVB sun exposure.[17]

4.2.2 *Microarray platforms in Merkel cell cancer*

There is currently very little information regarding microarray analysis and the global gene expression profiling of Merkel cell carcinoma. Van Gelle *et al.* used several Merkel cell carcinoma samples and compared them to small cell lung cancer, also a cancer of neuroendocrine origin. This analysis sought to analyze not only the differences between two kinds of neuroendocrine cancers but also attempted to distinguish between the classical Merkel cell carcinoma phenotype and some variant lines.[21] Unsupervised clustering highlighted the close genetic relationship between all of these neuroendocrine tumors, as they could not be separated according to gene expression profiles. It should be mentioned, however, that these arrays were quite tiny, and assessed less than 2000 clones, quite different from the larger genome wide arrays that are now available. However, even with this small number of genes, the use of supervised clustering demonstrated distinct transcriptional differences between small cell lung cancer and Merkel cell carcinoma, and between classical and variant Merkel cell carcinoma. A more recent study investigated the gene expression profiles of purified normal Merkel cells. Although this study did not address Merkel cell carcinoma directly, it did identify over 362 genes that were Merkel cell-specific. These included genes coding for neuropeptide receptors and suggested that the Merkel cell is responsive to glutamate and neuropeptides.[22] From a cancer standpoint, this study could be quite valuable, as comparing the genes identified in this study to the changes in the same genes that are associated with other skin or neuroendocrine cancers may reveal some clues as to the progression of Merkel cell carcinoma. For example, it is already known that in other skin cancers such as melanoma, mutations in glutamate receptors can lead to tumor progression.[23] Do these same mutations make Merkel cells malignant?

Finally, a tissue microarray study analyzed 43 markers in 15 patients who were disease-free after primary resection of their Merkel cell carcinoma, and 16 who had evidence of metastatic disease.[24] This study identified the over-expression of several matrix metalloproteases and related proteins including MMP-7, MMP10/2, TIMP3, VEGF, P38, as well as NF-Kappa B (stromal) and synaptophysin in advanced Merkel cell carcinoma. The expression of these angiogenic and metastatic proteins is intriguing, but it remains to be seen if their expression is a cause of Merkel cell carcinoma progression, or merely a response to it.

4.3 Signaling Pathways Involved in Merkel Cell Carcinoma

Genetic analyses often provide interesting and important directions for the analysis of signal transduction pathways in cancer and other diseases. Surprisingly little is known about the signal transduction mechanisms involved in Merkel cell carcinoma. It is clear that many of the common mechanisms involved in the pathogenesis of other tumors such as melanoma (another aggressive skin cancer) or small cell lung cancer (of neuroendocrine origin, and the most similar in phenotype to Merkel cell carcinoma), do not play a role in Merkel cell carcinoma progression. For example, there are no mutations in well-known oncogenes such as p53, c-KIT or RAS.[18,19,25] In this section we will analyze the potential role of some of the best known cancer-related pathways in Merkel cell carcinoma (Figure 1).

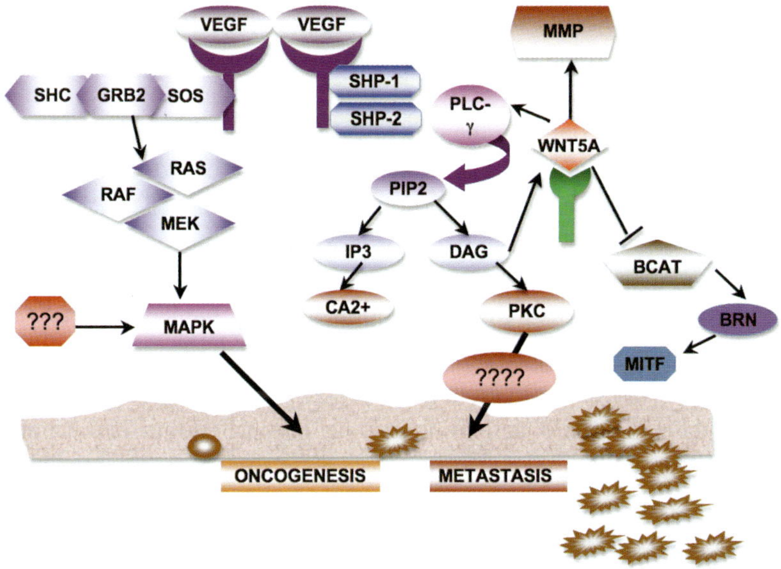

Figure 1. Pathways of potential importance in Merkel cell carcinoma development and progression. Activation of VEGF has been shown to be important for Merkel cell carcinoma progression. VEGF signalling can potentially activate both RAF/p38-MAPK pathways, and also activate non-canonical Wnt signaling via PKC, although no evidence exists for this. See text for details.

4.3.1 *RAS/RAF/MAPK*

RAS genes were first identified as viral genes with transforming potential, and were later confirmed as oncogenes when identified in human cells.[26] Three key family members include NRAS, HRAS and KRAS, and mutations in these are associated with the development of many types of cancers.[27] RAS proteins control a number of signaling cascades that affect motility, proliferation and apoptosis. The dysregulation of RAS genes results in the increased malignancy of many tumor types.[28] RAS signals to activate the MAP kinase pathway, and this occurs via two key effectors, RAF and PI3 kinase.[28] RAF may take one of three forms: ARAF, BRAF or CRAF, and its activation ultimately results in the activation of MAPK and ERK.[29] Mutations in BRAF are prevalent in melanoma.[30] However, BRAF mutations are also found in abundance in nevi,[31] implying that these mutations alone cannot promote malignancy. Indeed, it has been shown that the introduction of RAF into melanocytes can actually cause growth arrest and apoptosis.[32]

Houben *et al.* examined the role of RAF in Merkel cell carcinoma and found that, unlike melanoma, RAF mutations are virtually absent in Merkel cell carcinoma, and that despite expression of ERK, ERK remains inactive, as determined by its phosphorylation status.[25] Further, they demonstrate that silencing of RAF is essential for Merkel cell survival and progression to tumorigenicity.[33] In another study, however, p38-MAPK was activated in the majority of Merkel cell carcinomas, and its activation correlated to Merkel cell carcinoma progression.[24] It is unclear what the basis for the p38-MAPK activation may be, however it remains an intriguing finding, given the lack of signaling data in this cancer. It appears that RAF is likely not responsible for the p38-MAPK activation, as the introduction of activated RAF into Merkel cell carcinoma cells actually caused apoptosis.[33] These data underscore the difference between Merkel cell carcinoma and other aggressive skin cancers such as melanoma, in which RAF activation is key.

4.3.2 *The secreted Wingless type (Wnt) pathway*

The Wnt family of proteins consists of almost 20 Wnt proteins, which may signal via a variety of receptors and co-receptors. These receptors include frizzleds, LRPs and, most recently discovered, the tyrosine kinase receptor ROR2.[34] Wnt proteins have been implicated in cancer progression as they signal to activate some important signal transduction pathways, most notably β-catenin.[34] Wnts such as Wnt3A signal to activate disheveled, which in turn inhibits GSK3β. GSK3β exists in a complex with APC and Axin, and this complex is responsible for the phosphorylation of β-catenin, which in turns results in its ubiquitination and degradation.[35] Activating mutations of β-catenin have been shown to be important in the pathogenesis of a number of cancers, including melanoma and small cell lung cancer.[36] However, as with the RAS/RAF/MAPK pathway, no mutations in β-catenin (CTNNB1) have been found in Merkel cell carcinoma.[37] In addition, no mutations have been found in other commonly mutated genes in this pathway including APC.[37]

However, β-catenin may still play a role in this cancer, as the loss of the POU domain transcription factor Brn3 has been implicated in Merkel cell carcinoma progression.[38] β-catenin has previously been shown to activate MITF via Brn transcription factors,[39] promoting melanoma growth, and these data suggest that the role of β-catenin in Merkel cell carcinoma development should be further studied.

The other major Wnt signaling pathway involves the activation of PKC, via increases in Ca^{2+} release. This arm of the pathway is best characterized by Wnts such as Wnt5A.[40] Wnt5A has a very dichotomous role, acting as a tumor suppressor in some cancers[36] and as a promoter of tumorigenesis in others.[34] This may depend on which stage in the tumor it is expressed, and also its context to β-catenin. Wnt5A has been shown to suppress β-catenin,[41,42] so if it is expressed early in a tumor it may well suppress tumor growth. However, PKC activation has been shown to promote tumor metastasis, so if Wnt5A is expressed later in a tumor, it may contribute to malignant progression. In melanoma, Wnt5A over-expression contributes to increased malignancy.[43] This is mediated by the ability of Wnt5A to suppress metastasis suppressor genes such as Kiss-1, and also to cause an epithelial to mesenchymal transition via the upregulation of Snail, a transcriptional repressor.[9] Furthermore, Wnt5A can suppress the expression of melanoma differentiation antigens via the activation of PO_4-STAT3, making melanoma cells not only more invasive but also less susceptible to immune surveillance.[44] Whether or not Wnt5A, and the subsequent activation of PKC, plays a role in Merkel cell carcinoma remains to be determined. Given that Merkel cell carcinoma is of neuroendocrine origin, and that Wnts play key roles in the migration of cells from the neural crest to the skin, one would imagine that they may well play a role in Merkel cell carcinoma progression.

4.3.3 *VEGF and related proteins*

The vascular endothelial growth factor is important in the potentiation of angiogenesis in a malignant tumor. VEGF has been shown to induce upon conditions of hypoxia,[45] or when a tumor starts to outgrow its blood supply. In many cancers VEGF expression is a hallmark of increased malignancy and implies that the tumor is undergoing angiogenesis. A few isoforms of VEGF exist, VEGF-A, -B, -C, -D and other forms, including soluble VEGF receptors.[46] In different cancers, different isoforms are responsible for governing angiogenesis. In melanoma, VEGF-C appears to be the most significant mediator of angiogenesis, and most closely correlates to progression and decreased survival.[47,48] VEGF-C and -D are the two most increased isoforms in small cell lung cancer.[49] In Merkel cell carcinoma, a very high number of tumors express VEGF isoforms A (95%) and C (79%), and also the receptor VEGF-R2 (88%).[50] VEGF represents one of the few potential targets for clinical intervention in this disease identified to date.

4.3.4 *Matrix metalloproteinases*

Matrix metalloproteinases are enzymes that are responsible for the proteolytic dissolution of the basement membrane. Because of this, they are an important step in the metastatic dissemination of tumor cells. MT-MMP1, MMP1 and MMP2 have been the MMPs most closely associated with the progression of melanoma.[51] Interestingly, it is becoming clear that MMPs play an even more complex role than originally thought. Some MMPs may actually act as tumor suppressor genes, as demonstrated by an elegant study showing that the knockout of MMP8 in a mouse model increased the susceptibility to skin tumorigenesis.[52] The roles of MMPs in tumor growth and development remain unclear. In Merkel cell carcinoma, MMP7 is over-expressed in aggressive tumors, and correlates significantly with both VEGF and P38, both of which have been implicated in Merkel cell carcinoma progression, as discussed earlier.[24] Whether other MMPs are expressed and related to tumor suppression or metastasis in Merkel cell carcinoma remains to be seen.

4.4 Clinical Implications of Genomic Approaches to Merkel Cell Carcinoma

Gene expression profiling studies of Merkel cell cancers appear to be still in their infancy. However, the few studies that exist have already begun to provide us with information about potential targets and markers.

In particular, the tissue array analysis by Fernandez-Figueara *et al.* identified several markers that are upregulated in Merkel cell carcinoma.[24] Among these was VEGF, and further study on this topic highlighted VEGF-C and VEGF-R2. Inhibitors to VEGF have already met with some success in clinical trials for various cancers,[53–55] and this molecule may be a promising target for clinical intervention in Merkel cell carcinoma as well. The identification of glutamate as a marker of Merkel cell carcinoma may also have some implications for therapy as riluzole, a drug that has been shown to inhibit melanoma metastasis in animal models, appears to act by inhibiting glutamate release.[56] Although BRAF mutations are rare in this disease, the activation of p38-MAPk has been shown to be associated with Merkel cell carcinoma progression by a number of different groups. Drugs targeting this kinase may also have significant implications for Merkel cell carcinoma therapy. Finally, recent data implicating the polyoma virus MCPyV in Merkel cell carcinoma, as discussed elsewhere in this book, may also result in new approaches to the treatment of this disease. All in all, despite the paucity of gene expression profiling studies of this disease, those that exist have identified some promising targets for Merkel cell carcinoma therapy. It is hoped that in the future, larger scale analyses will uncover even more viable molecular targets as well as lead to a better understanding of the pathobiology of this disease.

References

1. Sidhu G.S., Chandra P., Cassai N.D. (2005). Merkel cells, normal and neoplastic: an update. *Ultrastruct Pathol* 29: 287–294.
2. Swann M.H., Yoon J. (2007). Merkel cell carcinoma. *Semin Oncol* 34: 51–56.
3. Velculescu V.E., Zhang L., Vogelstein B., Kinzler K.W. (1995). Serial analysis of gene expression. *Science* 270: 484–487.
4. Oostlander A.E., Meijer G.A., Ylstra B. (2004). Microarray-based comparative genomic hybridization and its applications in human genetics. *Clin Genet* 66: 488–495.
5. Komura D., Shen F., Ishikawa S., *et al.* (2006). Genome-wide detection of human copy number variations using high-density DNA oligonucleotide arrays. *Genome Res* 16: 1575–1584.

6. Greer B.T., Khan J. (2004). Diagnostic classification of cancer using DNA microarrays and artificial intelligence. *Ann N Y Acad Sci* 1020: 49–66.
7. Augustine C.K., Yoo J.S., Potti A., *et al.* (2009). Genomic and molecular profiling predicts response to temozolomide in melanoma. *Clin Cancer Res* 15: 502–510.
8. Packer L.M., Pavey S.J., Boyle G.M., *et al.* (2007). Gene expression profiling in melanoma identifies novel downstream effectors of p14ARF. *Int J Cancer* 121: 784–790.
9. Dissanayake S.K., Wade M., Johnson C.E., *et al.* (2007). The Wnt5A/protein kinase C pathway mediates motility in melanoma cells via the inhibition of metastasis suppressors and initiation of an epithelial to mesenchymal transition. *J Biol Chem* 282: 17259–17271.
10. Verona E.V., Elkahloun A.G., Yang J., *et al.* (2007). Transforming growth factor-beta signaling in prostate stromal cells supports prostate carcinoma growth by up-regulating stromal genes related to tissue remodeling. *Cancer Res* 67: 5737–5746.
11. Hayashi S., Yamaguchi Y. (2008). Estrogen signaling in cancer microenvironment and prediction of response to hormonal therapy. *J Steroid Biochem Mol Biol* 109: 201–206.
12. Decker N.K., Abdelmoneim S.S., Yaqoob U., *et al.* (2008). Nitric oxide regulates tumor cell cross-talk with stromal cells in the tumor microenvironment of the liver. *Am J Pathol* 173: 1002–1012.
13. Acharya C.R., Hsu D.S., Anders C.K., *et al.* (2008). Gene expression signatures, clinicopathological features, and individualized therapy in breast cancer. *JAMA* 299: 1574–1587.
14. Harle M., Arens N., Moll I., *et al.* (1996). Comparative genomic hybridization (CGH) discloses chromosomal and subchromosomal copy number changes in Merkel cell carcinomas. *J Cutan Pathol* 23: 391–397.
15. Larramendy M.L., Koljonen V., Bohling T., *et al.* (2004). Recurrent DNA copy number changes revealed by comparative genomic hybridization in primary Merkel cell carcinomas. *Mod Pathol* 17: 561–567.
16. Van Gele M., Leonard J.H., Van Roy N., *et al.* (2002). Combined karyotyping, CGH and M-FISH analysis allows detailed characterization of unidentified chromosomal rearrangements in Merkel cell carcinoma. *Int J Cancer* 101: 137–145.

17. Popp S., Waltering S., Herbst C., *et al.* (2002). UV-B-type mutations and chromosomal imbalances indicate common pathways for the development of Merkel and skin squamous cell carcinomas. *Int J Cancer* 99: 352–360.
18. Van Gele M., Leonard J.H., Van Roy N., *et al.* (2001). Frequent allelic loss at 10q23 but low incidence of PTEN mutations in Merkel cell carcinoma. *Int J Cancer* 92: 409–413.
19. Lassacher A., Heitzer E., Kerl H., Wolf P. (2008). p14ARF hypermethylation is common but INK4a-ARF locus or p53 mutations are rare in Merkel cell carcinoma. *J Invest Dermatol* 128: 1788–1796.
20. Lemos B., Nghiem P. (2007). Merkel cell carcinoma: more deaths but still no pathway to blame. *J Invest Dermatol* 127: 2100–2103.
21. Van Gele M., Boyle G.M., Cook A.L., *et al.* (2004). Gene-expression profiling reveals distinct expression patterns for Classic versus Variant Merkel cell phenotypes and new classifier genes to distinguish Merkel cell from small-cell lung carcinoma. *Oncogene* 23: 2732–2742.
22. Haeberle H., Fujiwara M., Chuang J., *et al.* (2004). Molecular profiling reveals synaptic release machinery in Merkel cells. *Proc Natl Acad Sci USA* 101: 14503–14508.
23. Pollock P.M., Cohen-Solal K., Sood R., *et al.* (2003). Melanoma mouse model implicates metabotropic glutamate signaling in melanocytic neoplasia. *Nat Genet* 34: 108–112.
24. Fernandez-Figueras M.T., Puig L., Musulen E., *et al.* (2007). Expression profiles associated with aggressive behavior in Merkel cell carcinoma. *Mod Pathol* 20: 90–101.
25. Houben R., Michel B., Vetter-Kauczok C.S., *et al.* (2006). Absence of classical MAP kinase pathway signalling in Merkel cell carcinoma. *J Invest Dermatol* 126: 1135–1142.
26. Bos J.L. (1989). Ras oncogenes in human cancer: a review. *Cancer Res* 49: 4682–4689.
27. Ehrhardt A., Ehrhardt G.R., Guo X., Schrader J.W. (2002). Ras and relatives — job sharing and networking keep an old family together. *Exp Hematol* 30: 1089–1106.
28. Rodriguez-Viciana P., Tetsu O., Oda K., *et al.* (2005). Cancer targets in the Ras pathway. *Cold Spring Harb Symp Quant Biol* 70: 461–467.

29. Meier F., Schittek B., Busch S., *et al.* (2005). The RAS/RAF/MEK/ERK and PI3K/AKT signaling pathways present molecular targets for the effective treatment of advanced melanoma. *Front Biosci* 10: 2986–3001.
30. Davies H., Bignell G.R., Cox C., *et al.* (2002). Mutations of the BRAF gene in human cancer. *Nature* 417: 949–954.
31. Pollock P.M., Meltzer P.S. (2002). A genome-based strategy uncovers frequent BRAF mutations in melanoma. *Cancer Cell* 2: 5–7.
32. Wajapeyee N., Serra R.W., Zhu X., *et al.* (2008). Oncogenic BRAF induces senescence and apoptosis through pathways mediated by the secreted protein IGFBP7. *Cell* 132: 363–374.
33. Houben R., Ortmann S., Schrama D., *et al.* (2007). Activation of the MAP kinase pathway induces apoptosis in the Merkel cell carcinoma cell line UISO. *J Invest Dermatol* 127: 2116–2122.
34. Weeraratna A.T. (2005). A Wnt-er wonderland — the complexity of Wnt signaling in melanoma. *Cancer Metastasis Rev* 24: 237–250.
35. Morin P.J., Weeraratna A.T. (2003). The APC tumor suppressor pathway. *Methods Mol Biol* 222: 21–40.
36. Morin P.J., Weeraratna A.T. (2003). Wnt signaling in human cancer. *Cancer Treat Res* 115: 169–187.
37. Liu S., Daa T., Kashima K., *et al.* (2007).The Wnt-signaling pathway is not implicated in tumorigenesis of Merkel cell carcinoma. *J Cutan Pathol* 34: 22–26.
38. Leonard J.H., Cook A.L., Van Gele M., *et al.* (2002). Proneural and proneuroendocrine transcription factor expression in cutaneous mechanoreceptor (Merkel) cells and Merkel cell carcinoma. *Int J Cancer* 101: 103–110.
39. Goodall J., Martinozzi S., Dexter T.J., *et al.* (2004). Brn-2 expression controls melanoma proliferation and is directly regulated by beta-catenin. *Mol Cell Biol* 24: 2915–2922.
40. Kuhl M. (2004). The WNT/calcium pathway: biochemical mediators, tools and future requirements. *Front Biosci* 9: 967–974.
41. Topol L., Jiang X., Choi H., *et al.* (2003). Wnt-5a inhibits the canonical Wnt pathway by promoting GSK-3independent beta-catenin degradation. *J Cell Biol* 162: 899–908.
42. Westfall T.A., Brimeyer R., Twedt J., *et al.* (2003). Wnt-5/pipetail functions in vertebrate axis formation as a negative regulator of Wnt/beta-catenin activity. *J Cell Biol* 162: 889–898.

43. Weeraratna A.T., Jiang Y., Hostetter G., *et al.* (2002). Wnt5a signaling directly affects cell motility and invasion of metastatic melanoma. *Cancer Cell* 1: 279–288.
44. Dissanayake S.K., Olkhanud P.B., O'Connell M.P., *et al.* (2008). Wnt5A regulates expression of tumor-associated antigens in melanoma via changes in signal transducers and activators of transcription 3 phosphorylation. *Cancer Res* 68: 10205–10214.
45. Rofstad E.K., Danielsen T. (1999). Hypoxia-induced metastasis of human melanoma cells: involvement of vascular endothelial growth factor-mediated angiogenesis. *Br J Cancer* 80: 1697–1707.
46. Roskoski R, Jr. (2007). Vascular endothelial growth factor (VEGF) signaling in tumor progression. *Crit Rev Oncol Hematol* 62: 179–213.
47. Brychtova S., Bezdekova M., Brychta T., Tichy M. (2008). The role of vascular endothelial growth factors and their receptors in malignant melanomas. *Neoplasma* 55: 273–279.
48. Boone B., Blokx W., De Bacquer D., *et al.* (2008). The role of VEGF-C staining in predicting regional metastasis in melanoma. *Virchows Arch* 453: 257–265.
49. Naumnik W., Izycki T., Swidzinska E., *et al.* (2007). Serum levels of VEGF-C, VEGF-D, and sVEGF-R2 in patients with lung cancer during chemotherapy. *Oncol Res* 16: 445–451.
50. Brunner M., Thurnher D., Pammer J., *et al.* (2008). Expression of VEGF-A/C, VEGF-R2, PDGF-alpha/beta, c-kit, EGFR, Her-2/Neu, Mcl-1 and Bmi-1 in Merkel cell carcinoma. *Mod Pathol* 21: 876–884.
51. Hofmann U.B., Westphal J.R., Van Muijen G.N., Ruiter D.J. (2000). Matrix metalloproteinases in human melanoma. *J Invest Dermatol* 115: 337–344.
52. Balbin M., Fueyo A., Tester A.M., *et al.* (2003). Loss of collagenase-2 confers increased skin tumor susceptibility to male mice. *Nat Genet* 35: 252–257.
53. Polyzos A. (2008). Activity of SU11248, a multitargeted inhibitor of vascular endothelial growth factor receptor and platelet-derived growth factor receptor, in patients with metastatic renal cell carcinoma and various other solid tumors. *J Steroid Biochem Mol Biol* 108: 261–266.
54. Choueiri T.K. (2008). Axitinib, a novel anti-angiogenic drug with promising activity in various solid tumors. *Curr Opin Investig Drugs* 9: 658–671.

55. Seiwert T.Y., Cohen E.E. (2008). Targeting angiogenesis in head and neck cancer. *Semin Oncol* 35: 274–285.
56. Namkoong J., Shin S.S., Lee H.J., *et al.* (2007). Metabotropic glutamate receptor 1 and glutamate signaling in human melanoma. *Cancer Res* 67: 2298–2305.

Chapter 5

Pathology of Merkel Cell Carcinoma

Jane L. Messina

The description of a unique cutaneous malignancy with a distinctive trabecular architecture by Cyril Toker in 1972 opened new insights into the diagnosis and treatment of the most aggressive primary neoplasm of the skin, now known as primary cutaneous neuroendocrine or Merkel cell carcinoma. In a mere 30 years, investigators have made significant discoveries in elucidating its cell of origin, etiology, distinctive pathologic features, as well as optimal surgical and medical treatment. This chapter will highlight current knowledge concerning the cellular origin of this tumor. The diagnostic workup of this tumor, including the role of adjunct techniques such as immunohistochemistry, electron microscopy, flow cytometry and cytopathology, will be discussed. The pathologic evaluation of both cutaneous and lymph node specimens will be addressed.

5.1 Histogenesis of Merkel Cell Carcinoma

In 1972, Toker described an unusual, distinctive neoplasm of the skin of putative sweat gland origin characterized by a trabecular, or column-like, growth pattern, which he named 'trabecular carcinoma.'[1] Since then, the tumor now known as Merkel cell carcinoma has gone by a variety of monikers, including cutaneous APUDoma, neuroendocrine tumor of the skin, primary small cell carcinoma of the skin, primary undifferentiated carcinoma of the skin, anaplastic carcinoma of the skin and 'murky cell' carcinoma.[2] Six years after its original description, the discovery of dense-core neurosecretory granules in three tumors studied by electron microscopy raised the possibility of a neuroendocrine origin, and the Merkel cell was proposed as the cell of origin.[3] In 1980, DeWoolf-Peters first proposed the name ‘Merkel cell carcinoma’ for this tumor.[4] Since this remains the most widely accepted explanation for the origin of this tumor, Merkel cell carcinoma is today the most commonly accepted terminology.

The exact function of the Merkel cell is not entirely clear. Merkel cells are found in the skin and some mucosal surfaces, and are thought be derived from neuroectodermal origin. In histologic sections of skin, they are optically clear, oval cells located within or close to the basal layer of the epidermis and within hair follicles, where they are most numerous. The Merkel cell appears to function as a cutaneous mechanoreceptor.[5] First described by Friedrich Sigmund Merkel in 1875 as ‘Tastzellen’ or ‘touch cells,’[6] the majority of the cells are intimately associated with a nerve terminal. Experimental evidence indicates that Merkel cells are directly involved in the transformation of mechanical stimuli to action potentials in afferent nerve fibers. While the vast majority of Merkel cells are intraepidermal, they are present in the dermis during embryogenesis, and they have reported to rarely be found in the dermis.[7]

Because Merkel cell carcinoma and Merkel cells share so many ultrastructural and immunohistochemical features, it seems likely that the Merkel cell is the origin of this tumor.[8] However, the differing locations of Merkel cells (epidermis) and Merkel cell carcinoma tumors (primarily arising in dermis) does raise some doubt concerning this hypothesis. Also, Merkel cells are most numerous in acral skin,[7] while Merkel cell carcinoma is most commonly located on the head and neck. Merkel cell carcinoma does not express vasoactive intestinal peptides and metenkephalin, which are expressed in Merkel cells. This has led to the proposal that Merkel cell carcinoma arises from a totipotential stem cell that acquires neuroendocrine characteristics during malignant transformation.[9] The same concept of precursor stem cells may explain the co-existence of Merkel cell carcinoma and squamous cell carcinoma of the skin.[10] Thus, at present, the exact cell of origin of this tumor remains controversial.

5.2 Light Microscopic Findings

Merkel cell carcinoma is composed of tumor cells with a 'small round blue cell' appearance, a pattern which is shared by other neuroectodermal tumors such as neuroendocrine carcinomas, especially of lung, peripheral neuroectodermal tumor, medulloblastoma and neuroblastoma, as well as malignant lymphoma, Ewing sarcoma, rhabdomyosarcoma, other poorly differentiated carcinoma, and the small cell variant of malignant melanoma. The tumor is nearly always dermally centered, beneath a Grenz zone of normal papillary dermis, and the epidermis is unaffected. The tumor cells are generally uniform and monotonous, with basophilic, smudged nuclei and dispersed nuclear chromatin that lacks nuclear detail (Figure 1). Nucleoli, if seen, are generally small and inconspicuous. Tumor cells have minimal cytoplasm without distinct cell borders. The tumor cells vary with respect to the degree of cohesiveness, from a completely dyscohesive sheet-like growth to prominent molding between the cytoplasm of adjacent cells. In rare instances, the cells may have plasmacytoid morphology, with an eccentric rim of eosinophilic cytoplasm. Artifactual clearing of the nuclear chromatin simulating 'Orphan Annie' nuclei of papillary thyroid carcinoma can also be observed. The tumor cells may rarely have large nuclei, simulating anaplastic or diffuse large cell lymphoma. Bizarre nuclei, multinucleate, or multilobated forms can be observed, resembling Touton giant cells or 'floret' cells as seen in fibrohistiocytic tumors. Warthin–Finkeldey-like cells may also be a feature.[11] Typically, numerous mitotic figures, up to ten per high-power field,[11] as well as apoptotic bodies, are seen (Figure 2).

Three histologic subtypes of Merkel cell carcinoma have been reported: intermediate, small cell and trabecular, but these variants have no known clinical relevance.[12] Also, most tumors display some heterogeneity in growth pattern, with two or more patterns of growth typically present. In all variants, the tumor is present in the dermis, beneath a normal epidermis and Grenz zone of normal dermis; pagetoid involvement of the epidermis is rare.[13,14] The intermediate variant is the most common subtype, characterized by diffuse, sheet-like growth of relatively larger cells with minimal cytoplasm and occasionally prominent nuclear molding (Figure 3). The small cell variant mostly closely resembles other small cell

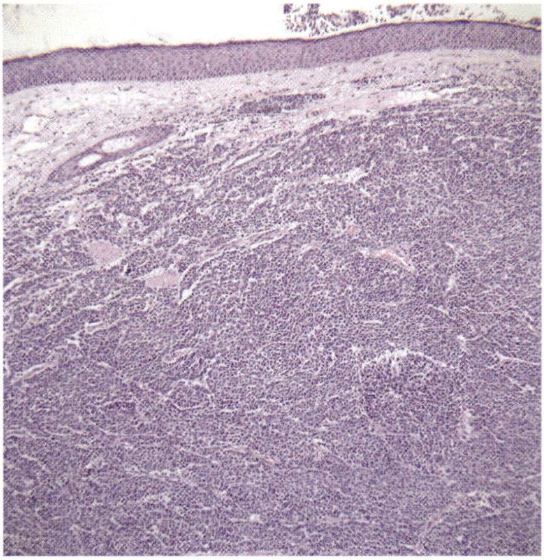

Figure 1. Low-power view of a primary Merkel cell carcinoma, showing 'small blue cell' tumor growth beneath a Grenz zone (H&E, 200×).

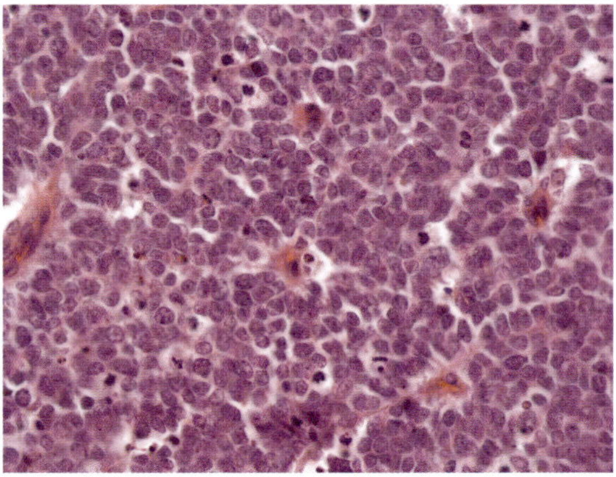

Figure 2. Typical high-power view of a primary Merkel cell carcinoma, showing numerous mitoses and apoptotic figures (H&E, 400×).

carcinomas (Figure 4), and in particular should be distinguished from the pulmonary neuroendocrine small cell carcinomas.[10] The small cell variant contains cells that are relatively small, round and dyscohesive, with hyperchromatic nuclei, minimal nuclear detail and minimal cytoplasm. These

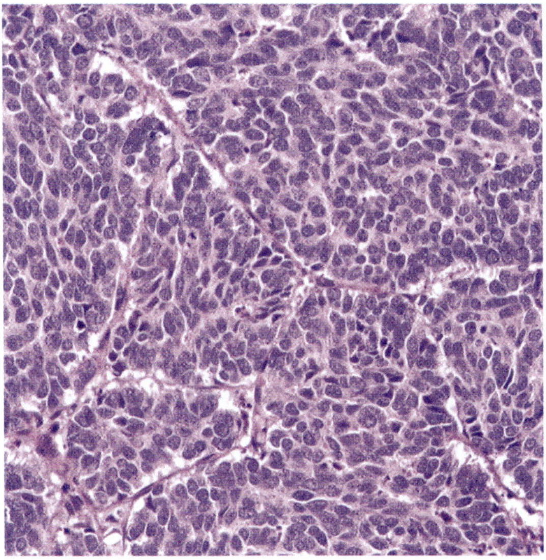

Figure 3. Intermediate cell growth pattern of Merkel cell carcinoma, showing fairly large uniform cells with occasional nuclear molding (H&E, 400×).

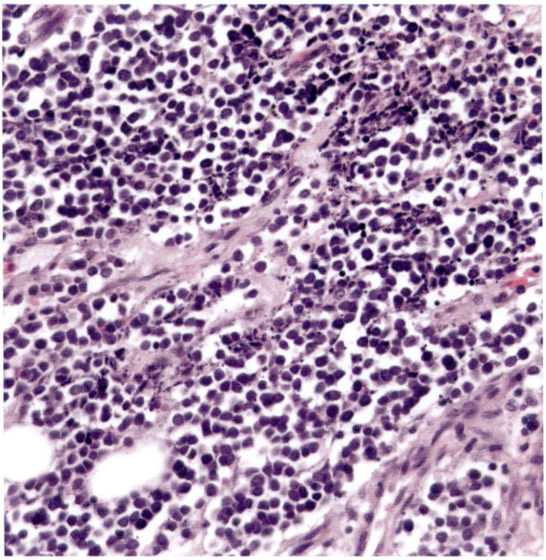

Figure 4. Small cell growth pattern of Merkel cell carcinoma. Note dyscohesive quality of tumor cells in this variant (H&E, 400×).

tumors are more often associated with irregular or geographic areas of necrosis. Encrustation of vessel walls by basophilic, stringy material originating from DNA of necrotic tumor cells (the so-called Azzopardi phenomenon) is most often seen in this variant. Although traditionally used as a feature to distinguish Merkel cell carcinoma from small cell carcinoma of the lung, in which it is more typically found, the Azzopardi phenomenon can be seen in up to 10% of Merkel cell carcinoma.[15] The trabecular variant is characterized by growth of columns of cells, two to three cell layers thick, oriented vertically or diagonally with respect to the epidermis (Figure 5). Trabecular tumors may have prominent spindling of the tumor cells, which often show prominent nuclear molding and visible nucleoli (Figure 6).[11]

Various types of stromal changes are seen in Merkel cell carcinoma. The stroma is usually delicate, with increased numbers of blood vessels. Similar to other neuroendocrine tumors, vascular proliferation may occasionally be a prominent feature. Vazmitel systemically examined vascular changes in a series of Merkel cell carcinoma and found some degree of

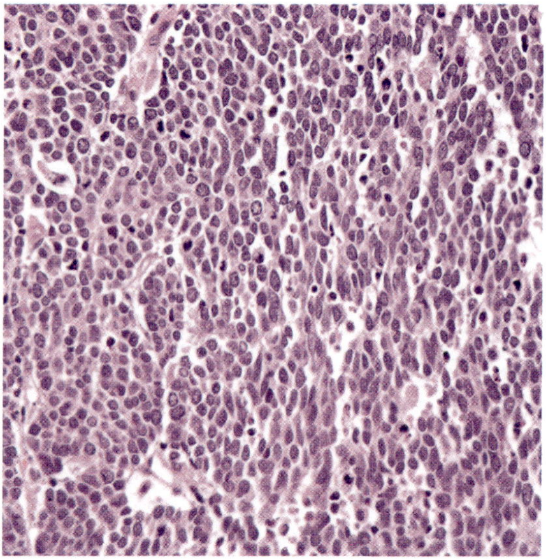

Figure 5. Trabecular growth pattern of Merkel cell carcinoma, demonstrating columns of tumor cells (H&E, 400×).

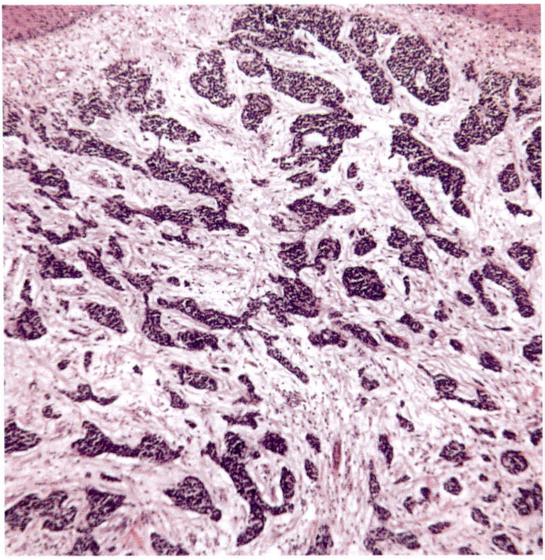

Figure 6. Extreme example of trabecular growth pattern with spindling of tumor cells (H&E, 100×).

vascular proliferation in 18/92 (20%) of cases studied. These changes were found to consist of six patterns: pericyte hyperplasia, pyogenic granuloma-like, hemangioendothelioma-like, epithelioid hemangioma-like, peliosis-like and follicular dendritic cell tumor-like. While the pathogenesis of these vascular changes is unclear, they are speculated to represent a response to endogenous tumor production of angiogenesis factors. In the same study, 18 tumors were examined by polymerase chain reaction for human herpesvirus-8 sequences, and all were negative.[16] In addition to vascular proliferation, a lymphoid response of varying intensity is usually seen (Figure 7). In some cases, this may cause confusion with a lymphoproliferative process.[11] There may be prominent mucinous change and retraction artifact, in up to 93% and 90% of tumors respectively, giving the tumor a histologic resemblance to basal cell carcinoma.[17] This prominent stromal retraction may often be mistaken for lymphatic invasion, but CD31 staining does not label the rim of the retracted space.[17] Deposition of amyloid-like material is rarely seen, and thought to originate from the numerous apoptotic cells that characterize Merkel cell carcinoma.[18]

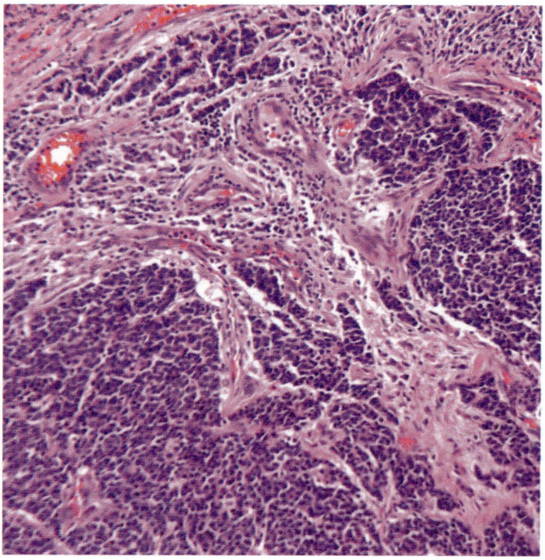

Figure 7. Dense lymphocytic infiltrate surrounding and infiltrating tumor islands (H&E, 400×).

Regression is a rare phenomenon in Merkel cell carcinoma, reported in 20 cases to date.[19,20] The phenomenon of regression may explain why approximately 10% of Merkel cell carcinomas present as metastatic disease of unknown primary origin.[21] Regression of Merkel cell carcinoma is thought to represent either a T cell immune-mediated reaction or a function of increased apoptosis, similar to that which occurs in melanoma. Regression may be either partial or complete. The latter is histologically characterized by the absence of tumor and the presence of scar and a dense lymphocytic infiltrate. Many of the described cases have occurred after biopsy of the primary tumor.[22] In a review of 16 cases of Merkel cell carcinoma regression reported prior to 2006, it was noted that patients who developed this phenomenon had a better prognosis than those without regression.[22] There are also reports of Merkel cell carcinoma undergoing regression after an improvement in the patient's immune status. In one report, an HIV-positive patient receiving antiretroviral therapy had a recovery of CD4 counts and regression of Merkel cell carcinoma.[23] Withdrawal of azathioprine induced regression of metastatic Merkel cell carcinoma in one patient.[24] In a case of Merkel cell carcinoma developing in a renal transplant patient, withdrawal of cyclosporine resulted in dramatic but temporary improvement of metastatic disease.[25]

Rarely, cells of Merkel cell carcinoma may be seen in the epidermis, with or without co-existing dermal Merkel cell carcinoma. Whether this represents and proves that the tumor originates from epidermal Merkel cells, or constitutes pagetoid spread from an underlying dermal tumor, is a matter of much controversy. In the setting of a typical dermal Merkel cell carcinoma, the epidermis may contain malignant tumor cells in up to 10% of cases.[26–29] In these cases, the mechanism of epidermal involvement is thought to represent transepidermal elimination of tumor cells, essentially a mechanical phenomenon related to heavy underlying tumor burden. There have been three reported cases of Merkel cell carcinoma present in the epidermis in the absence of underlying dermal component, although one later recurred as dermal Merkel cell carcinoma.[14,18,30] The term 'Merkel cell carcinoma *in situ*' has been proffered for this rare phenomenon.[13] In addition, there have been three reported cases of intraepidermal Merkel cell carcinoma admixed or concurrent with squamous cell carcinoma *in situ*. In two of these cases, however, the tumor recurred as dermal or metastatic Merkel cell carcinoma.[13] It is these latter cases, as well as the frequent co-existence of all form of Merkel cell carcinoma with squamous cell carcinoma *in situ*, that most strengthens the hypothesis that the tumor arises from a pluripotential stem cell in the epidermis, potentiated by the mutagenic effects of ultraviolet light and perhaps polyoma virus infection (see Chapter 3).

In fact, in one series, some form of squamous cell carcinoma was present in 37% of cases of typical, dermal Merkel cell carcinoma.[31] Usually, this takes the pattern of squamous cell carcinoma *in situ*, centered above the area of greatest dermal Merkel cell carcinoma growth. In this study of 27 Merkel cell carcinomas, 11 tumors (41%) were found to be in continuity or admixed with some form of other epithelial lesion, including two actinic keratoses, five squamous cell carcinomas *in situ*, three invasive squamous cell carcinomas (Figure 8) and one basal cell carcinoma.[31] Merkel cell carcinoma metastatic to a regional lymph node draining a squamous cell carcinoma in the absence of a primary Merkel cell carcinoma has even been reported.[32] While some may argue that this

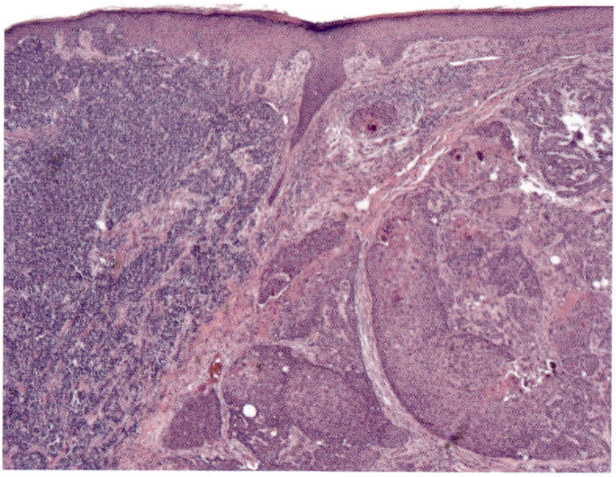

Figure 8. Primary Merkel cell carcinoma (left side of photomicrograph) demonstrating squamous differentiation (right side of photomicrograph; H&E, 200×).

co-existence represents a form of collision of tumors arising in sun-damaged skin, the predominance of associated squamous over the far more common basal cell carcinoma mitigates against this. It is far more likely that the not infrequent association of neuroendocrine and epithelial differentiation results from a tumor originating in an epidermal stem cell with the capacity to differentiate in two or more phenotypic directions.[31] Most importantly, this controversy should not detract from recognizing the limited clinical relevance of the finding of Merkel cell carcinoma co-existing with any epithelial tumor; the prognosis of the patient is similar to that of a pure Merkel cell carcinoma, irrespective of any secondary form of differentiation.[33]

In addition to the complex relationship with squamous cell carcinoma, Merkel cell carcinoma can show many other forms of aberrant differentiation. Small areas of squamous differentiation, taking the form of keratin pearls or whorls of squamous epithelium, are not uncommonly seen and usually constitute <10% of tumor volume. Other forms of epithelial differentiation include tubule formation, seen by either immunohistochemistry or electron microscopy, indicative of sweat gland differentiation,[26,34–36] as well as neuroectodermal differentiation. Rosette formation, which may resemble the Homer-Wright rosettes of neuroblastoma, has been reported (Figure 9).[27,31,37] Sarcomatous differentiation is even more unusual, and raises further questions concerning the histogenesis of these tumors

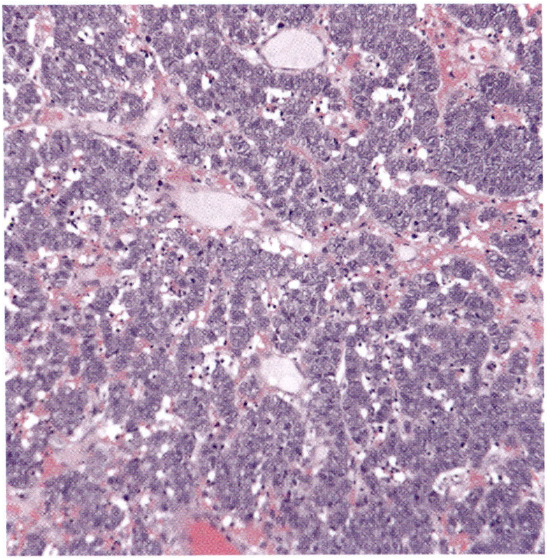

Figure 9. Ribbon and rosette-like growth pattern in primary Merkel cell carcinoma (H&E, 200×).

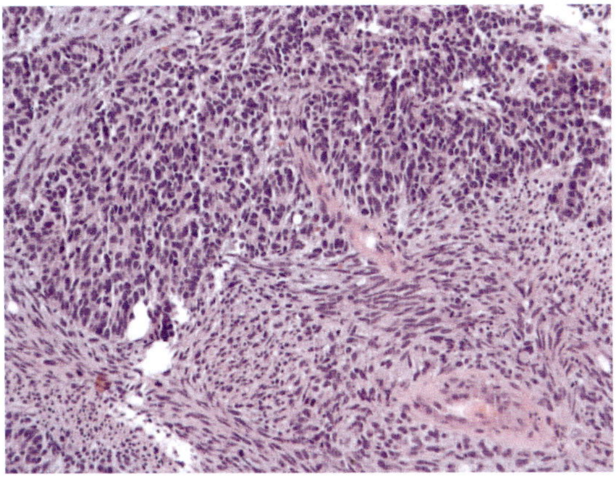

Figure 10. Sarcomatous transformation in Merkel cell carcinoma. In this example, the spindle cells were strongly S-100 positive, consistent with neurofibrosarcomatous transformation (H&E, 200×).

(Figure 10). Types of sarcomatous differentiation found as a component of Merkel cell carcinoma include rhabdomyosarcomatous,[38] atypical fibroxanthomatous with CD68 positivity,[39,40] leiomyosarcomatous[41] and fibrosarcomatous[33,42] differentiation. In some of these cases, the sarcomatous component first presented in the form of metastatic disease and was not present in the primary Merkel cell carcinoma. Areas of sarcomatous differentiation within Merkel cell carcinoma generally do not stain for the typical Merkel cell carcinoma markers such as cytokeratins or neuroendocrine markers. Other rare forms of aberrant differentiation include ganglion-cell[11] and melanocytic differentiation.[34]

5.3 Immunohistochemical Findings

Immunohistochemistry is an essential tool in the routine diagnostic workup of Merkel cell carcinoma. It is essential to differentiate Merkel cell carcinoma from other tumors in the histologic differential diagnosis, including small cell lung carcinoma, carcinoid tumor, anaplastic carcinoma, adnexal malignancies, malignant lymphoma, neuroblastoma and small cell forms of melanoma. Merkel cell carcinoma stains for both epithelial and neuroendocrine markers, but is negative for the lymphoid marker leukocyte common antigen and for melanoma markers S-100, HMB-45 and Melan-A. Several types of keratins react with Merkel cell carcinoma. The low molecular-weight cytokeratins 8, 18 and 20 appear to be the most consistently positive, each having a sensitivity of greater than 90%, but may react with other cutaneous carcinoma such as squamous and basal cell carcinoma. In one study, 100% of 25 Merkel cell carcinomas stained with cytokeratin CAM 5.2, and 20 demonstrated the 'paranuclear globular' or combined 'paranuclear globular'/diffuse pattern, and 17/25 (68%) stained with AE1/AE3 (Figure 11).[43] However, in the same study, CAM 5.2 reacted with 60% and 86% of small cell carcinomas of lung and esophagus respectively, while cytokeratin AE1/AE3 was found in 33% and 28% respectively.[43] Thus, CK 20 has been proposed as the cytokeratin marker best able to differentiate Merkel cell carcinoma from small cell lung carcinoma and other cutaneous carcinomas. CK20 is an intermediate filament protein whose expression is primarily restricted to gastric and intestinal epithelium, urothelium, taste buds of the tongue and Merkel cells.[44] CK20 staining in Merkel cell carcinoma has a characteristic perinuclear punctate or dot-like pattern of positivity (Figure 12). Cutaneous squamous cell carcinoma, basal cell carcinoma and melanoma are negative for CK20.[44] In a meta-analysis of 20 reports in the literature,

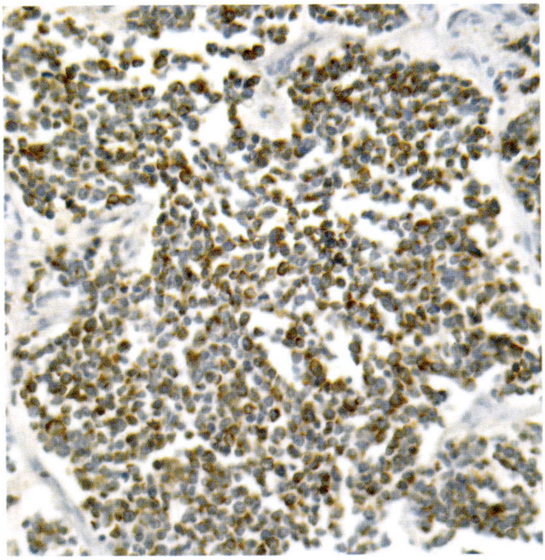

Figure 11. Membranous and perinuclear dot-like staining of Merkel cell carcinoma with AE1/AE3 cytokeratin (400×).

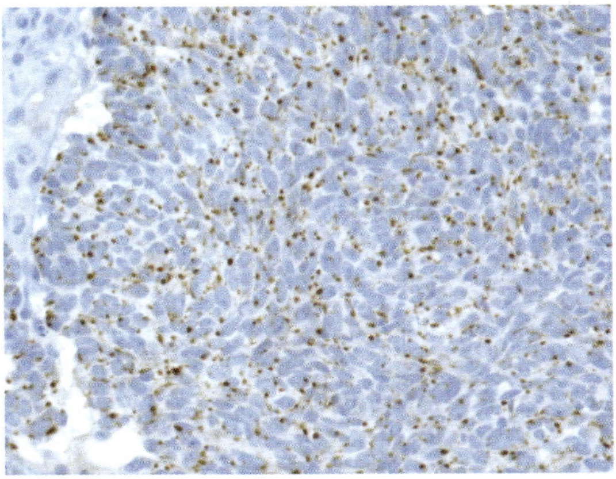

Figure 12. Exclusive perinuclear dot-like staining in Merkel cell carcinoma with cytokeratin 20 (400×).

Bobos *et al.* showed that CK20 expression has been reported in the majority of Merkel cell carcinomas tested, with 339 of 391 (87%) showing CK20 positivity, while only 14 of 302 (4.6%) of small cell lung carcinomas stained for this marker.[45] Due to the rare case of CK20 negative Merkel cell carcinoma, combined immunostaining with thyroid transcription factor-1 (TTF-1) and CK 20 has been advocated in distinguishing between Merkel cell carcinoma and small cell lung carcinoma.[46] TTF-1 is a homeodomain transcription factor expressed in the epithelial cells of the thyroid gland and lung. It is expressed in small cell and non-small cell carcinomas of the lung as well as pulmonary carcinoids, but there have been no reported cases of TTF-1 staining in 129 Merkel cell carcinoma cases combined from ten reports in the literature.[45] Others have advocated CK7 staining as a marker for pulmonary origin, but it is positive in up to 31% of Merkel cell carcinoma,[45,47] and in the author's opinion is not useful in the workup of Merkel cell carcinoma.

A variety of neuroendocrine markers have been demonstrated in Merkel cell carcinoma, and some recommend them as part of the diagnostic workup panel. Chromogranin-A is a sensitive marker for confirming the diagnosis of neuroendocrine tumors of a variety of origins, but was present in only 52% of Merkel cell carcinomas in one series.[48] Neuron-specific enolase is believed to be positive in almost all cases of Merkel cell carcinoma, although some studies have found it to be positive in only 50% of these tumors.[11] The specificity of neuron-specific enolase is also limited because melanoma may stain positively with this marker. Somatostatin can be positive in up to 33% of Merkel cell carcinomas.[49] Neurofilaments have been demonstrated in most Merkel cell carcinomas, and in 30% of cases shows the perinuclear dot-like pattern of staining similar to CK20. Interestingly, neurofilament is not found in small cell lung carcinoma and may thus be useful in excluding this diagnosis, similar to CK20.[45] CD56, or neural cell adhesion molecule, is expressed by a variety of neuroendocrine neoplasms and has been found in 40–100% of Merkel cell carcinomas.[50] CD56 positivity in crushed biopsies of Merkel cell carcinoma may rarely raise the possibility of a natural killer cell lymphoma, also CD56 positive, but keratin positivity would exclude this diagnosis.[51] Finally, synaptophysin is seen even less frequently, in one series only staining 21% of tumors.[48] Interestingly, despite the presence of neurosecretory granules in tumor cells, polypeptide hormones have not been demonstrated by immunohistochemical staining to any significant degree. In one study, insulin, calcitonin, and somatostatin were demonstrated in $< 5\%$ of cases.[48] In another, 1/15 cases stained for ACTH, but all were negative for bombesin, met-enkephalin, calcitonin, gastrin and somatostatin.[49] Thus, considering the variable sensitivity of neuroendocrine markers and their lack of specificity in excluding non-cutaneous neuroendocrine carcinoma, their role as part of the routine diagnostic workup of Merkel cell carcinoma is limited.

Overall, immunohistochemistry plays a vital role in the accurate diagnosis of Merkel cell carcinoma. A panel of immunohistochemical stains is suggested to confirm the diagnosis and exclude the other entities in the differential diagnosis. In our routine practice, we employ an initial panel of broad-spectrum keratin (AE1/AE3 or Cam 5.2), CK20, and TTF-1. A CK20-dot-like positive/TTF-1 negative result in a tumor morphologically consistent with Merkel cell carcinoma establishes the diagnosis. If CK20 is negative, but broad-spectrum keratin demonstrates dot-like positivity, chromogranin and synaptophysin are performed for confirmation of neuroendocrine differentiation.

5.4 Surgical Pathology of Sentinel Lymph Nodes

Sentinel lymph node biopsy has become an established part of the surgical treatment for Merkel cell carcinoma (see Chapter 10). In a compilation of the 14 studies published on patients undergoing sentinel node biopsy, metastases were found in 29/93 (30%) of patients.[52] Similar to the experience with melanoma and breast carcinoma, immunohistochemistry plays an essential role in the evaluation of these nodes for micrometastatic disease. In the first report on its utility, immunohistochemistry for CAM 5.2, CK20 and chromogranin was performed on lymph nodes from 26 patients; five had metastatic disease. In two of the five patients, the micrometastatic disease was detected by immunohistochemistry; all three antibodies stained both cases.[53] Su and colleagues found immunohistochemistry using CAM 5.2 and CK20 identified metastases in 5/23 (22%) of sentinel nodes tested in 4/10 (40%) of patients. In this study, neurofilament and chromogranin stained only one of five positive lymph nodes, and are not recommended for sentinel node evaluation.[54]

In our practice, we use CAM 5.2 to evaluate all sentinel nodes excised from patients with Merkel cell carcinoma. Despite the presence of some background positivity with this antibody, it has a stronger, crisper dot-like

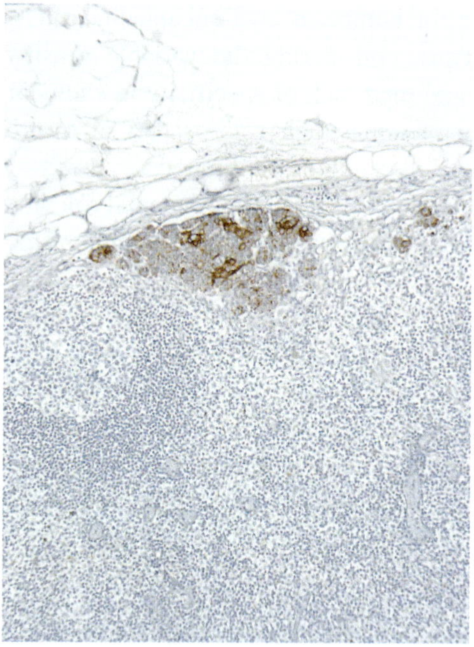

Figure 13. Sentinel lymph node demonstrating subcapsular cluster of cells positive for AE1/AE3 cytokeratin (100×).

staining pattern than CK20, which may not stain 100% of tumor cells in small deposits of micrometastatic disease. Patterns of metastatic disease in lymph nodes range from the presence of scattered individual tumor cells to small clusters (Figures 13 and 14) to large sheets. In the former, it is often difficult to identify the tumor cells, even retrospectively, on H&E stains. However, due to the specificity of the immunostaining pattern it is possible to render a diagnosis of metastatic disease on the basis of the immunostains alone. The significance of this micrometastatic disease in the sentinel node is not totally clear, and its implications for further treatment such as complete nodal dissection remain to be fully defined.

5.5 Ultrastructural Findings

Normal Merkel cells possess many of the ultrastructural features of Merkel cell carcinoma. In human skin, Merkel cells are present in the

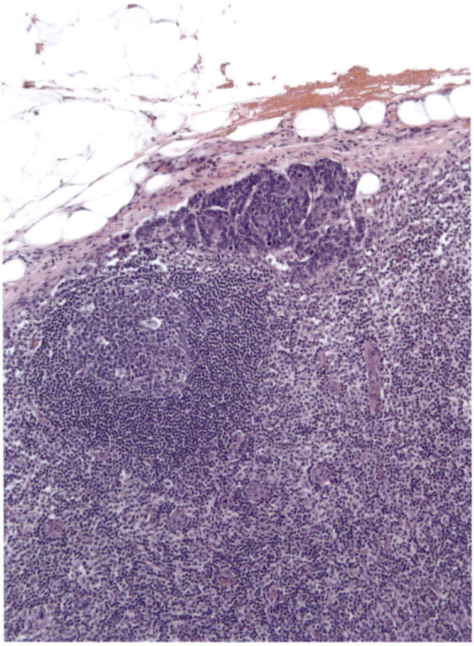

Figure 14. Same cluster of cells from Figure 13. Note similarity of the metastases to normal lymph node (H&E, 100×).

basal layer of the epidermis. They are also found in hair follicles and in oral mucosa. Except in birds, where they are located in the dermis, Merkel cells in all other vertebrates are located in the epidermis.[55] In the epidermis, Merkel cells can be distinguished from other 'clear cells' such as melanocytes or Langerhan cells by electron microscopy, where these cells are oval in shape and measure 10–15 μm in the long axis. They may be present in clusters in the basal layer of the epidermis, in close contact with nerve terminals. Merkel cells possess spike-like protrusions, and they interdigitate with the surrounding keratinocytes.[7] The desmosomes are much smaller than those between neighboring keratinocytes.[55] The nuclei of Merkel cells are large and lobulated. The cytoplasm contains neurofilaments, intermediate cytokeratin filaments, and many large (50–110 nm) dense-core vesicles accumulated near the junction with the nerve fiber.[7]

Although electron microscopy rarely plays a role in the diagnosis of Merkel cell carcinoma today because of the routine use of reliable immunohistochemical stains, it was instrumental in first defining the origin of this tumor and distinguishing it from tumors in the histologic differential diagnosis.[1] Ultrastructurally, all Merkel cell carcinomas are characterized by the presence intercellular junctions. The tumor cells contain ball-like collections of intermediate filaments adjacent to the nucleus, which are the genesis of the characteristic dot-like positivity for various keratins seen on immunohistochemical stains. The cells also contain numerous cytoplasmic dense-core membrane-bound secretory granules and rigid, cytoplasmic spinous processes.[55] These processes or 'spikes' are thought to represent the only ultrastructural characteristic absolutely diagnostic of Merkel cell carcinoma, since the foregoing may also be found in other neuroendocrine tumors.[56] The three histologic subtypes of Merkel cell carcinoma do demonstrate some differences in their electron microscopic findings; the trabecular type possesses numerous desmosomes, neurosecretory granules and perinuclear filaments, while the intermediate type is poor in desmosomes and granules but often contains numerous filaments. The small type also shows poorly formed junctions and rare neurosecretory granules, but the spike-like cytoplasmic dendritic projections may be prominent.[55]

5.6 Cytopathology

Fine needle aspiration cytology can be quite helpful in the initial diagnostic workup of a patient with suspected Merkel cell carcinoma. It is particularly useful in the staging and follow-up of patients with a known diagnosis of Merkel cell carcinoma. In general, the findings are those of a poorly differentiated carcinoma and often overlap with those of other neuroendocrine tumors as well as malignant lymphoma, similar to the light microscopic findings. Typically, aspirates are highly cellular and reveal loosely clustered or dissociated single cells. Tumor cells possess monomorphic, round to oval, regularly contoured nuclei, scant cytoplasm, and fine chromatin with multiple small, inconspicuous nucleoli.[57,58] Occasionally, unusual findings include a spectrum of pleomorphism ranging from moderately complex nuclear membranes with cleaves, indentations and protrusions to large, markedly bizarre, convoluted nuclei and multinucleate tumor cells.[59] Nuclear molding and rosettes are infrequent findings.[58] In one report of two cases studied with three aspirates, hematoxylin and eosin staining of alcohol-fixed smears revealed that some of the tumor cells possessed 'intermediate filament buttons.' These were described as homogeneous, pale pink, well-circumscribed round or oval buttons of cytoplasm present in a perinuclear location, seen in both intact cells as well as loose in the aspirate smears.[60] Due to the frequency of other tumors being associated with Merkel cell carcinoma, especially squamous cell carcinoma, aspirates should be examined carefully with this possibility in mind.[58] Immunohistochemical confirmation remains the gold standard for diagnosis, and may be performed on cell block material if the specimen is adequately cellular.

5.7 Flow Cytometry

While flow cytometry is not used as part of the routine workup for Merkel cell carcinoma, it is occasionally performed on these tumors when the working diagnosis includes malignant lymphoma. Neuroendocrine tumors such as Merkel cell carcinoma have a distinct flow cytometric pattern; the finding of CD56 expression in the presence of negative immunostaining with other lymphoid markers.[61] A potential pitfall of flow cytometry is the rare finding of TdT immunoreactivity in Merkel cell carcinoma. This marker stains lymphoblastic lymphoma, which may lack CD45 or CD20. Buresh *et al.* analyzed 26 tumors and identified TdT in 19/26 (73%) of Merkel cell carcinomas. The staining intensity was variable but was often moderate to strong and present in a significant percentage of cells.[62]

5.8 Conclusion

Great advances have been made in the pathologic diagnosis of Merkel cell carcinoma, enabling better understanding of the origin of this tumor. Electron microscopy, while no longer in routine use diagnostically, was instrumental in elucidating the possible origin of this tumor. Immunohistochemical staining has become essential in both the initial diagnosis of a tumor suspected to represent Merkel cell carcinoma, as well as evaluation of subsequent surgical material, especially nodal specimens. It has also revealed divergent differentiation that continues to fuel the debate concerning the histogenesis of Merkel cell carcinoma. Further studies examining the relationship of pathologic features, such as tumor size and depth, immunologic response and growth pattern, may contribute to prediction of prognosis in this rare but deadly tumor.

References

1. Toker C. (1972). Trabecular carcinoma of the skin. *Arch Dermatol* 105: 107–110.
2. Haag M.L., Glass L., Fenske N.A. (1995). Merkel cell carcinoma. Diagnosis and treatment. *Dermatol Surg* 21: 669–683.
3. Tang C.K., Toker C. (1978). Trabecular carcinoma of the skin: an ultrastructural study. *Cancer* 42: 2311–2321.
4. De Wolf-Peeters C. Marien K., Mebis J., *et al.* (1980). A cutaneous APUDoma or Merkel cell tumor? A morphologically recognizable tumor with a biological and histological malignant aspect in contrast with its clinical behavior. *Cancer* 46: 1810–1816.
5. Winkelmann R. (1977). The Merkel cell system and a comparison between it and the neurosecretory or APUD cell system. *J Invest Dermatol* 69: 41–46.
6. Merkel F. (1875). Tastzellen and Tastkoerperchen bei den Hausthieren und beim Menschen. *Arch Mikrosc Anat* 11: 636–652.
7. Halata Z., Grim M., Bauman K. (2003). Friedrich Sigmund Merkel and his "Merkel Cell", morphology, development, and physiology: review and new results. *Anat Rec A Discov Mol Cell Evol Biol* 71: 225–239.
8. Warner T., Uno H., Hafez G., *et al.* (1983). Merkel cells and Merkel cell tumors. Ultrastructure, immunocytochemistry and review of the literature. *Cancer* 51: 238–245.
9. Hoefler H., Kerl H., Rauch H.J., Denk H. (1984). New immunocytochemical observations with diagnostic significance in cutaneous neuroendocrine carcinoma. *Am J Dermatopathol* 6: 525–530.
10. Pectasides D., Pectasides M., Economopoulos T. (2006). Merkel cell cancer of the skin. *Ann Oncol* 17: 1489–1495.

11. Plaza J.A., Suster S. (2006). The Toker tumor: spectrum of morphologic features in primary neuroendocrine carcinomas of the skin (Merkel cell carcinoma). *Ann Diagn Pathol* 10: 376–385.
12. Pilotti S., Rilke F., Lombardi L. (1982). Neuroendocrine (Merkel cell) carcinoma of the skin. *Am J Surg Pathol* 6: 243–254.
13. Al-Ahmadie H.A., Mutasim D.F., Mutema G.K. (2004). A case of intraepidermal Merkel cell carcinoma within squamous cell carcinoma in-situ: Merkel cell carcinoma in-situ? *Am J Dermatopathol* 26: 230–233.
14. Ferringer T., Rogers H.C., Metcalf J.S. (2005). Merkel cell carcinoma in situ. *J Cutan Pathol* 32: 162–165.
15. Vazmitel M., Michal M., Kazakov D.V. (2007). Merkel cell carcinoma and Azzopardi phenomenon. *Am J Dermatopathol* 29: 314–315.
16. Vazmitel, M., Michal M., Shelekova K.V., *et al.* (2008). Vascular changes in Merkel cell carcinoma based on a histopathological study of 92 cases. *Am J Dermatopathol* 30: 106–111.
17. Ball N.J., Tanhuanco-Kho G. (2007). Merkel cell carcinoma frequently shows histologic features of basal cell carcinoma: a study of 30 cases. *J Cutan Pathol* 34: 612–619.
18. Hashimoto K., Lee M.W., D'Annunzio D.R., *et al.* (1998). Pagetoid Merkel cell carcinoma: epidermal origin of the tumor. *J Cutan Pathol* 25: 572–579.
19. Connelly T., Cribier B., Brown T.J., Yanguas I. (2000). Complete spontaneous regression of Merkel cell carcinoma: a review of the 10 reported cases. *Dermatol Surg* 26: 853–856.
20. Sais G., Admella C., Soler T. (2002). Spontaneous regression in primary cutaneous neuroendocrine (Merkel cell) carcinoma: a rare immune phenomenon? *J Eur Acad Dermatol Venereol* 16: 81–94.
21. Poulsen M. (2004). Merkel-cell carcinoma of the skin. *Lancet Oncol* 5: 593–599.
22. Vesely M.J., Murray D.J., Neligan P.C., *et al.* (2008). Complete spontaneous regression in Merkel cell carcinoma. *J Plast Reconstr Aesthet Surg* 61: 165–171.
23. Burack J., Altschuler E. (2003). Sustained remission of metastatic Merkel cell carcinoma with treatment of HIV infection. *J R Soc Med* 96: 238–239.

24. Muirhead R., Ritchie D. (2007). Partial regression of Merkel cell carcinoma in response to withdrawal of azathioprine in an immunosuppression-induced case of metastatic Merkel cell carcinoma. *Clin Oncol R Coll Radiol* 19: 96.
25. Friedlaender M.M., Rubinger D., Rosenbaum A.E., *et al.* (2002). Temporary regression of Merkel cell carcinoma metastases after cessation of cyclosporine. *Transplantation* 73: 1849–1850.
26. Smith K.J., Skelton H.G., Holland T.T., *et al.* (1993). Neuroendocrine (Merkel cell) carcinoma with an intraepidermal component. *Am J Dermatopathol* 15: 528–533.
27. Rocamora A., Badía N., Vives R., *et al.* (1987). Epidermotropic primary neuroendocrine (Merkel cell) carcinoma of the skin with Pautrier-like microabscesses. *J Am Acad Dermatol* 16: 1163–1168.
28. Skelton H., Smith K.J., Hitchcock C.L. *et al.* (1997). Merkel cell carcinoma: analysis of clinical, histologic and immunohistologic features of 132 cases with relation to survival. *J Am Acad Dermatol* 37: 734–739.
29. Gilman S., Morrison R., Hurt M. (1991). Epidermotropic neuroendocrine carcinoma. Immunohistochemical differentiation from simulators, including malignant melanoma. *J Cutan Pathol* 18: 120–127.
30. Brown H.A., Sawyer D.M., Woo T. (2000). Intraepidermal Merkel cell carcinoma with no dermal involvement. *Am J Dermatopathol* 22: 65–69.
31. Walsh N. (2000) Primary neuroendocrine (Merkel cell) carcinoma of the skin: morphologic diversity and implications thereof. *Hum Pathol* 32: 680.
32. Gomez L., Silva E., DiMaio S., *et al.* (1983). Association between neuroendocrine (Merkel cell) carcinoma and squamous carcinoma of the skin. *Am J Surg Pathol* 7: 171–177.
33. Hwang J.H., Alanen K., Dabbs J.D., *et al.* (2008). Merkel cell carcinoma with squamous and sarcomatous differentiation. *J Cutan Pathol* 35: 955–959.
34. Isimbaldi G., Sironi M., Taccagni G., *et al.* (1993). Tripartite differentiation (squamous, glandular and melanocytic) of a primary cutaneous neuroendocrine carcinoma. *Am J Dermatopathol* 15: 260–264.
35. Scurry J., Brand A., Planner R., *et al.* (1996). Vulvar Merkel cell tumor with glandular and squamous differentiation. *Gynecol Oncol* 62: 292–297.
36. Gould E., Albores-Saavedra J., Dubner B, *et al.* (1998). Eccrine and squamous differentiation in Merkel cell carcinoma: an immunohistochemical study. *Am J Surg Pathol* 12: 768–772.

37. Silva E.G., Mackay B., Goepfert H., *et al.* (1984). Endocrine carcinoma of the skin (Merkel cell carcinoma). *Pathol Annu* 19: 1–30.
38. Fernandez-Figueras M.T., Puig L., Gilaberte M., *et al.* (2002). Merkel cell (primary neuroendocrine) carcinoma of the skin with nodal metastasis showing rhabdomyosarcomatous differentiation. *J Cutan Pathol* 29: 619–622.
39. Boutilier R., Desormeau L., Cragg F., *et al.* (2001). Merkel cell carcinoma: squamous and atypical fibroxanthoma-like differentiation in successive local tumor recurrences. *Am J Dermatopathol* 23: 46–49.
40. Youker S., Billingsley E. (1986). Combined Merkel cell carcinoma and atypical fibroxanthoma. *J Cutan Med Surg* 9: 6–9.
41. Cooper L., Debono R., Alsanjari N., Al-Nafussi A. (2000). Merkel cell tumour with leiomyosarcomatous differentiation. *Histopathology* 36: 540–543.
42. Tan K.B., Murali R., Karim R.Z., *et al.* (2008). Merkel cell carcinoma with fibrosarcomatous differentiation. *Pathology* 40: 314–316.
43. Johansson L., Tennvall J., Akerman M. (1990). Immunohistochemical examination of 25 cases of Merkel cell carcinoma: a comparison with small cell carcinoma of the lung and oesophagus, and a review of the literature. *APMIS* 98: 741–752.
44. Moll I., Löwe A., Laufer J., Franke W.W. (1992). Cytokeratin 20 in human carcinomas. A new histodiagnostic marker detected by monoclonal antibodies. *Am J Pathol* 140: 427–447.
45. Bobos M., Hytiroglou P., Kostopoulos I., *et al.* (2006). Immunohistochemical distinction between Merkel cell carcinoma and small cell carcinoma of the lung. *Am J Dermatopathol* 28: 99–104.
46. Hanly A., Elgart G., Jorda M., *et al.* (2000). Analysis of thyroid transcription factor-1 and cytokeratin 20 separates Merkel cell carcinoma from small cell carcinoma of lung. *J Cutan Pathol* 27: 118–120.
47. Wang N., Zee S., Zarbo R., *et al.* (1995). Coordinate expression of cytokeratins 7 and 20 defines unique subsets of carcinomas. *Appl Immunohistochem* 3: 99–107.
48. Visscher D., Cooper P.H., Zarbo R.J., Crissman J.D. (1989). Cutaneous neuroendocrine (Merkel cell) carcinoma: an immunophenotypic, clinicopathologic, and flow cytometric study. *Mod Pathol* 2: 331–338.
49. Layfield L., Ulich T., Liao S., *et al.* (1986). Neuroendocrine carcinoma of the skin: an immunohistochemical study of tumor markers and neuroendocrine products. *J Cutan Pathol* 13: 268–273.

50. Kurokawa M., Nabeshima K., Akiyama Y., *et al.* (2003). CD56: a useful marker for diagnosing Merkel cell carcinoma. *J Dermatol Sci* 31: 219–224.
51. McNiff J.M., Cowper S.E., Lazova R., *et al.* (2005). CD56 staining in Merkel cell carcinoma and natural killer-cell lymphoma: magic bullet, diagnostic pitfall, or both? *J Cutan Pathol* 32: 541–545.
52. Blom A., Kolb F., Lumbroso J., *et al.* (2003). Significance of sentinel lymph node biopsy in Merkel cell carcinoma. Analysis of 11 cases. *Ann Dermatol Venereol* 130: 417–422.
53. Allen P.J., Busam K., Hill A.D., *et al.* (2001). Immunohistochemical analysis of sentinel lymph nodes from patients with Merkel cell carcinoma. *Cancer* 92: 1650–1655.
54. Su L.D., Lowe L., Bradford C.R., *et al.* (2002). Immunostaining for cytokeratin 20 improves detection of micrometastatic Merkel cell carcinoma in sentinel lymph nodes. *J Am Acad Dermatol* 46: 661–666.
55. Sidhu G.S., Chandra P., Cassai N.D. (2005). Merkel cells, normal and neoplastic: an update. *Ultrastruct Pathol* 29: 287–294.
56. Sidhu G.S., Feiner H., Flotte T.J., *et al.* (1980). Merkel cell neoplasms. Histology, electron microscopy, biology, and histogenesis. *Am J Dermatopathol* 2: 101–119.
57. Dey P., Jogai S., Amir T., Temim L. (2004). Fine-needle aspiration cytology of Merkel cell carcinoma. *Diagn Cytopathol* 31: 364–365.
58. Collins B.T., Elmberger P.G., Tani E.M., *et al.* (1998). Fine-needle aspiration of Merkel cell carcinoma of the skin with cytomorphology and immunocytochemical correlation. *Diagn Cytopathol* 18: 251–257.
59. Hallman J.R., Shaw J.A., Geisinger K.R., *et al.* (2000). Cytomorphologic features of Merkel cell carcinoma in fine needle aspiration biopsies. A study of two atypical cases. *Acta Cytol* 44: 185–193.
60. Domagala W., Weber K., Osborn M. (1987). Neuroendocrine (Merkel-cell) carcinoma of the skin. Cytology, intermediate filament typing and ultrastructure of tumor cells in fine needle aspirates. *Acta Cytol* 31: 267–275.
61. Farinola M.A., Weir E.G., Ali S.Z. (2003). CD56 expression of neuroendocrine neoplasms on immunophenotyping by flow cytometry: a novel diagnostic approach to fine-needle aspiration biopsy. *Cancer* 99: 240–246.
62. Buresh C.J., Oliai B.R., Miller R.T. (2008). Reactivity with TdT in Merkel cell carcinoma: a potential diagnostic pitfall. *Am J Clin Pathol* 129: 894–898.

Chapter 6

Clinical Recognition and Diagnosis of Merkel Cell Carcinoma

Mary H. Lien, L. Frank Glass and Neil Alan Fenske

This chapter discusses the clinical characteristics of Merkel cell carcinoma in order to serve as a reference tool for clinicians in determining when a biopsy may be warranted. Merkel cell carcinoma is a challenging tumor to diagnose because it frequently mimics a number of benign dermatologic tumors.[1] Its characteristic asymptomatic nature, coupled with its usual pattern of rapid growth and frequent presentation with regional or distant metastases, partly explains its high mortality rate. Therefore, high clinical suspicion and early detection of this neoplasm may lead to a better prognosis and an improved outcome.

6.1 Clinical Features

The clinical diagnosis of Merkel cell carcinoma is difficult secondary to both the long list of differential diagnoses that clinically mimic Merkel cell carcinoma as well as the fact that the incidence of Merkel cell carcinoma is very low. Primary Merkel cell carcinoma usually presents as a rapidly growing, red or purple cutaneous or subcutaneous lesion.[2–4] In one recent series, the most frequent presenting color was reddish-pink (56%, Figure 1), followed by a bluish or violaceous hue (26%, Figure 2) and then flesh-colored (16%).[2]

The surface of Merkel cell carcinoma tumors tend to be shiny, often with overlying telangectiasias, and the epidermis may be intact or ulcerated

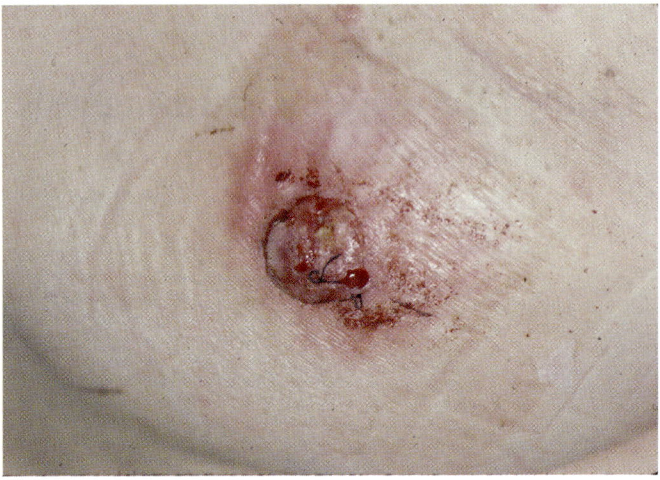

Figure 1. Typical reddish-pink primary Merkel cell tumor with surrounding erythema. Sutures are present in an incisional biopsy site.

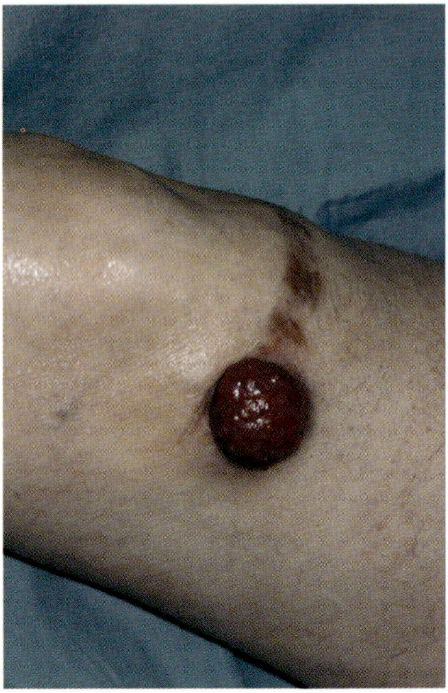

Figure 2. Violaceous Merkel cell carcinoma on the lower extremity.

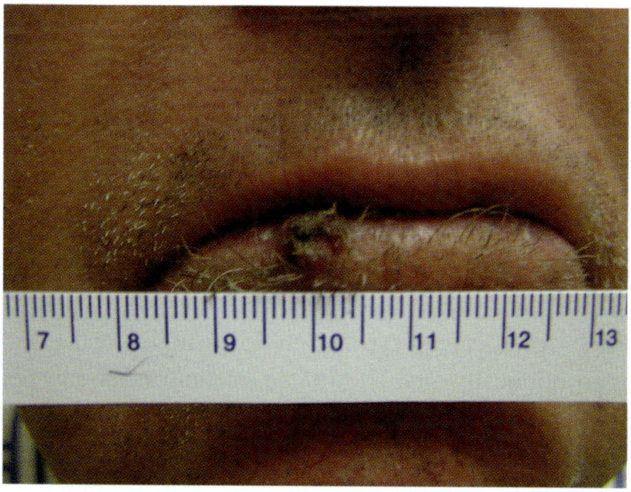

(A)

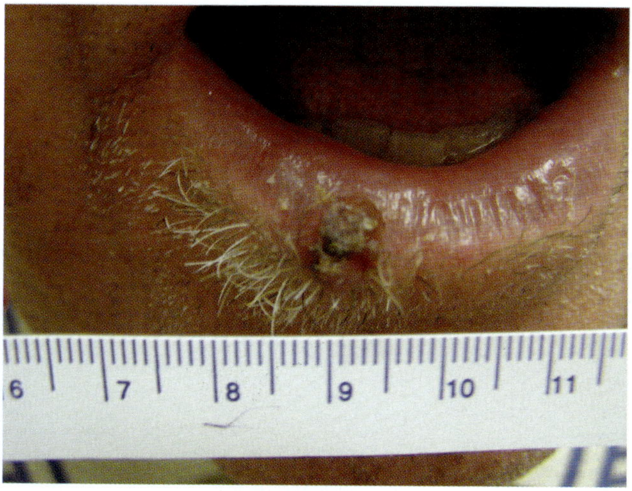

(B)

Figure 3. Ulcerated primary Merkel cell carcinoma on the lower lip.

(Figure 3).[2,3] Most primary Merkel cell carcinomas present as solitary tumors, but there have been rare reports of multiple primary Merkel cell tumors; in-transit and/or satellite lesions and regional or distant metastases in the absence of a known primary tumor have also been seen as presenting complaints in Merkel cell carcinoma patients.[3]

6.2 Anatomic Distribution

Most frequently, Merkel cell carcinoma presents on the head and neck (Figures 3–5) or extremities.[2–6] A literature review of 1024 patients demonstrated that 40.6% of tumors arose on the head and neck, followed by the extremities (33%), trunk (23%) and unknown sites (3.4%).[5] A recent study comprising 195 patients reported the head and neck to be the site of origin of 29% of cases, with 45% on the extremities (lower extremity 24%, upper extremity (21%), and relatively few on the trunk (8%), buttock (5%) or vulva (0.5%).[2] Allen *et al.* reported on 251 patients and also found the extremities to be the favored site (38%), leading head and neck (29%), buttocks (14%), trunk (7%) and unknown sites (12%).[7] Merkel cell carcinoma has been reported to involve the regional nodes without a known primary site in up to 14% of cases (unknown primary tumor).[2] There are additional publications reporting varying percentages of head and neck involvement, ranging from 41% (England) to 70% (Texas) and even up to 84% in one study from Canada.[8–10] Such differences have been postulated to result from varying sun exposures and climates due to differing geographic locations,[4] but may also reflect referral bias.

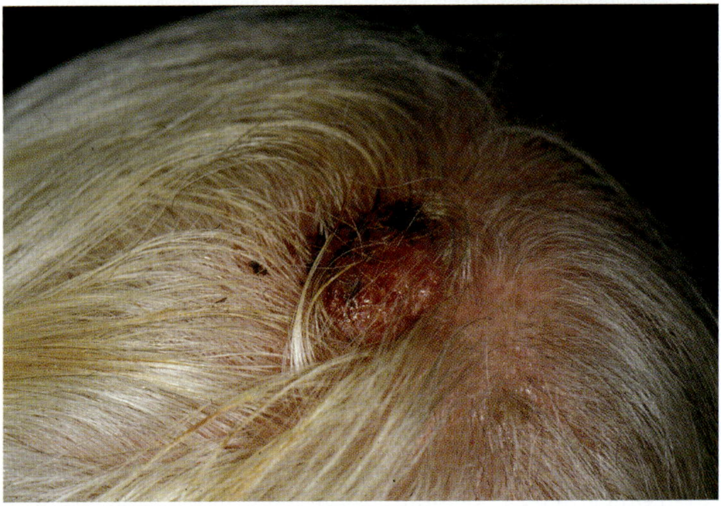

Figure 4. Primary Merkel cell carcinoma on the scalp.

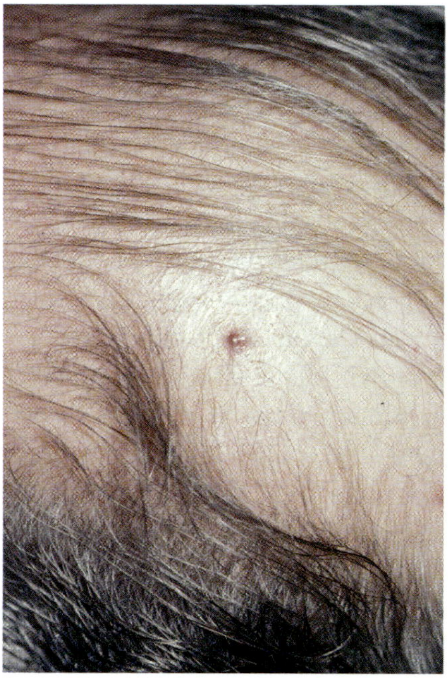

Figure 5. Small primary Merkel cell carcinoma on the sun-exposed scalp.

6.3 'AEIOU' Acronym for Merkel Cell Carcinoma

Based on previously published observations regarding the anatomic distribution, clinical presentation, and the predilection of Merkel cell carcinoma for certain patient populations, an acronym was recently proposed by Heath *et al.* to incorporate the five most common clinical features of Merkel cell carcinoma: **AEIOU**, which stands for **A**symptomatic/lack of tenderness, **E**xpanding rapidly (<3 months), **I**mmunosuppression, **O**lder than 50 years, and location on an **U**ltraviolet-exposed site.[2]

The first criteria, specifically defined as '*asymptomatic/lack of tenderness*,' is an important guiding feature. Numerous studies have remarked on the typical painless presentation of primary Merkel cell carcinoma.[3,4,6] In a recent study involving 89 patients, the majority (88%) of the primary Merkel cell carcinoma lesions were asymptomatic.[2]

Indeed, it is this observed absence of tenderness or pain which may alert the clinician that further evaluation may be warranted. For example, an inflamed cyst — one of the most common differential diagnoses of a rapidly enlarging erythematous/pink nodule — would likely be painful, therefore differentiating it from the typical presentation of a much less frequent primary Merkel cell carcinoma.

The second feature, '*rapid expansion*,' would also help to distinguish this cancer from most lesions sharing similar nondescript features. In one study of 91 patients with Merkel cell carcinoma, 63% were noted to experience rapid growth of their tumor within three months of the diagnosis.[2] The diameter of the primary tumor at presentation was less than 1 cm in 21%, 1–2 cm in 43%, and greater than 2 cm in 35%.[2] Other studies reported mean tumor sizes of 2 cm (661 patients; range 0.3–15 cm); 2.7 cm (16 patients; range 0.7–7.3 cm); and 1.3 cm (251 patients; range 0.2–14 cm).[4,5,7] Few series actually document the pre-diagnosis growth rate of primary Merkel cell tumors, however, and this is a subjective assessment in almost all cases.

The third clinical characteristic, '*immunosuppression*,' is a significant risk factor for Merkel cell carcinoma. In the US population with Merkel cell carcinoma, the most common causes of immunosuppression are HIV, followed by chronic lymphocytic leukemia (CLL) and solid organ transplantation.[11,12] In fact, Friedlaender *et al.* reported on a patient status post two living-donor kidney transplants on post-transplant immunosuppression therapy who had regression of his distant and symptomatic bony Merkel cell metastases after his cyclosporine therapy was discontinued and his immune system was allowed to recover.[13] There are some reports that suggest that Merkel cell carcinoma develops in immunosuppressed patients at a younger age (mean age of 53 years at diagnosis) compared to non-immunocompromised subjects.[14] In this study, the authors found that 5% of Merkel cell carcinomas in the non-immunosuppressed population presented before 50 years of age, whereas 29% of the Merkel cell carcinomas in the immunocompromised population presented before 50 years of age.[14] However, a more contemporary publication showed that the mean age of presentation of immunocompromised patients was comparable to that of immunocompetent patients (65 years versus 67 years, respectively).[2]

The fourth criteria, '*older than 50 years*,' stemmed from the demographics of the study population, which mirrored those of other published series. Merkel cell carcinoma predominantly affects the elderly caucasian male population (incidence rate per 100,000 of 0.23 for caucasians and 0.01 for blacks).[7] Previous reviews have reported the median age of patients diagnosed with Merkel cell carcinoma to range from 68–70 years.[2,4,15,16] A literature review of 1024 patients demonstrated a mean patient age of 69 years (range 18–98).[5] The study by Heath *et al.* listed the median age of patients developing Merkel cell carcinoma to be 69 years (range 34–97).[2]

Previous studies suggested that males were affected much more frequently than females. Incidence rates of 0.65 and 0.26 cases per 100,000 person-years, respectively were reported in a large study from 2001 ($n = 1124$, $p = 0.05$).[17] In another study, the percentage of affected males (60%) exceeded that of females (40%).[7] Moreover, recently published data involving 62 patients corroborated that males were affected more frequently than females with a ratio of 58.5% male to 41.5% female.[2]

Another risk factor for developing Merkel cell carcinoma is the fifth criterion, '*ultraviolet light exposure*,' as demonstrated by the increased prevalence of these tumors in sun-exposed body regions. Utilizing SEER registry data, Agelli and Clegg demonstrated a link between geographic UVB radiation indices and the age-adjusted incidence of Merkel cell carcinoma in Caucasian patients.[18] Furthermore, Lunder and Stern reported a 100-fold increase in the incidence of Merkel cell carcinoma in psoriatic patients treated with psoralen and UVA (PUVA) irradiation therapy.[19] However, as demonstrated by Heath *et al.*, although 81% of the Merkel cell carcinomas had developed on sun-exposed skin, the disease can still arise in the absence of significant sun exposure.

In the Heath *et al.* publication, after analyzing the incidence of all five variables in a population of 62 Merkel cell carcinoma patients, it was shown that 89% of patients met three or more of the clinical criteria, 52% met four or more criteria, and 7% met all five criteria.[2] The authors concluded that these criteria may be useful in providing a systematic algorithm to guide clinicians in recognizing Merkel cell carcinoma. On the other hand, it is clear that the overwhelming majority of Merkel cell carcinomas do not manifest all five AEIOU criteria, while an exceedingly large number of benign lesions will manifest some or most of these same criteria. Thus, while this and other mnemonics may help keep the possibility of Merkel cell carcinoma in mind, at present there are no criteria that can be considered to definitively establish the diagnosis of this disease.

6.4 Differential Diagnoses

Generally, Merkel cell carcinoma is not initially considered in the differential diagnoses of a skin lesion. Due to its nondescript appearance, there are multiple other lesions in the differential diagnosis for Merkel cell carcinoma (Table 1). In the Heath *et al.* study, the majority (56%) of the 106 patients were initially diagnosed as benign growths. In fact, a correct presumptive diagnosis of Merkel cell carcinoma was made in only two cases in their

Table 1. Common differential diagnoses of Merkel cell carcinoma.

Benign tumors
Epidermoid cyst
Acneiform lesion
Lipoma
Dermatofibroma/fibroma
Vascular lesion
Malignant tumors
Amelanotic melanoma
Non-melanoma skin carcinomas (basal cell carcinomas, squamous cell carcinomas)
Lymphoma
Metastatic carcinoma
Sarcoma
Miscellaneous cutaneous lesions
Adnexal tumors
Pyogenic granuloma
Carcinoid
Retinoblastoma
Neuroblastoma
Leukemia cutis
Pilomatrixoma

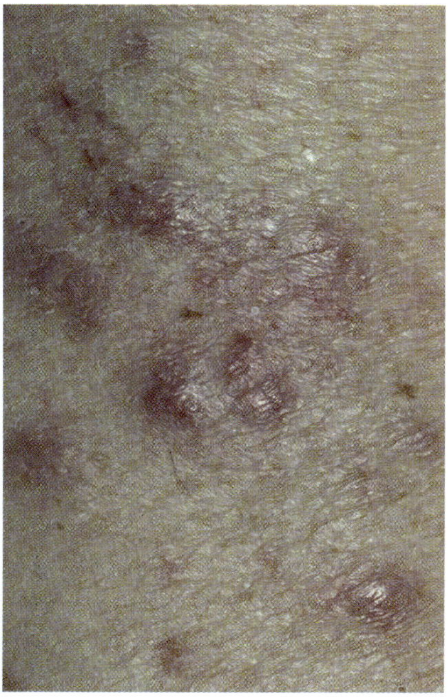

Figure 6. Acneiform presentation of multifocal Merkel cell carcinoma on the lower extremity.

series,[2] and in most series in no patient! Topping the presumptive diagnosis list was cyst/acneiform lesion (32%) (see Figure 6), followed by lipoma (6%), dermatofibroma or fibroma (4%) and vascular lesions (4%).[2,3,6] The remainder (36%) of the differential diagnoses constituted malignant neoplasms, of which non-melanoma skin carcinoma was the most common (19%), followed by lymphoma (6%), metastatic carcinoma (2%) and sarcoma (2%).[2–4,6] Other cutaneous tumors which may be clinically mistaken for Merkel cell carcinoma include: melanoma, adnexal tumors, basal cell carcinoma, squamous cell carcinoma, pyogenic granuloma, carcinoid, retinoblastoma, neuroblastoma, pilomatrixoma and leukemia cutis.[2–4,6]

6.5 Diagnostic Workup

Since Merkel cell carcinoma may often be misdiagnosed due to its nonspecific clinical presentation, the AEIOU acronym can be utilized to assist clinicians in recognizing the features of Merkel cell carcinoma, and to determine when a biopsy is warranted. Typically, an excisional, punch or deep shave biopsy is used to obtain tissue for histopathologic examination. Biopsies, especially if they are excisional, should be oriented in line with the axis of the extremity or with Langer's lines of skin tension, so that if the diagnosis of Merkel cell carcinoma is correct and the patient is referred for wide excision the re-excision will be easier to perform and less likely to require a skin graft for closure. Once the biopsy is performed, the tissue specimen should be placed in formalin and prepared for standard hematoxylin and eosin staining as well as special immunohistochemical staining. The details of the pathologic analysis of Merkel cell carcinoma are presented in Chapter 5.

6.6 Summary

In conclusion, Merkel cell carcinoma is a rare cutaneous neoplasm that presents with varied clinical features that may confound its diagnosis. Its nondescript appearance and similarity to many benign cutaneous tumors frequently delay its correct diagnosis. Early diagnosis may achieve a better prognosis for this rare but devastating neoplasm, but improved criteria for the recognition of this tumor are clearly needed.

References

1. Toker C. (1972). Trabecular carcinoma of the skin. *Arch Dermatol* 105: 107–110.
2. Heath M., Jaimes N., Lemos B., *et al.* (2008). Clinical characteristics of Merkel cell carcinoma at diagnosis in 195 patients: the AEIOU features. *J Am Acad Dermatol* 58: 375–381.
3. Ratner D., Nelson B.R., Brown M.D., Johnson T.M. (1993). Merkel cell carcinoma. *J Am Acad Dermatol* 29(Pt1): 143–156.
4. Tai P.T., Yu E., Tonita J., Gilchrist J. (2000). Merkel cell carcinoma of the skin. *J Cutan Med Surg* 4: 186–195.
5. Medina-Franco H., Urist M.M., Fiveash J., *et al.* (2001). Multimodality treatment of Merkel cell carcinoma: case series and literature review of 1024 cases. *Ann Surg Oncol* 8: 204–208.

6. Bichakjian C.K., Lowe L., Lao C.D., *et al.* (2007). Merkel cell carcinoma: critical review with guidelines for multidisciplinary management. *Cancer* 110: 1–12.
7. Allen P.J., Bowne W.B., Jaques D.P., *et al.* (2005). Merkel cell carcinoma: prognosis and treatment of patients from a single institution. *J Clin Oncol* 23: 2300–2309.
8. Savage P., Constenia D., Fisher C., *et al.* (1997). The natural history and management of Merkel cell carcinoma of the skin: a review of 22 patients treated at the Royal Marsden Hospital. *Clin Oncol (R Coll Radiol)* 9: 164–167.
9. Morrison W.H., Peters L.J., Silva E.G., *et al.* (1990). The essential role of radiation therapy in securing locoregional control of Merkel cell carcinoma. *Int J Radiat Oncol Biol Phys* 19: 583–591.
10. Tai P.T., Yu E., Winquist E., *et al.* (2000). Chemotherapy in neuroendocrine/ Merkel cell carcinoma of the skin: case series and review of 204 cases. *J Clin Oncol* 18: 2493–2499.
11. Miller R.W., Rabkin C.S. (1999). Merkel cell carcinoma and melanoma: etiological similarities and differences. *Cancer Epidemiol Biomarkers Prev* 8: 153–158.
12. Engels E.A., Frisch M., Goedert J.J., *et al.* (2002). Merkel cell carcinoma and HIV infection. *Lancet* 359: 497–498.
13. Friedlaender M.M., Rubinger D., Rosenbaum E., *et al.* (2002). Temporary regression of Merkel cell carcinoma metastases after cessation of cyclosporine. *Transplantation* 73: 1849–1850.
14. Penn I., First M.R. (1999). Merkel's cell carcinoma in organ recipients: report of 41 cases. *Transplantation* 68: 1717–1721.
15. Shaw J.H., Rumball E. (1991). Merkel cell tumour: clinical behaviour and treatment. *Br J Surg* 78: 138–142.
16. Hitchcock C.L., Bland K.I., Laney R.G. 3rd, *et al.* (2008). Neuroendocrine (Merkel cell) carcinoma of the skin. Its natural history, diagnosis, and treatment. *Ann Surg* 207: 201–207.
17. Hodgson N.C. (2005). Merkel cell carcinoma: changing incidence trends. *J Surg Oncol* 89: 1–4.
18. Agelli M., Clegg L.X. (2003). Epidemiology of primary Merkel cell carcinoma in the United States. *J Am Acad Dermatol* 49: 832–841.
19. Lunder E.J., Stern R.S. (1998). Merkel-cell carcinomas in patients treated with methoxsalen and ultraviolet A radiation. *N Engl J Med* 339: 1247–1248.

Chapter 7

Current Staging Systems for Merkel Cell Carcinoma

Bianca D. Lemos and Paul Nghiem

Because of its increasing incidence and high mortality rate, Merkel cell carcinoma has recently been recognized as deserving of attention and a staging system distinct from melanoma and other non-melanoma skin cancers. Until recently, the American Joint Committee on Cancer (AJCC), the official staging entity in the United States, did not have a specific staging system for Merkel cell carcinoma but rather included it with 82 other non-melanoma skin cancers in a single generic skin cancer staging model. There are five existing staging systems for Merkel cell carcinoma at the current time (Table 1). All five of these staging systems are published and in use in the literature, but none have been independently validated. This situation leads to confusion among patients, medical providers and researchers. Thus, there is a need for a consensus staging system for Merkel cell carcinoma to improve communication and care of patients. There is now significant data to suggest that microscopic nodal evaluation is very important in predicting outcome among patients who present with clinically negative nodes because clinical exam falsely under-stages one-third of such patients as they actually have microscopic nodal disease. Microscopic versus clinical nodal staging has been incorporated into the new consensus staging system for Merkel cell carcinoma in the most recent version (7th edition) of the AJCC *Cancer Staging Manual* as discussed below.

Table 1. Summary of five published staging systems for Merkel cell carcinoma.[2–6]

Year (Author)	Stage I	Stage II	Stage III	Stage IV
1991 (Yiengpruksawan, *et al.*)	• Local	• Nodal	• Metastatic	—
1999 (Allen, *et al.*)	• IA: Local <2cm • IB: Local ≥2cm	• Nodal	• Metastatic	—
2002 (AJCC, 6th edition)	• Local ≤2cm	• Local >2cm	• Local extradermal deep invasion • Nodal	• Metastatic
2005 (Allen, *et al.*)	• Local <2cm	• Local ≥2cm	• Nodal	• Metastatic
2007 (Clark, *et al.*)	• Local ≤1cm	• IIA: Local ≤1cm and 1–2 positive regional lymph nodes • IIB: Local ≥2cm	• >2 positive lymph nodes	• Metastatic

7.1 Existing Staging Systems for Merkel Cell Carcinoma

Like many cancers, staging is exceedingly important in Merkel cell carcinoma because there is a significant survival difference based on extent of disease at presentation. Survival can be as high as 90% for local disease, ranges from 50–60% for nodal disease, and drops to below 25% for metastatic disease (Figure 1).[1] Up to this time, staging of Merkel cell carcinoma has been based primarily on the extent of disease at presentation (local vs. nodal vs. metastatic disease). Primary tumor size has also been used to separate stages in some systems, and the number of involved lymph nodes has been used in one system.

The first staging system for Merkel cell carcinoma, published in 1991, was based on a cohort of 70 patients at Memorial Sloan-Kettering Cancer Center.[2] It was a three-tiered system with separate stages for local (stage I), nodal (stage II) and metastatic (stage III) disease. As this system did not include a stage IV, it is unconventional compared to most other systems in which stage IV typically designates metastatic disease.

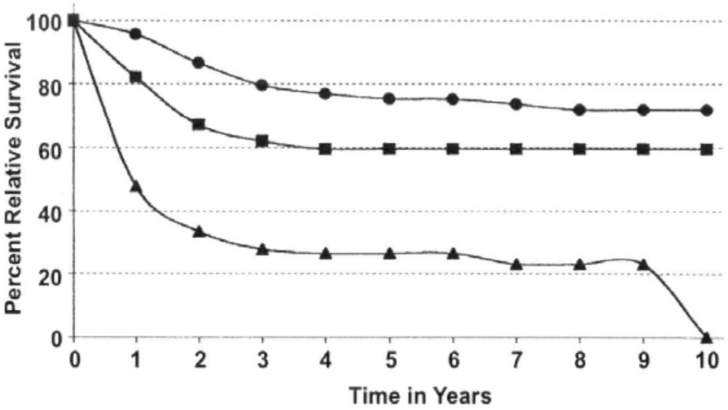

Figure 1. Relative survival by stage of Merkel cell carcinoma (circle, localized; square, regional; triangle, distant metastasis). SEER Program (cases from 1973–99). Reprinted with permission.[1]

Eight years later, the same group published a subsequent staging system for Merkel cell carcinoma with more patients (109).[3] Extent of disease continued to be the primary predictor of survival. For local disease, however, tumor size was found to be an independent predictor of survival. Thus, two substages were created for stage I (local) disease with primary tumors <2 cm designated as stage Ia and primary tumors ≥2 cm designated as stage Ib. Up to the present time, these three-tiered systems derived at Memorial Sloan-Kettering Cancer Center are the staging systems most frequently cited throughout the literature.

In 2005, an expanded Memorial Sloan-Kettering Cancer Center cohort of 251 patients was published.[4] This third staging system shifted to a more conventional four-tiered system. Stages Ia and Ib were converted to stages I and II, respectively, where only local disease was present. Stage III became nodal disease, and stage IV represented metastatic disease. This staging model is consistent with that of most other cancers.

Recently, a new staging system was published based on 110 head and neck Merkel cell carcinoma patients at three institutions in Australia and Canada.[5] This system differed significantly from the prior systems in that the cutoffs for tumor size were different and the number of positive lymph nodes was included in the staging model. In this new system, stage I includes local disease with primary tumors less than or equal to 1 cm.

Stage II is subdivided into 2 substages: stage IIa includes patients with tumors ≤1 cm and with 1–2 positive regional lymph nodes, and stage IIb designates patients with tumors ≥2 cm. Stage III disease is for patients with more than two positive regional lymph nodes, regardless of tumor size, and stage IV indicates metastatic disease. This system is unique in that it allows for some node positive disease to be in stage II, and it uses different cut-off values of primary tumor size compared with the prior three staging systems. In addition, this model was created using head and neck patients only and therefore may not be applicable to Merkel cell carcinoma found on other body sites.

In addition to these four staging systems published in the literature, the AJCC, the official entity for staging of all cancers in the US, has a system that includes Merkel cell carcinoma published in their 2002, 6th edition *Cancer Staging Manual*.[6] This system, however, is not specific for Merkel cell carcinoma but rather has Merkel cell carcinoma grouped with 82 other non-melanoma skin cancers in a chapter titled 'Carcinoma of the Skin.' The staging system in this chapter is similar to the 2005 system developed at Memorial Sloan-Kettering Cancer Center with the exception of putting local disease with primary tumors of exactly 2.0 cm in stage I rather than in stage II and the inclusion of deeply invasive tumors (into cartilage, skeletal muscle or bone) in stage III. A revised AJCC system specific for Merkel cell carcinoma has been published in the next edition of the AJCC *Cancer Staging Manual* (see Table 2).

7.2 Toward a Consensus TNM Staging System

Sentinel lymph node biopsy, while not previously incorporated into any staging system for Merkel cell carcinoma, has an important role in this cancer. Gupta *et al.* found that, of patients staged by clinical nodal examination only, one-third in fact had microscopic nodal disease after a sentinel lymph node biopsy was carried out (Figure 2).[7] The importance of sentinel lymph node biopsy is further emphasized in the Memorial Sloan-Kettering Cancer Center cohort that found disease-specific survival to be significantly better for local disease if node negativity was established by pathologic lymph node examination rather than by clinical examination alone (Figure 3).[4]

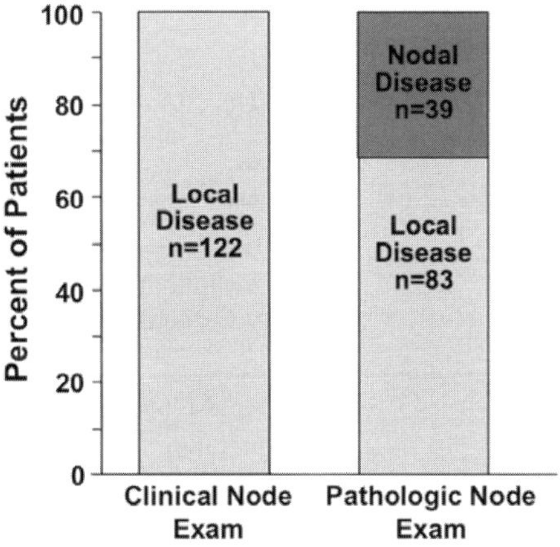

Figure 2. Impact of sentinel lymph node biopsy on staging; 122 patients were thought to have only local disease after clinical node examination alone. All patients subsequently underwent sentinel lymph node biopsy. Microscopic nodal metastases were found in 39 patients (32%). Adapted from Gupta *et al.*, 2006.[7]

These studies highlight the importance of the routine use of sentinel lymph node biopsy in Merkel cell carcinoma as there is an approximately 30% likelihood of a microscopically positive node among Merkel cell carcinoma patients presenting with clinically negative lymph nodes. Because of the importance of pathologic nodal exam and impact on survival in Merkel cell carcinoma, the AJCC has proposed a new staging system for Merkel cell carcinoma that will incorporate the method of nodal staging (clinical vs. pathologic evaluation) for the next version (7th edition) of the *Cancer Staging Manual* (Table 2). In melanoma, at least some patients presenting with thin lesions are not considered candidates for sentinel node biopsy.[8] The suggestion has recently been made that small diameter tumors (≤1.0 cm) have a low risk of nodal metastasis and may not require sentinel node biopsy.[9] This observation has not been substantiated, and while others have found a trend for greater likelihood of finding a positive sentinel node as tumor diameter enlarges,[7] there is as yet little corroborative evidence to support withholding sentinel node biopsy based on any diameter (or thickness) cutoff.

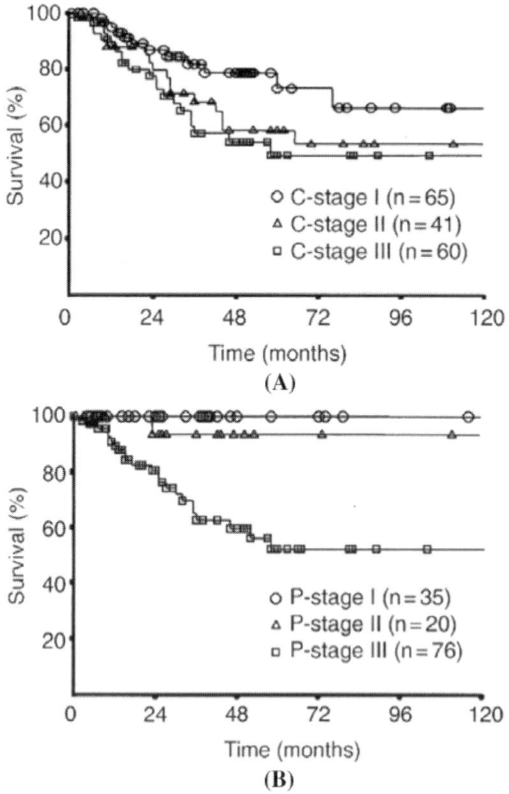

Figure 3. Disease-specific survival among Merkel cell carcinoma patients who underwent **(A)** clinical nodal staging (C-stage) and **(B)** pathologic nodal staging (P-stage) by sentinel lymph node biopsy, elective lymph node dissection, or therapeutic nodal staging. Stages were as follows: I = local disease, primary tumor <2 cm; II = local disease, primary tumor ≥2 cm; III = nodal disease. Differences between C-stage and P-stage were statistically significant for stages I and II: stage I, $p = 0.01$; stage II, $p = 0.01$; and stage III, $p = 0.81$. From Allen *et al.*, 2005.[4] Reprinted with permission.

7.3 Prognostic Factors and Staging Beyond TNM

Tumor, node and metastasis, or 'TNM,' criteria are the most established parameters used for staging cancers and predicting survival. TNM staging is a clean method of putting patients into discrete categories to predict survival

Table 2. New AJCC staging system for Merkel cell carcinoma.[24]

T	N	M
Tx, Primary tumor cannot be assessed	**Nx**, Regional nodes cannot be assessed	**Mx**, Distant metastasis cannot be assessed
T0, No primary tumor	**N0**, No regional node metastasis*	**M0**, No distant metastasis
Tis, *In situ* primary tumor	**cN0**, Nodes not clinically detectable*	**M1**, Distant metastasis
T1, Primary tumor ≤2 cm	**cN1**, Nodes clinically detectable*	**M1a**, To skin, subcutaneous tissues or distant lymph nodes
T2, Primary tumor >2 but ≤5 cm	**pN0,** Nodes negative by pathologic exam	**M1b**, To lung
T3, Primary tumor >5 cm	**pNx**, Nodes not examined pathologically	**M1c**, To all other visceral sites
T4, Primary tumor invades bone, muscle, fascia, or cartilage	**N1a**, Micrometastasis**	
	N1b, Macrometastasis***	
	N2, In-transit metastasis ****	

Stage	Stage grouping		
0	Tis	N0	M0
IA	T1	pN0	M0
IB	T1	cN0	M0
IIA	T2/T3	pN0	M0
IIB	T2/T3	cN0	M0
IIC	T4	N0	M0
IIIA	Any T	N1a	M0
IIIB	Any T	N1b/N2	M0
IV	Any T	Any N	M1

* N0 denotes negative nodes by clinical, pathologic or both types of exam. Clinical detection of nodal disease may be via inspection, palpation and/or imaging; cN0 is used only for patients who did not undergo pathologic node staging.

** Micrometastases are diagnosed after sentinel or elective lymphadenectomy.

*** Macrometastases are defined as clinically detectable nodal metastases confirmed pathologically by biopsy or therapeutic lymphadenectomy.

**** In-transit metastasis is a tumor distinct from the primary lesion and located either (1) between the primary lesion and the draining regional lymph nodes or (2) distal to the primary lesion.

and is useful for designing trials and guiding management decisions. However, parameters have been found that have an impact on survival in Merkel cell carcinoma but cannot readily be incorporated into a TNM model.

Several histologic parameters have been identified as potentially predictive of survival in Merkel cell carcinoma. Breslow thickness in Merkel cell carcinoma and its relationship to patient outcome has been evaluated in a number of studies.[10–14] Results of these studies have been mixed, but the largest and most recent study did find an association with poorer survival and thicker tumors.[14] An analysis of thickness and its association with lymph node positivity has shown an association,[15] but it remains to be seen whether this has predictive value for nodal metastasis in Merkel cell carcinoma as it does for melanoma. The absence of lymphovascular invasion and nodular (compared to infiltrative) growth pattern of the primary tumor have each been found to confer improved prognosis in a multivariate analysis of 156 patients, but these findings have yet to be confirmed in an independent set of patients.[14]

Molecular prognostic features also show promise for relevance in Merkel cell carcinoma. Expression of p63, an epidermal/basal cell differentiation marker, has been associated with poor survival in one study of 47 patients.[16] In that study, p63 expression was associated with overall survival of $<10\%$ while absence of expression conferred $>90\%$ overall survival ($p < 0.0001$). The recent identification of the Merkel cell polyomavirus may lead to a discovery of differences in survival between virus-positive and virus-negative tumors, although no significant effect has yet been observed.[17,18]

Another variable of importance for its impact on survival in Merkel cell carcinoma is the presence of profound immune suppression such as HIV, chronic lymphocytic leukemia or solid organ transplantation. One study found that solid organ transplant recipients presented with more advanced disease at diagnosis and had worse survival than other Merkel cell carcinoma patients who were not transplant recipients.[19] Factors such as patient gender, age and tumor location may also have small but independent effects on survival. Incorporation of continuous variables such as tumor size, number of positive lymph nodes and site of metastasis will likely improve the prognostic accuracy of a more complete staging system in the future.

The best way to incorporate multiple non-TNM variables and to weight them appropriately for their independent predictive value is through a nomogram.[20] A nomogram is a graphical representation of a mathematical model that characterizes relationships between multiple predictive factors and an outcome, such as survival after a cancer diagnosis. In a nomogram, weighted values (derived from multivariate survival models) are assigned to predictive factors, and these are combined to predict disease outcomes in a way that is easily understood by patients and clinicians. A cancer prognostic nomogram overcomes the shortcomings of a traditional categorical TNM staging system and allows capture of multiple independently predictive features into a single model to predict prognosis more accurately for a given patient.

Nomograms currently exist for predicting recurrence in prostate cancer[21] and the likelihood of non-sentinel lymph node metastases in breast cancer.[22] A major advantage of the nomogram system is that it allows the incorporation of continuous variables (such as primary tumor size) rather than a categorical system which forces each case to be placed into a 'bin' such as ≤2.0 cm or >2.0 cm tumor size. Another advantage of nomograms is that they can readily be updated if a new variable is to be added. Because nomograms can incorporate more predictive factors in more realistic forms than is possible with traditional categorical staging systems, they can often yield better predictions of outcome.[23]

The future of Merkel cell carcinoma staging will eventually include the development of a nomogram to predict survival in Merkel cell carcinoma patients. It ideally would incorporate weighted factors for the TNM features in the categorical AJCC system as well as additional clinical, histologic and molecular features found to be independently predictive in Merkel cell carcinoma.

References

1. Agelli M., Clegg L.X. (2003). Epidemiology of primary Merkel cell carcinoma in the United States. *J Am Acad Dermatol* 49: 832–841.
2. Yiengpruksawan A., Coit D.G., Thaler H.T., *et al.* (1991). Merkel cell carcinoma. Prognosis and management. *Arch Surg* 126: 1514–1519.

3. Allen P.J., Zhang Z.F., Coit D.G. (1999). Surgical management of Merkel cell carcinoma. *Ann Surg* 229: 97–105.
4. Allen P.J., Bowne W.B., Jaques D.P., *et al.* (2005). Merkel cell carcinoma: prognosis and treatment of patients from a single institution. *J Clin Oncol* 23: 2300–2309.
5. Clark J.R., Veness M.J., Gilbert R., *et al.* (2007). Merkel cell carcinoma of the head and neck: Is adjuvant radiotherapy necessary? *Head Neck* 29: 249–257.
6. *AJCC Cancer Staging Manual*, 6th Ed. Springer, Chicago, 2002.
7. Gupta S.G., Wang L.C., Penas P.F., *et al.* (2006). Sentinel lymph node biopsy for evaluation and treatment of patients with Merkel cell carcinoma: the Dana–Farber experience and meta-analysis of the literature. *Arch Dermatol* 142: 685–690.
8. Lens M.B., Dawes M., Newton-Bishop J.A., Goodacre T. (2002). Tumour thickness as a predictor of occult lymph node metastases in patients with stage I and II melanoma undergoing sentinel lymph node biopsy. *Br J Surg* 89: 1223–1227.
9. Stokes J.B., Graw K.S., Dengel L.T., *et al.* (2009). Patients with Merkel cell carcinoma tumors ≤ 1.0 cm in diameter are unlikely to harbor regional lymph node metastases. *J Clin Oncol* 27: 3772–3777.
10. Llombart B., Monteagudo C., Lopez-Guerrero J.A., *et al.* (2005). Clinicopathological and immunohistochemical analysis of 20 cases of Merkel cell carcinoma in search of prognostic markers. *Histopathology* 46: 622–634.
11. Skelton H.G., Smith K.J., Hitchcock C.L., *et al.* (1997). Merkel cell carcinoma: analysis of clinical, histologic, and immunohistologic features of 132 cases with relation to survival. *J Am Acad Dermatol* 37: 734–739.
12. Sandel H.D., Day T., Richardson M.S., *et al.* (2006). Merkel cell carcinoma: does tumor size or depth of invasion correlate with recurrence, metastasis, or patient survival? *Laryngoscope* 116: 791–795.
13. Goldberg S.R., Neifeld J.P., Frable W.J. (2007). Prognostic value of tumor thickness in patients with Merkel cell carcinoma. *J Surg Oncol* 95: 618–622.
14. Andea A.A., Coit D.G., Amin B., Busam K.J. (2008). Merkel cell carcinoma: histologic features and prognosis. *Cancer* 113: 2549–2558.
15. Meredith K.L., Zager J.S., Messina J.L., *et al.* (2007). Management options for sentinel node positive Merkel cell carcinoma. *Ann Surg Oncol* 14(2 suppl): 29–30.

16. Asioli S., Righi A., Volante M., *et al.* (2007). p63 expression as a new prognostic marker in Merkel cell carcinoma. *Cancer* 110: 640–647.
17. Garneski K.M., Warcola A.H., Feng Q., *et al.* (2009). Merkel cell polyomavirus is more frequently present in North American than Australian Merkel cell carcinoma tumors. *J Invest Dermatol* 129: 246–248.
18. Becker J.C., Houben R., Ugurel S., *et al.* (2009). MC polyomavirus is frequently present in Merkel cell carcinoma of European patients. *J Invest Dermatol* 129: 248–250.
19. Penn I., First M.R. (1999). Merkel's cell carcinoma in organ recipients: report of 41 cases. *Transplantation* 68: 1717–1721.
20. Kattan M.W., Scardino P.T. (2007). Evidence for the usefulness of nomograms. *Nat Clin Pract Urol* 4: 638–639.
21. Pal A., Provenzano E., Duffy S.W., *et al.* (2008). A model for predicting non-sentinel lymph node metastatic disease when the sentinel lymph node is positive. *Br J Surg* 95: 302–309.
22. Stephenson A.J., Scardino P.T., Eastham J.A., *et al.* (2006). Preoperative nomogram predicting the 10-year probability of prostate cancer recurrence after radical prostatectomy. *J Natl Cancer Inst* 98: 715–717.
23. Bochner B.H., Kattan M.W., Vora K.C. (2006). Postoperative nomogram predicting risk of recurrence after radical cystectomy for bladder cancer. *J Clin Oncol* 24: 3967–3972.
24. *AJCC Cancer Staging Manual*, 7th Ed. Springer, Chicago, 2010.

Chapter 8

New Prognostic Factors in Merkel Cell Carcinoma

Charles Knapp, Jonathan S. Zager, Jane L. Messina and Vernon K. Sondak

8.1 Introduction

Despite recent research into the behavior and prognosis of Merkel cell carcinoma, there is a relative paucity of evidence regarding the pathologic prognostic markers for this tumor. Chapters 5 and 7 discuss the pathologic evaluation of Merkel cell carcinoma and the currently utilized staging systems, respectively. In this chapter, we will attempt to summarize and review the literature on potential prognostic and predictive factors for Merkel cell carcinoma, as well as to note the manifold deficits in the current available evidence base and offer suggestions for future studies in these areas.

The 'standard' clinicopathologic prognostic factors for Merkel cell carcinoma, detailed in Chapter 7, are: tumor diameter, using 2 cm as the cut-off between 'small' and 'large' tumors; clinical and pathologic regional lymph node status; and the presence or absence of metastases beyond the regional nodes. Unlike melanoma, these factors are relatively poor at categorizing patients into 'low', 'intermediate' and 'high' risk groups. In particular, no low-risk group akin to melanoma patients with thin primary lesions — where the risk of nodal metastasis and death from melanoma is exceedingly small — has ever been defined for Merkel cell carcinoma. Virtually no prospective studies have been conducted in localized Merkel cell carcinoma. Worse yet, few if any of the retrospective or correlative studies done to date were inclusive of all or even most potential prognostic factors, used multivariate analytic techniques, and had uniform staging and treatment and long-term follow-up of patients.

8.2 Standard Histologic Features

Perhaps the largest study to date to characterize the histopathologic prognostic features of Merkel cell carcinoma involved 251 cases.[1] Based on a review of Memorial Sloan-Kettering Cancer Center's Merkel cell carcinoma database, Allen *et al.* found that the overall five-year disease-specific survival rate was 64%. They concluded that patients with histologically negative regional lymph nodes had very favorable long-term survival (97% disease-specific survival at five years) with the only patient in this group who died of disease having a primary tumor ≥2 cm in diameter. In contrast, patients with clinically negative but histologically positive nodes had a five-year survival rate of 62%, and patients who presented with clinically positive nodes had a five-year survival rate of 49%. When factors associated with survival were analyzed in a multivariate Cox model, the only independent predictor of survival was pathologic nodal status.[1]

Several years after the Allen *et al.* report, another review of the Memorial Sloan-Kettering Merkel cell carcinoma was published by Andea *et al.*[2] This study involved 156 patients who had adequate assessment of histologic parameters and verified clinical follow-up, and investigated the impact of tumor thickness, tumor size, tumor growth pattern, lymphovascular invasion, tumor-infiltrating lymphocytes, tumor necrosis, ulceration and solar elastosis on prognosis. In contrast to the study of only three years earlier, the disease-specific survival for patients with histologically node-negative disease was 82.5% and patients with stage I disease (tumors <2 cm and negative lymph nodes) had a five-year survival rate of 86%. Within the stage I group, with a median follow-up of 51 months, none of the patients with tumors <5 mm thick died of disease at five years compared to an 80% five-year survival rate for patients who had tumors that measured >5 mm. This difference, however, was not statistically significant.

Andea *et al.* did find that the presence of a nodular growth pattern, more superficial tumors (dermis/subcutis versus deeper), the absence of lymphovascular invasion and the presence of tumor-infiltrating lymphocytes were all associated with statistically significantly longer survival for node-negative patients. But on multivariate analysis of the entire cohort of patients, only stage, tumor growth pattern and lymphovascular invasion correlated independently with survival.[2] The finding that the histologic appearance of the primary tumor itself has prognostic significance was also made by Skelton *et al.*, who evaluated prognostic factors for survival in 85 patients whose Merkel cell carcinoma was evaluated at the Armed Forces Institute of Pathology and who were known to have either died of disease or to be alive without disease at a median of 55 months. These patients were almost all treated in an earlier era, before the routine use of sentinel node biopsy, and as a referral series these cases were treated in a completely non-standard fashion. On univariate analysis, tumor diameter, tumor cell size ('small' versus 'intermediate', see Chapter 5, Figures 3 and 4) and mitotic rate (≤ 5 vs. 6 to 10 vs. >10 mitoses/high power field) were significantly correlated with survival. The authors went on to create separate multivariate models for the small and intermediate cell size tumor groups: no other factors were found to significantly impact survival in the small cell group but mitotic rate retained significance for the intermediate cell size group. Tumor diameter was not independently significant for either cell size group.[3]

Although all three of these studies had the advantage of relying on expert pathology to evaluate the histologic features of the primary tumor, it is readily apparent that none of them evaluated the same set of parameters or dealt with comparably staged and treated patients. Difficulty drawing conclusions is magnified even further in review articles that evaluate smaller series with less uniform and potentially less reliable pathologic evaluation.[4] Nonetheless, given the relatively limited prognostic value of tumor diameter and clinical nodal status, and the importance of pathologic microstaging in prognostication in melanoma, considerable interest remains in finding histologic correlates of survival in Merkel cell carcinoma. Tumor thickness, measured in a manner analogous to Breslow's thickness for melanoma, remains an area of active investigation, and it is hoped that as larger studies of pathologically staged patients become available, a more reliable determination of its value in Merkel cell carcinoma can be obtained. To foster future studies, we and others recommend a standardized set of histologic features be developed to allow uniform pathology reporting for all primary Merkel cell carcinomas and sentinel node biopsies.[5]

8.3 Immunohistochemical Staining

Given the limited role standard histopathologic factors have played to date in defining prognosis in patients with Merkel cell carcinoma, attempts have been undertaken to find associations between immunohistochemical assessments of protein expression and increased or decreased likelihood of tumor metastasis or survival. The literature on immunohistochemical prognostic markers in Merkel cell carcinoma suffers from all of the limitations that plague studies of standard histopathologic features, and is characterized by small studies that rarely account for all or even most other potential confounding prognostic factors.

In 1993, Micali *et al.* analyzed eight patients with Merkel cell carcinoma and concluded that 'immunohistology' did not correlate with outcome.[6] Kennedy *et al.* assessed 15 cases of Merkel cell carcinoma for staining with antibodies to bcl-2 (associated with resistance to apoptosis) and p53 (a critical cell cycle regulatory protein).[7] They found moderate to strong staining for p53 in five cases, and moderate to strong staining for bcl-2 in ten cases, but no relationship between immunohistochemistry results and survival.[7] Mott *et al.*, in addition to assessing multiple histologic features, evaluated cytokeratin 20 and neural cell adhesion molecule expression and found no correlation between staining intensity and recurrence or survival.[8] Feinmesser *et al.* looked at the expression of the antiapoptotic proteins bcl-2 and bax, as well as p53, in Merkel cell carcinoma.[9] While they could not establish a link with either response to treatment or survival, Feinmesser did suggest the possibility of tumor cell resistance to apoptosis-inducing agents due to their significant rate of bcl-2 positivity (76%).[9]

The relationship between expression of cell cycle regulatory proteins p27(Kip1) and p45(Skp2), along with the proliferation marker Ki67, and Merkel cell carcinoma prognosis was investigated by Fernandez-Figueras *et al.* in 24 Merkel cell carcinomas.[10] Expression of p27(Kip1) and p45(Skp2) was seen in Merkel cell carcinoma and also in small cell neuroendocrine carcinomas of the lung and urinary bladder. Fernandez-Figueras *et al.* concluded that these molecules did not have a significant impact on the prognosis of either Merkel cell carcinoma or these other neuroendocrine tumors.[10] However, the authors found increased Ki67 expression to be significantly correlated with a higher risk of recurrence in Merkel cell carcinoma in a univariate analysis.[10] Llombart *et al.* evaluated Ki67 expression along with other histopathologic and immunochemical factors in 20 cases of Merkel cell carcinoma, and found that the presence of >50% of Ki67 positive tumor cells was significantly associated with a decreased disease-free interval on univariate analysis, but only 'absent' lymphocytic infiltration was an independent prognostic factor for disease-free interval on multivariate analysis.[11]

Tucci *et al.* looked at the staining patterns of Ki67, bcl-2, p53, survivin, p16 and CXCR4 — all proteins with roles in cell proliferation, survival and apoptosis — in 12 cases of primary Merkel cell carcinoma.[12] The authors categorized patients as 'poor prognosis' if they were stage II or III, or if they were stage I but had recurred. Using that definition, they found that bcl-2 expression was statistically significantly correlated with poor prognosis, and Ki67 and survivin were associated with poor prognosis but not significantly so. No expression of CXCR4 was found in the samples tested.[12] Kim and McNiff tested 19 cases of Merkel cell carcinoma (18 primary tumors and one metastasis) with antibodies to survivin; clinical follow-up information was available in 15 cases (79%). All 19 cases demonstrated strong immunoreactivity for survivin; localization of the protein was classified as predominately nuclear (eight cases), cytoplasmic (four cases) or mixed (three cases). Seven of the eight patients with predominantly nuclear staining developed metastatic disease or died, while all four cases with predominately cytoplasmic survivin localization were disease free.[13]

Asioli *et al.* studied 47 cases of Merkel cell carcinoma; 27 represented localized primary tumors, 18 lymphatic metastases and two distant metastases. The authors found that the expression of p63, a member of the p53 family whose gene is frequently amplified and/or overexpressed in human cancers, was significantly associated with worse overall survival ($p < 0.0001$). Multivariate analysis showed p63 expression to be a strong independent prognostic factor (hazard ratio 22.2) along with disease stage and the presence of Ki-67 staining.[14] Although this study suffers from a relatively small number of cases, the large magnitude of the impact of p63 expression on survival combined with the independent significance on multivariate analysis offers the possibility that p63 might actually be a relevant prognostic marker in Merkel cell carcinoma. It is certainly one marker that has emerged as worthy of further study.

E-cadherin is a cellular protein which functions in normal intercellular adhesion. Loss of E-cadherin has been recognized in several malignant tumors, and is thought to be associated with a higher rate of tumor invasion due to loss of adhesion to adjacent cells.[15] Han *et al.* found that E-cadherin was the most frequently expressed cadherin in Merkel cell carcinoma, followed by N- and then P-cadherin. Interestingly, they found that the N-cadherin was localized to the nucleus instead of present in the cytoplasm.[16] Tanaka *et al.*, however, while confirming reduced cytoplasmic E-cadherin in Merkel cell carcinoma, found nuclear localization of E-cadherin in only four of 31 cases.[17] More recently, Panelos *et al.* investigated 31 Merkel cell carcinoma specimens for immunoreactivity for E-cadherin, along with Notch-1 and β-catenin. As in other studies, E-cadherin membranous expression was low, with only one of 26 cases found positive in more than 50% of cells. But nuclear expression was observed in only three of 26 cases. Cytoplasmic and membrane Notch-1 expression in more than 50% of cells was observed in 30 of 31 Merkel cell carcinomas. β-catenin membrane-associated staining was also seen in 30 of 31 cases, but nuclear β-catenin was seen only in two cases.[18]

Measures of angiogenesis have received increasing attention as prognostic markers in a variety of malignancies. A study of angiogenesis in Merkel cell carcinoma was conducted by Ng *et al.*, who stained 36 cases of Merkel cell carcinoma with an antibody to the endothelial marker CD34. Increased vascular density measured using this antibody was statistically significantly associated with worse survival, as was tumor size, lymphovascular invasion and tumor mast cell count. Specifically, the investigators found that a one-unit increase in total vessel score was associated with a 3.9 times increase in the risk of death.[19]

Brunner *et al.* determined the expression of a number of molecules which could be potentially targeted for treatment, including c-kit, Mcl-1, Bmi-1, vascular endothelial growth factor (VEGF)-A, VEGF-C, VEGF-receptor 2 (VEGF-R2), platelet derived growth factor (PDGF)-α, PDGF-β, epidermal growth factor receptor (EGFR) and Her-2/Neu. Using immunohistochemical staining of a tissue microarray containing 32 samples from 29 Merkel cell carcinoma patients, they found that the majority of tumors stained with relatively low intensity for all of these markers except for EGFR and Her-2/Neu, which were completely absent, and PDGF-β and c-kit, which stained more strongly.[20] The finding of prominent c-kit staining supported a similar observation by Su *et al.*, who found staining in 95% of 22 cases, but saw no correlation with outcome.[21] Brunner's group extracted DNA from c-kit positive samples and performed direct DNA sequencing to analyze for exon 9 and 11 mutations, but no mutations were found. The authors concluded that tumor expression of these markers could be used to select patients for trials of the promising agents that target them.[20] The results also highlight that immunohistochemical staining, as in the case of c-kit, may not predict the presence of mutations that are responsive to targeted therapies — in this case explaining the observed lack of responsiveness of Merkel cell tumors to imatinib (see Chapter 16).

In a subsequent study from the same group, Brunner *et al.* used a tissue microarray with 28 samples from 25 patients to study hedgehog signaling molecules, which are important in a variety of malignancies including basal cell carcinoma. These proteins were frequently over-expressed, and expression of high levels of Patched and Indian hedgehog were both independently correlated with improved outcome (Patched with overall survival and Indian hedgehog with recurrence-free survival) in multivariate analysis.[22]

Recognizing the sample-size limitations of the foregoing types of investigations, investigators at our institution created a tissue microarray containing cores from 227 tumors from 86 patients — 110 primary, 73 nodal and 44 metastatic (Figure 1). In an initial study, the tumors were stained with antibodies to bcl-2, CXCR4, survivin and E-cadherin, and image analysis utilized to compare staining between primary, regional and metastatic disease. Similar to other investigators' findings, a high proportion

Figure 1. Immunohistochemically-stained Merkel cell carcinoma tissue microarray showing cored samples of primary lesions in the left upper region, lymph node metastases in the right upper region, and distant metastases in the lower portion of the block (anti-CXCR4).

of tumors of all stages stained strongly for bcl-2. E-cadherin staining was weak, focal and did not differ significantly between the three sites. While these findings have yet to be correlated with clinical outcome, there was a statistically significant increase in immunoreactivity for both CXCR4 and survivin (nuclear and cytoplasmic) in nodal metastases compared to primary and metastatic sites (Figures 2A–2C).[23]

As noted above, the body of research involving pathologic and immunohistochemical prognosis of Merkel cell carcinoma is relatively sparse. Larger and more controlled studies must still be conducted, as the opportunities for research involving new and as yet untested immunohistochemical markers are vast. In particular, the advent of tissue microarray technology paves the way for much larger studies using formalin-fixed, paraffin-embedded tissue that can be collected from multiple institutions and analyzed for expression of multiple different proteins.[24]

(A)

(B)

(C)

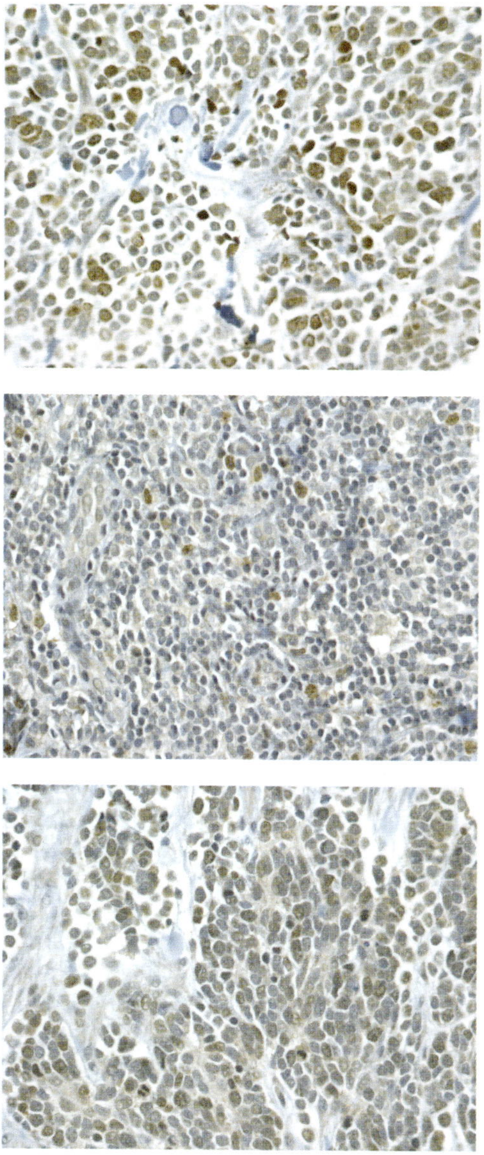

Figure 2. **(A)** Tissue microarray core sample from a Merkel cell carcinoma metastatic to a lymph node, showing strong nuclear and cytoplasmic staining for survivin (Novus Biologicals, Littleton, CO, 400×). **(B)** Tissue microarray core sample from a primary Merkel cell carcinoma showing focal nuclear staining and weak cytoplasmic staining for survivin (400×). **(C)** Tissue microarray core sample from a metastatic Merkel cell carcinoma deposit, showing weak nuclear and cytoplasmic staining for survivin (400×).

8.4 Viral Infection and Prognosis

The discovery that viral gene sequences were integrally incorporated into the genome of a significant percentage of Merkel cell carcinomas, described in detail in Chapter 3, was revolutionary for our understanding of the pathogenesis of this tumor. Soon after this discovery, a series of studies were undertaken to determine if the presence of viral genes were associated with outcome. The evidence from these studies has been conflicting, with some data suggesting that patients with viral gene positive Merkel cell carcinoma experience better survival, some not showing a difference, and some indicating worse survival for virus positive cases. In favor of an association with favorable outcome was the study by Bhatia *et al.* in which patients with ≥ 0.06 viral copies per cell experienced higher median survival than those with ≤ 0.0035 viral copies per cell (86 months versus 20 months, $p = 0.015$).[25] Sihto *et al.* studied 114 Finnish Merkel cell carcinoma patients and found the five-year survival to be 45% for patients with virus positive tumors compared to 13% for those with virus negative tumors ($p < 0.001$).[26] After adjusting for gender and the presence of nodal metastases, the presence of viral DNA was significantly associated with improved survival (hazard ratio 0.42, 95% confidence interval 0.25–0.71). In contrast, Garneski *et al.* evaluated the outcome for 30 Merkel cell carcinoma patients based on the presence or absence of viral sequences by real-time quantitative PCR. Using Kaplan–Meier analysis, no survival difference was noted between virus-positive and virus-negative tumors.[27] Becker *et al.* analyzed 75 samples from 53 Merkel cell carcinoma patients for the presence of Merkel cell polyomavirus by real-time PCR. Their clinical follow-up data suggested that patients whose tumors contained the viral genome displayed a more aggressive behavior, but after stratifying for tumor stage there was no statistically significant difference between the groups.[28]

It is clear from the above data that further investigation in larger cohorts of patients, preferably prospectively treated and well characterized in terms of known clinicopathologic prognostic factors, is needed before any association between viral status and outcome in Merkel cell carcinoma can conclusively be established or excluded. This is undoubtedly worth pursuing, however, particularly given the observation that viral infection with human papillomavirus in head and neck cancers has been a predictor of improved prognosis and superior response to chemotherapy and radiation therapy.[29] Efforts to study the relationship between detection of viral DNA incorporation and outcome in a disease as rare as Merkel cell carcinoma will undoubtedly be improved by techniques that more reliably detect viral DNA or protein products, particularly in paraffin-embedded tissue.[30,31]

8.5 Genetic Abnormalities and Prognosis

The evolving role of gene expression profiling in the study of Merkel cell carcinoma is described in Chapter 4. In a growing number of tumor types, common and rare, expression profiling has shown promise for identifying prognostic and predictive signatures, and even for predicting sites of metastases among tumors that have spread.[32,33] As yet, however, very little is known in terms of correlating gene expression profiles with any outcome parameter in Merkel cell carcinoma.

Comparative genomic hybridization (CGH) is another approach to evaluating genetic abnormalities — in this case at the chromosomal level — in cancers. Paulson *et al.* performed high-resolution comparative genomic hybridization on 25 Merkel cell carcinoma tumor samples from 23 patients using a high-density oligonucleotide microarray. Some samples were from fresh-frozen tumors while others were from formalin-fixed paraffin embedded specimens, and both primary tumors and metastases were studied. Importantly, for those patients in whom both a primary and metastasis were profiled, the signatures were considered to be nearly identical, suggesting that sampling a primary tumor may be useful to understand metastases with this technique. Merkel cell cancers of all types frequently carried extra copies of chromosomes 1, 3q, 5p, and 6 and lost chromosomes 3p, 4, 5q, 7, 10 and 13. As has been seen with other types of cancer, tumors with fewer genomic aberrations were associated with better survival. Also of interest, considering the conflicting data about viral infection and outcome, tumors from 13 of 22 patients had detectable Merkel cell polyomavirus DNA and these tumors had fewer genomic deletions.[34] Using array CGH, Sastre-Garau *et al.* analyzed ten Merkel cell carcinomas, all of which had been found to contain viral DNA sequences. Three of the ten samples analyzed did not show any chromosomal imbalance on array CGH; imbalances seen in at least two cases included gains of 1q (two cases), 6p (three cases), and 11 (two cases), and loss of 17p (two cases). No correlation was found between these chromosome rearrangements and the viral integration sites.[35]

8.6 Predictors of Response to Therapy

As discussed in Section 8.3 above, gene expression and/or mutation not only may convey prognostic information but can also serve to predict response to therapy as well.[36] Caution must be exercised in trying to extrapolate from other tumor types, as was seen when imatinib was used in Merkel cell carcinoma (see Chapter 16) based on significant levels of protein expression of c-kit. In gastrointestinal stromal tumors, such protein expression detected immunohistochemically usually indicates the presence of imatinib-responsive gene mutations resulting in constitutive expression of the c-kit gene.[37] The potential of this approach, however, is indicated by a recent report of three patients with disseminated Merkel cell carcinoma treated on a clinical trial of the tyrosine kinase inhibitor pazopanib, which targets vascular endothelial growth factor receptor-1, -2 and -3; platelet-derived growth factor receptor-α and -β; and c-kit. One of the three patients had a dramatic partial response that lasted a total of six months. The authors found a 1432 T > C (ser478pro) mutation in the PDGFR-α gene in all three patients' tumor samples, but also in their germline DNA. They postulate that such mutations could be related to susceptibility to Merkel cell carcinoma development as well as possibly predictive of response to targeted therapy against PDGFR-α.[38]

8.7 Prospects for the Future

We clearly still have a long way to go if we are to improve prognostication for patients with Merkel cell carcinoma. We have even further to go before we can reliably predict responsiveness to therapy in this disease. Nonetheless, the rapid progression of basic scientific knowledge about this disease allows us at least cautious optimism for the future. Given the rarity of this tumor, progress will necessitate collaborative efforts including prospective studies on patients diagnosed and treated in a uniform manner.

References

1. Allen P.J., Bowne W.B., Jaques D.P., *et al.* (2005). Merkel cell carcinoma: prognosis and treatment of patients from a single institution. *J Clin Oncol* 23: 2300–2309.
2. Andea A.A., Coit D.G., Busam K.J. (2008). Merkel cell carcinoma: histologic features and prognosis. *Cancer* 113: 2549–2558.
3. Skelton H.G., Smith K.J., Hitchcock C.L., *et al.* (1997). Merkel cell carcinoma: analysis of clinical, histologic, and immunohistologic features of 132 cases with relation to survival. *J Am Acad Dermatol* 37: 734–739.
4. Bickle K., Glass L.F., Messina J.L., *et al.* (2004). Merkel cell carcinoma: a clinical, histopathologic, and immunohistochemical review. *Semin Cutan Med Surg* 23: 46–53.
5. Brown J.A., Smoller B.R. (2009). Merkel cell carcinoma: what is it, what will it do and where will it go? What role should the pathologist play in reporting this information? *J Cutan Pathol* 36: 924–927.
6. Micali G., Ferraú F., Innocenzi D. (1993). Primary Merkel cell tumor: a clinical analysis of eight cases. *Int J Dermatol* 32: 345–349.
7. Kennedy M.M., Blessing K., King G., Kerr K.M. (1996). Expression of bcl-2 and p53 in Merkel cell carcinoma. An immunohistochemical study. *Am J Dermatopathol* 18: 273–277.
8. Mott R.T., Smoller B.R., Morgan M.B. (2004). Merkel cell carcinoma: a clinicopathologic study with prognostic implications. *J Cutan Pathol* 31: 217–223.
9. Feinmesser M., Halpern M., Fenig E., *et al.* (1999). Expression of the apoptosis-related oncogenes bcl-2, bax, and p53 in Merkel cell carcinoma: can they predict treatment response and clinical outcome? *Hum Pathol* 30: 1367–1372.
10. Fernández-Figueras M.T., Puig L., Musulen E., *et al.* (2005). Prognostic significance of p27Kip1, p45Skp2 and Ki67 expression profiles in Merkel cell carcinoma, extracutaneous small cell carcinoma, and cutaneous squamous cell carcinoma. *Histopathology* 46: 614–621.

11. Llombart B., Monteagudo C., López–Guerrero J.A., *et al.* (2005). Clinicopathological and immunohistochemical analysis of 20 cases of Merkel cell carcinoma in search of prognostic markers. *Histopathology* 45: 622–634.
12. Tucci M.G., Lucarini G., Ciangiacomi M, *et al.* (2006). Immunohistochemical study of apoptosis markers and involvement of chemokine CXCR4 in skin Merkel cell carcinoma. *J Eur Acad Dermatol Venereol* 20: 1220–1225.
13. Kim J., McNiff J.M. (2008). Nuclear expression of survivin portends a poor prognosis in Merkel cell carcinoma. *Mod Pathol* 21: 764–769.
14. Asioli S., Righi A., Volante M., *et al.* (2007). p63 expression as a new prognostic marker in Merkel cell carcinoma. *Cancer* 110: 640–647.
15. Chetty R., Serra S. (2008). Nuclear E-cadherin immunoexpression: from biology to potential applications in diagnostic pathology. *Adv Anat Pathol* 15: 234–240.
16. Han A.C., Soler A.P., Tang C.K., *et al.* (2000). Nuclear localization of E-cadherin expression in Merkel cell carcinoma. *Arch Pathol Lab Med* 124: 1147–1151.
17. Tanaka Y., Sano T., Qian Z.R., Hirokawa M. (2004). Expression of adhesion molecules and cytokeratin 20 in Merkel cell carcinomas. *Endocr Pathol* 15: 117–129.
18. Panelos J., Batistatou A., Paglierani M., *et al.* (2009). Expression of Notch-1 and alteration of the E-cadherin/beta-catenin cell adhesion complex are observed in primary cutaneous neuroendocrine carcinoma (Merkel cell carcinoma). *Mod Pathol* 22: 959–968.
19. Ng L., Beer T.W., Murray K. (2008). Vascular density has prognostic value in Merkel cell carcinoma. *Am J Dermatopathol* 30: 442–445.
20. Brunner M., Thurnher D., Pammer J., *et al.* (2008). Expression of VEGF-A/C, VEGF-R2, PDGF-alpha/beta, c-kit, EGFR, Her-2/Neu, Mcl-1 and Bmi-1 in Merkel cell carcinoma. *Mod Pathol* 21: 876–884.
21. Su L.D., Fullen D.R., Lowe L., *et al.* (2002). CD117 (KIT receptor) expression in Merkel cell carcinoma. *Am J Dermatopathol* 24: 289–293.
22. Brunner M., Thurnher D., Pammer J., *et al.* (2010). Expression of hedgehog signaling molecules in Merkel cell carcinoma. *Head Neck* 32: 333–340.
23. Knapp C.F., Sayegh Z., Schell M., *et al.* (2009). Potential markers of progression and prognosis in Merkel cell carcinoma: an immunohistochemical

study using a tissue microarray. American Society of Dermatopathology, poster presentation.

24. Camp R.L., Neumeister V., Rimm D.L. (2008). A decade of tissue microarrays: progress in the discovery and validation of cancer biomarkers. *J Clin Oncol* 2008 26: 5630–5637.
25. Bhatia K., Goedert J.J., Modali R., *et al.* (2010). Merkel cell carcinoma subgroups by Merkel cell polyomavirus DNA relative abundance and oncogene expression. *Int J Cancer* 126: 2240–2246.
26. Sihto H., Kukko H., Koljonen V., *et al.* (2009). Clinical factors associated with Merkel cell polyomavirus infection in Merkel cell carcinoma. *J Natl Cancer Inst* 101: 938–945.
27. Garneski K.M., Warcola A.H., Feng Q., *et al.* (2009). Merkel cell polyomavirus is more frequently present in North American than Australian Merkel cell carcinoma tumors. *J Invest Dermatol* 129: 246–248.
28. Becker J.C., Houben R., Ugurel S., *et al.* (2009). MC polyomavirus is frequently present in Merkel cell carcinoma of European patients. *J Invest Dermatol* 129: 248–250.
29. Fakhry C., Westra W.H., Li S., *et al.* (2008). Improved survival of patients with human papillomavirus-positive head and neck squamous cell carcinoma in a prospective clinical trial. *J Natl Cancer Inst* 100: 261–269.
30. The Rockville Merkel Cell Carcinoma Group. (2009). Merkel cell carcinoma: Recent progress and current priorities on etiology, pathogenesis, and clinical management. *J Clin Oncol* 27: 4021–4026.
31. Duncavage E.J., Zehnbauer B.A., Pfeifer J.D. (2009). Prevalence of Merkel cell polyomavirus in Merkel cell carcinoma. *Mod Pathol* 22: 516–521.
32. Haqq C., Nosrati M., Sudilovksy D., *et al.* (2005). The gene expression signatures of melanoma progression. *Proc Natl Acad Sci USA* 102: 6092–6097.
33. Michiels S., Koscielny S., Hill C. (2007). Interpretation of microarray data in cancer. *Br J Cancer* 96: 1155–1158.
34. Paulson K.G., Lemos B.D., Feng B., *et al.* (2009). Array-CGH reveals recurrent genomic changes in Merkel cell carcinoma including amplification of L-Myc. *J Invest Dermatol* 129: 1547–1555.
35. Sastre-Garau X., Peter M., Avril M.F., *et al.* (2009). Merkel cell carcinoma of the skin: pathological and molecular evidence for a causative role of MCV in oncogenesis. *J Pathol* 218: 48–56.
36. Yeatman T.J. (2009). Predictive biomarkers: identification and verification. *J Clin Oncol* 27: 2743–2744.

37. Renouf D.J., Wilson L., Blanke C.D. (2009). Successes and challenges in translational research: the development of targeted therapy for gastrointestinal stromal tumors. *Clin Cancer Res* 15: 3908–3911.
38. Davids M., Charlton A., Ng S.S., *et al.* (2009). Response to a novel multi-targeted tyrosine kinase inhibitor pazopanib in metastatic Merkel cell carcinoma. *J Clin Oncol* 27: e97–e100.

Chapter 9

Imaging of Merkel Cell Carcinoma

Simon Brodsky, Jonathan S. Zager and Claudia G. Berman

9.1 Introduction

The staging of Merkel cell carcinoma is in flux, and there is no consensus as to the best use of imaging modalities in the workup or staging of localized or metastatic Merkel cell carcinoma. At the present time, the Memorial-Sloan Kettering and AJCC staging systems are most frequently used (see Chapter 7).[1] These systems classify Merkel cell carcinoma based on tumor size, lymph node status and the presence or absence of distant metastases. Stage I is distinguished from stage II disease based on the size of the primary tumor (T1, primary 2 cm or less versus T2, primary larger than 2 cm); node-positive disease is stage III. The presence of distant metastatic disease constitutes stage IV. The new 7th edition of the AJCC staging manual incorporates a distinction between macroscopic and microscopic nodal disease, reflecting the significance of detecting occult nodal metastases via sentinel lymph node biopsy. In this chapter we will discuss the initial imaging of localized Merkel cell carcinoma, including the use of localizing studies for sentinel lymph node biopsy, as well as follow-up imaging and the evaluation of patients with known or suspected metastatic disease.

9.2 Initial Imaging of Clinically Node-Negative Primary Merkel Cell Carcinoma

To date, there is no consensus in the literature as to how, and how extensively, patients with localized primary Merkel cell carcinoma should be evaluated prior to surgical intervention. Most patients present without evidence of regional or distant metastases, and extensive imaging prior to surgery has not been shown to have a high yield of findings that will alter management. We feel that the most important aspect of management of patients with clinically localized Merkel cell carcinoma is evaluation of the regional nodal basins with sentinel lymph node biopsy. Of course, any patient who is experiencing symptomatology that would suggest the presence of distant metastases should be evaluated with CT, CT/PET fusion or magnetic resonance imaging as clinically indicated. Given the fact that most patients with Merkel cell carcinoma are older individuals, and many have comorbidities that could impact their risk for general anesthesia, a PA and lateral chest X-ray may be included as part of the preoperative evaluation.

Those patients who present with very large, fungating or bulky primary tumors without evidence of regional nodal metastases, as well as those with clinically evident nodal metastases are at much higher risk of harboring distant metastases, and preoperative imaging is used routinely, as described subsequently.

9.3 Regional Nodal Evaluation — Sentinel Lymph Node Biopsy

Clinical studies, albeit with relatively small numbers of patients, have demonstrated the reliability of sentinel lymph node biopsy in identifying regional nodal metastases in patients presenting with clinically localized Merkel cell carcinoma. Messina and colleagues reported the utility of sentinel lymph node biopsy in Merkel cell carcinoma back in 1997.[2] The authors reported that two of 12 (16%) patients with clinically negative regional nodal basins had a positive sentinel node biopsy, and the remaining ten node-negative patients had not experienced a nodal recurrence in a maximum follow-up period of 26 months. Numerous other studies have substantiated the prognostic role of sentinel lymph node biopsy in Merkel cell carcinoma, but results differ in the number of false-negative biopsies, that is, patients in whom a regional relapse develops despite a negative sentinel node.[3–5] Based on the available data, about one-third of patients with clinically localized Merkel cell carcinoma are found to have nodal metastases on sentinel lymph node biopsy.[6] Incidentally, among these patients, CT had a sensitivity of only 20% in identifying regional nodal disease that was detected on sentinel lymph node biopsy.

Sentinel lymph node biopsy provides the unique capacity to detect *microscopic* nodal disease. As is the case with melanoma, we must presume that no currently available 'macroscopic' imaging technique, such as CT or ^{18}F-fluorodeoxyglucose PET scanning or ^{111}In-octreotide imaging, or any foreseeable alternative, will approach the sensitivity of sentinel lymph node biopsy in the critical function of detecting microscopic node metastasis harbored in clinically negative regional lymph nodes. Sentinel lymph node biopsy for Merkel cell carcinoma is routinely performed using lymphoscintigraphy to identify the regional basin(s) draining the primary site and to identify for the surgeon the number and location of sentinel nodes (Figure 1).

Our standard procedure for sentinel node identification in Merkel cell carcinoma is as follows: A standard large field-of-view camera is used, deploying a low energy, high resolution, parallel hole collimator and a 20% energy window centered at the 140keV ^{99m}technetium energy peak. ^{99m}Tc-labeled sulfur colloid is filtered within two hours of injection using a 0.2 micron filter. Patients with trunk and extremity lesions receive 450 μCi of filtered ^{99m}Tc-labeled sulfur colloid intradermally in four equal aliquots around the lesion or near the center of a biopsy scar. The amount of colloid injected is reduced in head, neck and facial lesions to 250 μCi to minimize the degree to which radiation at the injection site conceals the nearby lymph node basins. This lesser amount of radiopharmaceutical is used whenever the primary tumor is judged to be close to a regional lymph node basin. The total volume of injectate of the radiopharmaceutical varies with the amount of activity used. The 250 μCi doses are in a total volume 0.5–1.0 ml, while the 450 μCi doses are in a total volume of 2 ml using normal saline as the diluent.

The patient is then positioned with the injection site under the gamma camera in the supine position to determine the lymphatic drainage pattern. Cine imaging can be helpful to differentiate lymph nodes from areas of

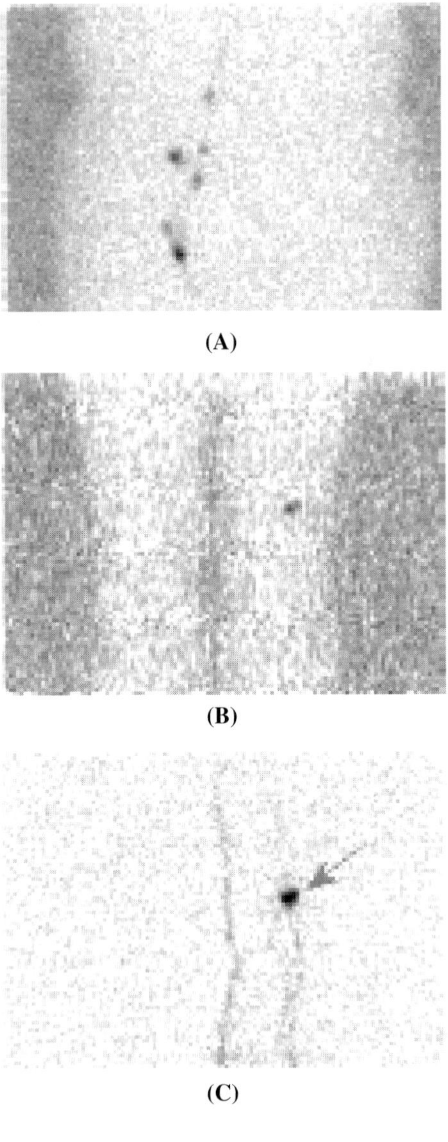

Figure 1. ^{99m}Tc-sulfur colloid lymphoscintigraphy from a patient with a Merkel cell carcinoma involving the right foot. A ^{57}Cobalt flood source is positioned beneath the patient to delineate body contour. **(A)** An image of the pelvis shows drainage to right inguinal and pelvic lymph nodes. **(B)** A posterior image of the mid-legs shows drainage to an ipsilateral popliteal node. **(C)** A posterior image of the mid-legs, taken with optimized visualization of the lymphatic channels, demonstrates two distinct lymphatic channels: one leading to the popliteal node and the other draining more proximally to the groin and pelvis.

stasis in the channel and to identify in-transit lymph nodes. Since more than one basin can provide lymphatic drainage, it is important that all potential drainage basins are imaged in multiple projections. Localization of lymph nodes with regard to normal structures is aided by performing a transmission image using a ^{57}Cobalt flood sheet and outlining anatomical landmarks with a technetium or cobalt pen (Figure 2). Oblique and/or lateral views may also be important for anatomic localization (Figure 2C–2F and Figure 3).

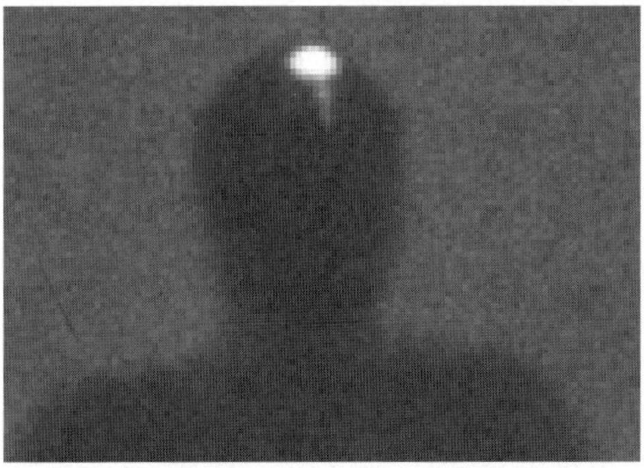

(A)

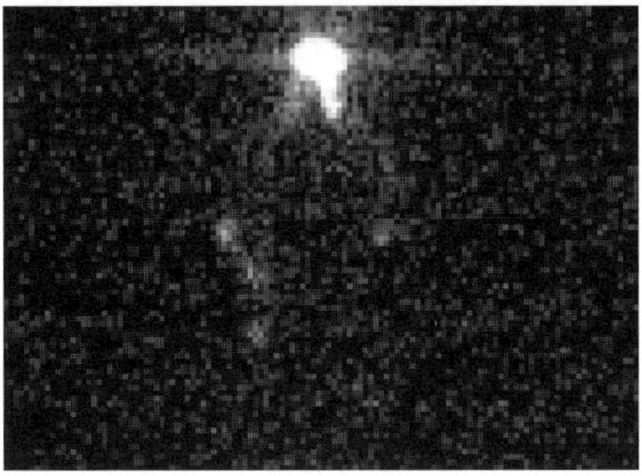

(B)

Figure 2. ^{99m}Tc-sulfur colloid lymphoscintigraphy from a patient with a Merkel cell carcinoma arising in the midline of the scalp. **(A)** Early image of the head and neck shows tracer at the primary site only. **(B)** A slightly later image shows drainage to bilateral cervical lymph nodes. (**C** and **D**, next page). Improved anatomic delineation is achieved with right anterior oblique and (**E** and **F**, subsequent page) left anterior oblique images. Note outlining of the ear, anterior border of the sternocleidomastoid and clavicle with a radioactive pen for additional localization in (C) and (E).

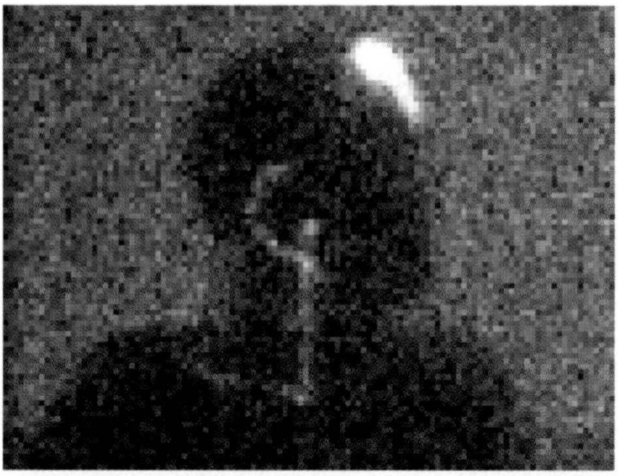

(C)

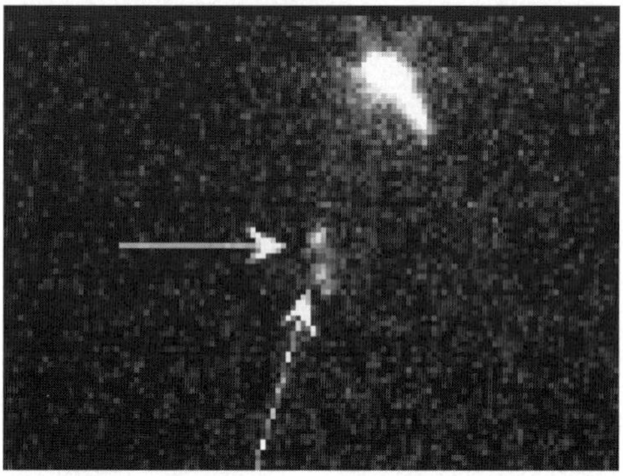

(D)

Figure 2. (*Continued*)

Lymphoscintigraphy in the head and neck area, where a large proportion of Merkel cell carcinomas present, requires particular care and attention to technique. Stadelmann and colleagues have examined their single institution series of 74 patients undergoing preoperative head and neck lymphoscintigraphy for Merkel cell carcinoma or melanoma.[7] In five of their patients (three midline scalp primaries, two cheek primaries) preoperative lymphoscintigraphy failed to identify *any* draining nodal basin, for a localization failure rate of nearly 7%. Intraoperative gamma probe examination failed to detect any areas of radionuclide localization in these

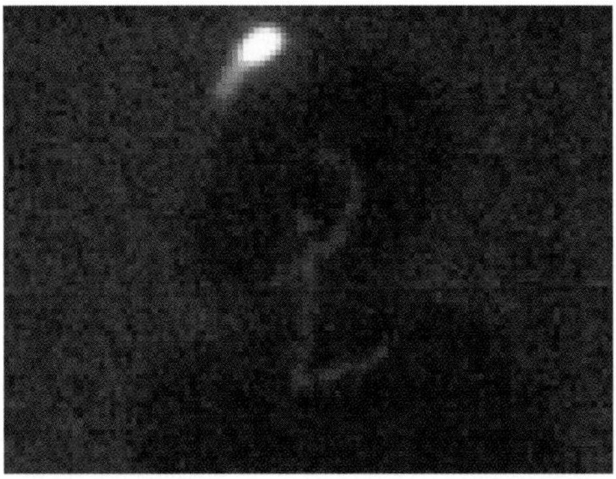

(E)

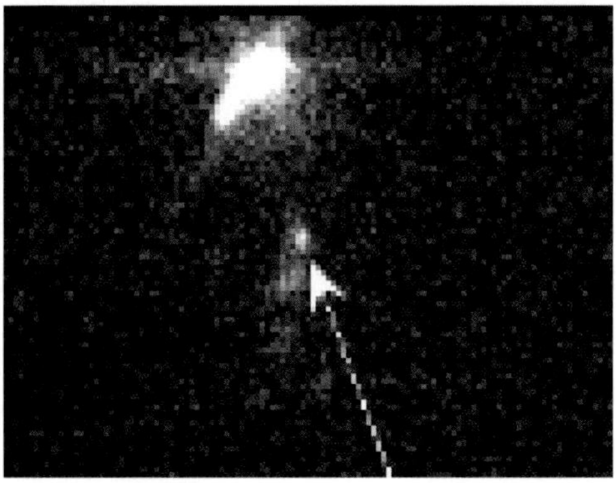

(F)

Figure 2. (*Continued*)

patients, and hence sentinel lymph node biopsy was not performed in any of them. Consistent with this is an intriguing recent report showing discordant nodal basins in approximately one-third of head and neck melanoma or Merkel cell carcinoma patients in whom two lymphoscintigraphic studies were performed on different days prior to sentinel node surgery.[8] Failure to localize to a regional nodal basin despite two consecutive studies was seen in 10% of these patients, consistent with the above and other reports.[9] This 7–10% SLN localization failure rate is not unique to head and neck Merkel cell carcinomas. It was also seen in sentinel

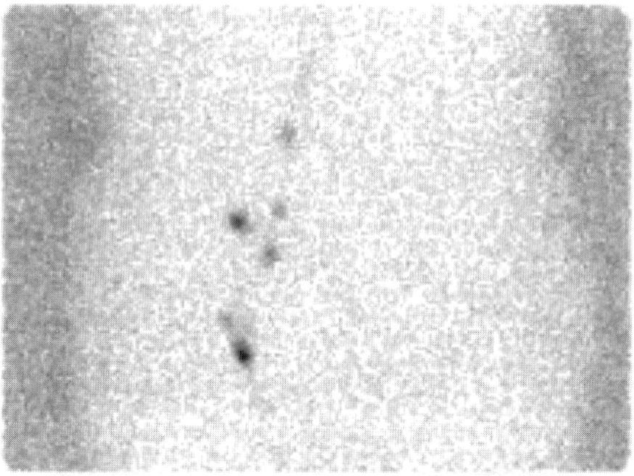

(A)

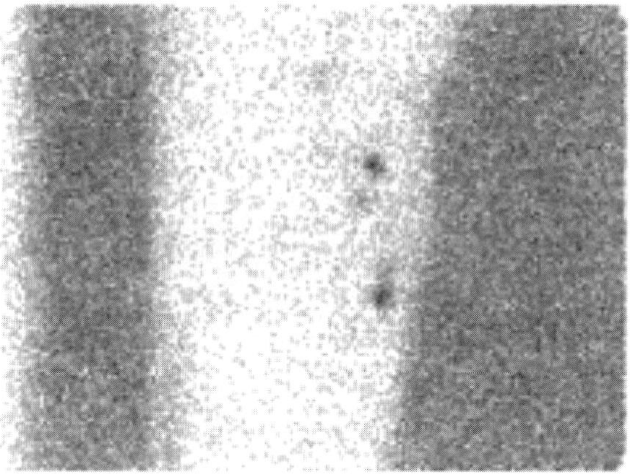

(B)

Figure 3. ^{99m}Tc-sulfur colloid lymphoscintigraphy demonstrating drainage to ipsilateral inguinal and pelvic nodes from a distal leg primary Merkel cell carcinoma. **(A)** Anterior view. **(B)** Lateral view, which allows for localization of lymph node depth relative to the skin. The determination of whether a node is located in the inguinal nodes or the pelvis is best made on this view.

lymph node biopsy for head and neck melanomas, where a study by Doting *et al.*[10] showed that only 33 of 36 patients had a successful sentinel lymph node biopsy of a head and neck melanoma, indicating a 8% failure in identifying the SLN in their small series.

In our experience however, using the techniques outlined above, failure to visualize a sentinel node is very infrequent even for head and neck primaries, occurring in only about 1% of cases. The most likely explanations for non-localization would be the close proximity of the primary tumor to the sentinel node and obstruction of the node by tumor preventing radiotracer uptake, but this cannot explain all cases (Figure 4).[11] Sometimes intraoperative evaluation using vital blue dye and a hand-held gamma detector once the primary has been removed can identify a sentinel node that was obscured by the radioactivity at the primary site. Reports in melanoma have suggested that SPECT lymphoscintigraphy may improve the localization of nodes close to the primary site, and this may ultimately

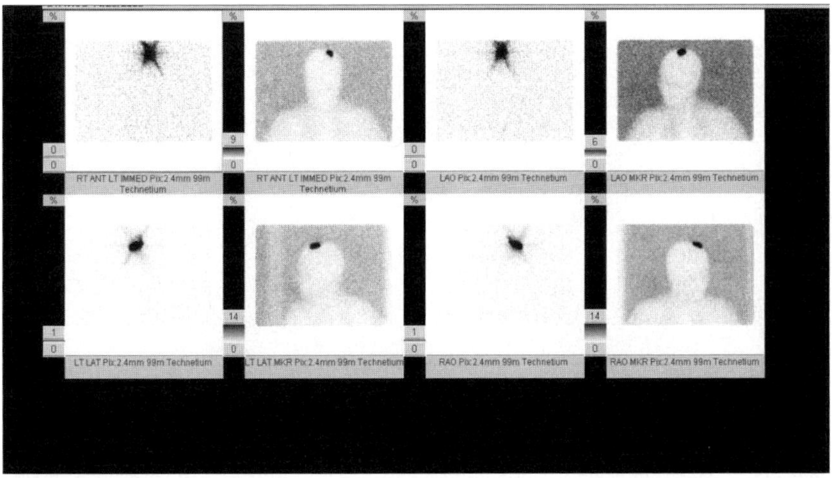

(A)

Figure 4. **(A)** Multiple views from a ^{99m}Tc-sulfur colloid lymphoscintigraphy from a patient with a 1 cm diameter, 3.4 mm thick Merkel cell carcinoma located just to the left of midline on the vertex of the scalp. No drainage is seen to parotid or cervical nodes. Intraoperative evaluation of the nodes with a hand-held gamma detector failed to identify any evidence of a sentinel node, and a postoperative whole-body PET-CT scan as well as ultrasounds of the parotid glands and cervical nodes bilaterally were normal. Approximately five months later, a follow-up cervical ultrasound identified an abnormal 8 mm lymph node in the left neck. (**B** and **C**, next page) PET-CT scan confirmed this lesion to be hypermetabolic. Ultrasound-guided aspiration cytology demonstrated metastatic Merkel cell carcinoma.

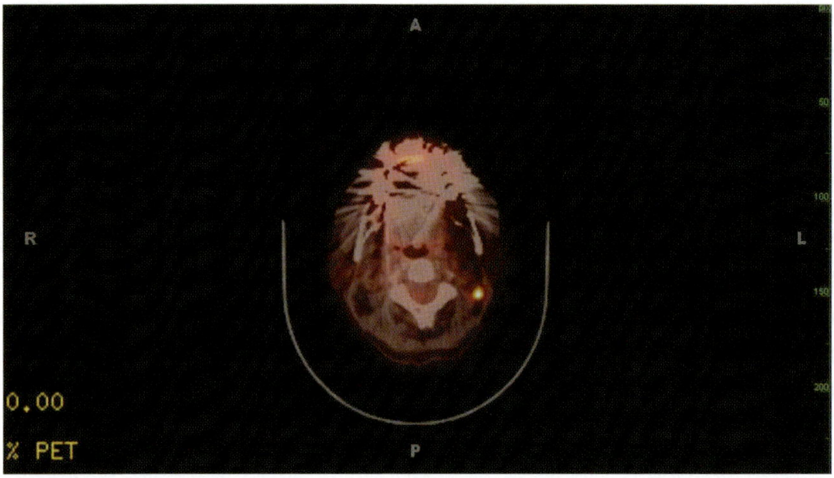

(B)

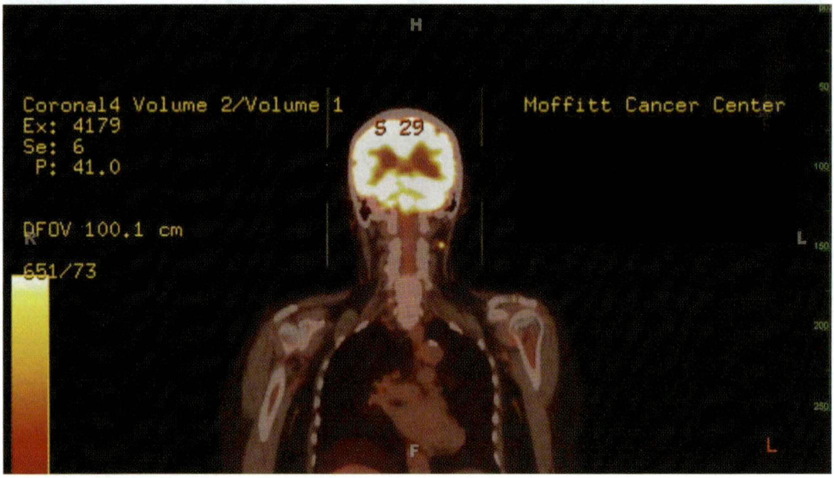

(C)

Figure 4. (*Continued*)

prove to have particular value in head and neck primary tumors.[12] Close clinical follow-up is indicated for any patient in whom lymphoscintigraphy and intraoperative evaluation fails to identify a sentinel node; as discussed below, ultrasound may have a role to play in these patients.[11]

9.4 The Role of Ultrasound in Evaluating Regional Nodal Basins

Increasingly, ultrasound is being used to evaluate regional nodal basins in breast cancer and melanoma,[11,13–16] and the experience we and others have gained with ultrasound in these malignancies has prompted us to extend its use to selected patients with Merkel cell carcinoma. Most centers with experience with preoperative ultrasound evaluation of clinically negative nodal basins for melanoma, including our own, have consistently shown that sentinel node biopsy is much more sensitive for detecting nodal metastasis than ultrasound.[16–19] Nonetheless, some elderly or infirm patients with clinically node-negative Merkel cell carcinoma are at high risk for severe perioperative complications from general anesthesia (which is usually required for sentinel lymph node biopsy). In these patients, we now prefer to evaluate the regional nodal basin using pre-operative high resolution ultrasound, and if that shows no evidence of nodal metastases, we perform an excision of the primary tumor under local anesthesia. We would then routinely follow these nodal basins with serial ultrasounds at each follow-up visit on an every three- to six-month basis. We also use nodal ultrasound to evaluate patients with questionable findings on physical examination not amenable to percutaneous fine needle aspiration cytology during follow-up visits. Nodal ultrasound may also be performed prior to sentinel node biopsy in an attempt to identify macroscopic nodal metastases and facilitate 'one-stage' procedures where the primary excision and nodal dissection are carried out at the same sitting. Which patients, if any, are at high enough risk of having identifiable nodal metastases to justify such an approach remains an unresolved question.

9.5 Imaging of Patients with Stage III Disease

In cases where regional lymph nodes are suspected to be involved based on physical examination, fine needle aspiration cytology is the preferred approach to confirm the diagnosis prior to definitive treatment. Ultrasound guidance is frequently employed to maximize the likelihood of accurately sampling the suspect node. After a diagnosis of a positive lymph node, whether it is clinically evident on initial presentation, as a result of a positive sentinel lymph node biopsy, or at the time of regional nodal recurrence, we will routinely image these patients with high-resolution cross-sectional body imaging, using contrast-enhanced CT scans and/or PET scanning. For patients with microscopic disease found on sentinel lymph node biopsy, this imaging is often deferred until completion lymph node dissection has been performed. Patients with clinically evident nodal disease routinely undergo imaging to rule out distant metastases before definitive surgical and/or radiation treatment.

9.6 Imaging Modalities to Evaluate Metastatic Merkel Cell Carcinoma

There is no established consensus regarding the optimum imaging modalities to identify distant metastatic disease in patients with Merkel cell carcinoma. Most often, based on analogy to cutaneous melanoma and also to small cell lung cancer, imaging consists of contrast-enhanced CT scans or whole body PET scanning. CT abnormalities that have been described among patients with metastatic Merkel cell carcinoma correspond precisely to the imaging characteristics typical more generally of metastatic malignancy.[20] Nuclear medicine imaging agents specific for neuroendocrine cancers, particularly ^{111}In-octreotide, can also be used.

9.6.1 *^{18}FDG PET/CT fusion scanning*

For small cell lung cancer, which shares histologic and clinical features with Merkel cell carcinoma, ^{18}F-fluorodeoxyglucose PET/CT scanning has emerged as the preferred screening modality for distant metastasis.[21] The utility of PET/CT fusion scanning in Merkel cell carcinoma patients for screening high-risk patients, staging patients with documented regional or distant disease, as well as assessing the response to therapy has been well described in the literature. Unfortunately due to the rarity of the disease, there are no large series published nor are there randomized trials comparing one modality to another for the aforementioned clinical scenarios.

The clinical value of ^{18}F-fluorodeoxyglucose PET and CT fusion scanning in Merkel cell carcinoma has recently been discussed by Belhocine and colleagues.[22] In their small series, four patients were imaged for initial staging and seven for recurrence detection. The findings were compared to those obtained from other simultaneous radiologic and clinical findings. It was the authors' impression that PET/CT was clinically helpful in the majority of the patients studied. Documented false negative results are provided for an instance of brain metastasis and another of regional nodal metastasis. The authors, as have others,[23] stress inclusion of the complete extremities to not miss the occasional distant subcutaneous or bony extremity metastases seen in this disease.

Using whole body PET/CT fusion scanning as a screening modality in high-risk Merkel cell carcinoma patients has been described by numerous investigators.[24-26] Peloshek *et al.*[25] describe the comparison of PET/CT and conventional CT findings in patients with Merkel cell carcinoma. Iagaru *et al.*[26] describe their use of PET/CT as an initial screening modality or for restaging in a small series of patients with Merkel cell carcinoma. The authors mention that findings were seen in 50% of the patients that had imaging, and these findings were confirmed as Merkel cell carcinoma on histopathological examination. One patient had a hot spot in the sigmoid colon that was biopsied and proven to be a colon adenocarcinoma. Two patients (33% of their series) who had negative initial PET/CT scans continue to have negative exams on subsequent follow-up over one year after diagnosis.

PET/CT fusion scanning is not only useful in determining the extent of disease at diagnosis, but it has been proven useful to gauge the response to therapy in patients with distant disease.[27]

It is therefore our experience and practice to utilize ^{18}F-fluorodeoxyglucose PET/CT as the primary imaging modality in patients with regional or distant metastases of Merkel cell carcinoma (Figures 4 to 6).[28] High-resolution CT, including triple-phase contrast-enhanced CT for suspected liver metastasis, as well as magnetic resonance imaging (MRI) and occasionally somatostatin receptor scintigraphy with ^{111}In-octreotide, remain useful for clinical problem solving in special circumstances.

9.6.2 ^{111}*Indium octreotide scanning*

Functional nuclear medicine imaging for Merkel cell carcinoma is available utilizing neuroendocrine-specific tagged moieties as well as

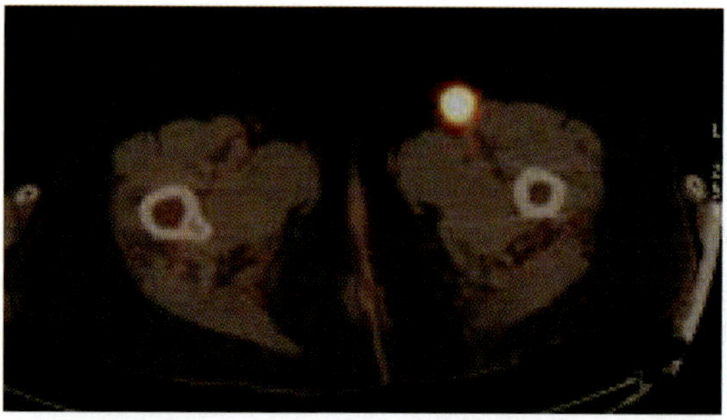

(A)

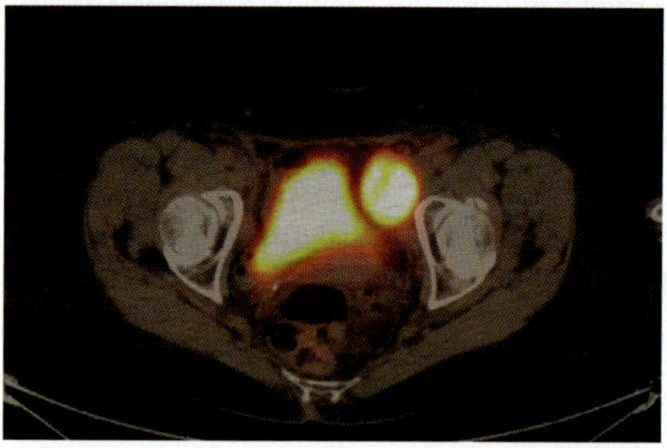

(B)

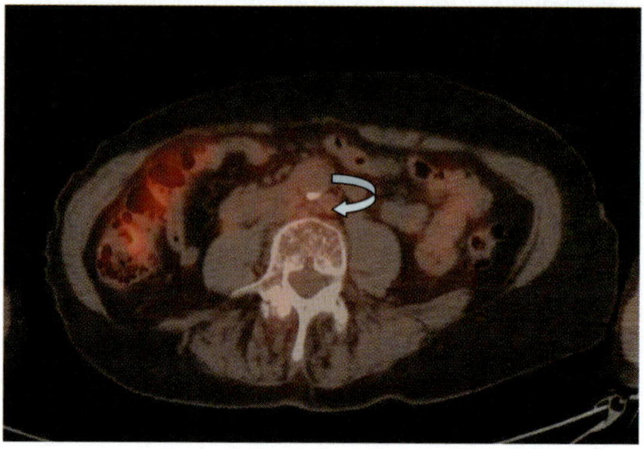

(C)

Figure 5. ^{18}F-fluorodeoxyglucose PET scan images from a patient with metastatic Merkel cell carcinoma to lymph nodes in the groin and pelvis. **(A)** Increased uptake of the radiotracer was present in lymph node metastases in the left groin and **(B)** external iliac nodal basins. **(C)** A slightly enlarged but PET-negative para-aortic lymph node (arrow) was seen and proved to be histologically negative.

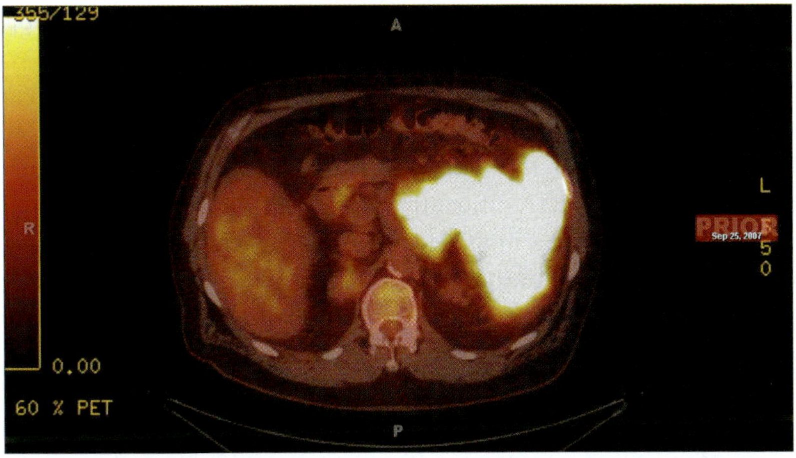

(A)

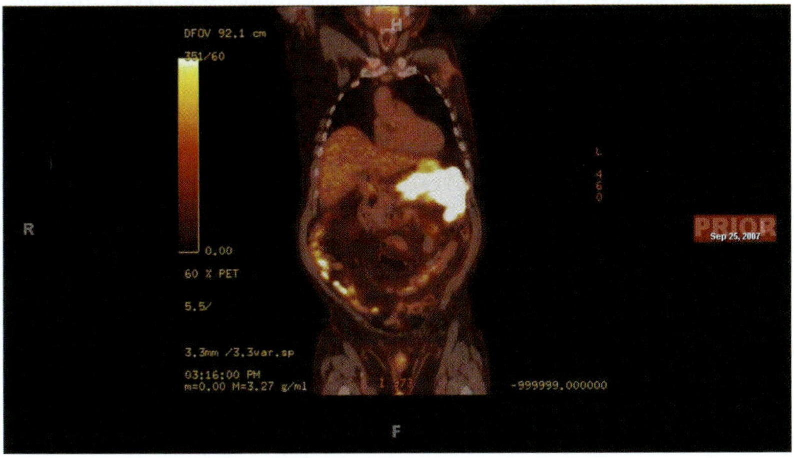

(B)

Figure 6. ^{18}F-fluorodeoxyglucose PET scan images from a patient with widespread metastatic Merkel cell carcinoma. Axial **(A)** and coronal **(B)** views demonstrate a large, hypermetabolic mass in the left upper quadrant of the abdomen, but also abnormal activity in the right lower quadrant consistent with peritoneal implants.

non-specific tagged metabolic indicator molecules. In the former instance, ^{111}Indium octreotide scintigraphy is readily available and supersedes less specific agents previously employed such as ^{123}Iodine-MIBG.[29]

The first clinical use of the radiolabeled somatostatin analogue ^{111}In-octreotide as a nuclear medicine imaging agent in patients with Merkel cell carcinoma was undertaken in Rotterdam in the early 1990s.[30] In this small series, somatostatin receptor scintigraphy with radiolabeled octreotide was able to identify all tumor deposits seen by ultrasound or CT and, significantly, was able to identify nodal disease not detected by CT one month prior to the development of clinically apparent adenopathy. Additionally, imaged disease in another patient regressed on serial octreotide imaging following apparently effective systemic chemotherapy.

A more recent, somewhat larger study from the Institut Gustave Roussy describes their seven-year experience with 20 patients.[31] While the specificity was high (96%) utilizing histopathology as the standard, sensitivity was low, only 78%. In particular, skin and liver metastases were not identified, in the latter case at least in part because of high background activity within the liver. It is the conclusion of these authors as well as others publishing more recently that somatostatin receptor scintigraphy with radiolabeled octreotide is not a reliable technology for clinical decision making.[32] We resort to octreotide scanning only rarely, chiefly when other tools for identifying metastases are equivocal or impractical.

9.6.3 *Magnetic resonance imaging*

MRI, in Merkel cell carcinoma as in other malignancies, is best utilized to identify otherwise clinically and radiographically indistinct soft tissue abnormalities, especially in brain and bone marrow. It affords the most accurate method for determining the presence of metastatic disease in these tissues. Brain metastases are rare in Merkel cell carcinoma but do occur on occasion (Figure 7) and have been described in the literature.[33] Their incidence as a first site of metastasis is not clear, and appears to be much less commonplace as an initial site of metastasis compared to melanoma and small cell lung cancer. In our practice, we do not obtain MRI of the brain in the absence of suggestive symptoms, even in patients with documented metastatic disease beyond the regional nodes.[34]

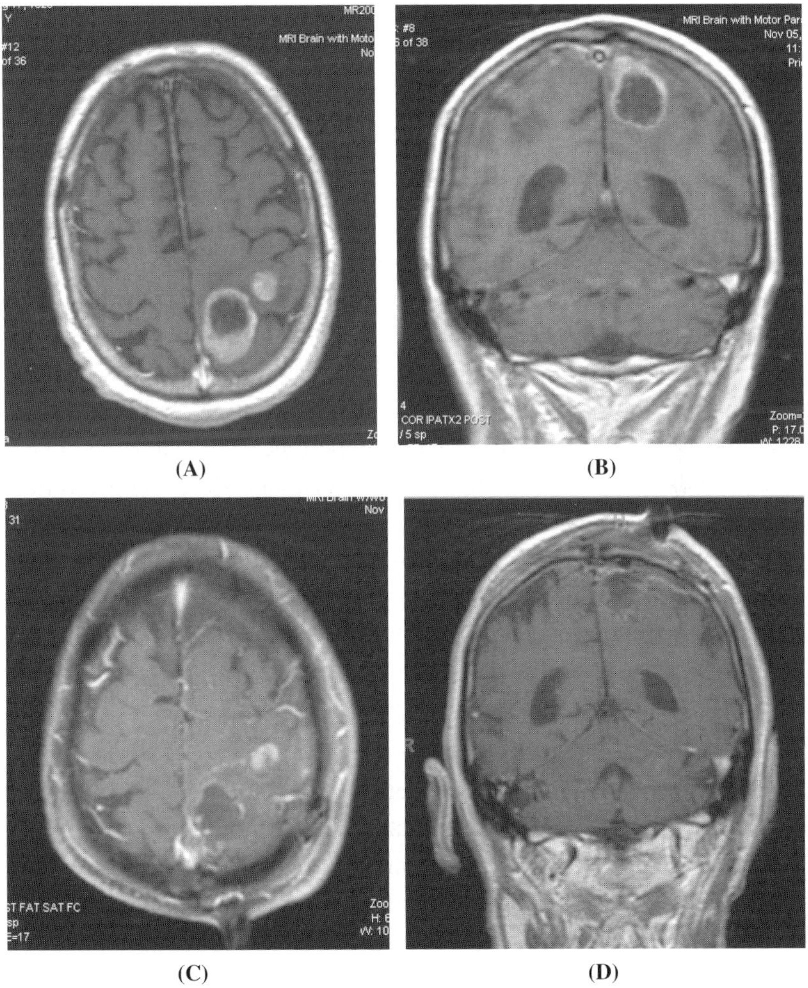

Figure 7. (**A**) T1 axial post-contrast MR scan shows a large Merkel cell carcinoma metastasis in the mesial left parietal lobe with peripheral contrast enhancement and associated edema. A second enhancing lesion is seen anterior and lateral to the larger lesion. (**B**) T1 coronal post-contrast MR scan shows the large mesial left parietal lesion with peripheral enhancement and vasogenic edema. (**C**) T1 axial post-contrast MR scan following resection of the mesial left parietal lobe lesion shows a post-operative CSF collection and a small amount of peripheral enhancement. The smaller enhancing lesion in the left parietal lobe persists. (**D**) T1 coronal post contrast MR scan following resection of the mesial left parietal lobe lesion shows a post-operative CSF collection and a small amount of peripheral enhancement. Post-craniotomy changes are also evident.

9.7 Merkel Cell Carcinoma from Unknown Primary Sites

Merkel cell carcinoma occasionally presents with metastatic disease involving lymph nodes or distant sites in the absence of a clinically evident cutaneous primary tumor. As is the case with metastatic melanoma from an unknown primary site, regression of the primary tumor or removal or ablation of the primary without obtaining a correct histologic diagnosis likely explain most such cases. In cases of apparent unknown primary Merkel cell carcinoma, however, one must also consider the possibility of unrecognized small cell lung carcinoma or another neuroendocrine primary, particular in instances where there is histologic uncertainty of the diagnosis, as with CK-20 negative or TTF-1 positive immunohistochemistry. While in our experience an extensive imaging workup rarely adds to the identification of primary Merkel cell carcinoma in unknown primary cases, PET/CT and/or high resolution chest CT scanning, coupled when needed with ^{111}In-octreotide imaging, can be valuable to exclude an unrecognized primary lung small cell cancer or intraabdominal neuroendocrine primary tumor.[35]

9.8 Follow-Up

The median time to recurrence of Merkel cell carcinoma after unsuccessful surgical treatment is approximately eight months. Up to 90% of recurrences will occur within five years.[36,37] We pay particular attention to nodal basins at risk for relapse, and employ nodal ultrasound every three to six months for surveillance of those patients who did not have sentinel lymph node biopsy (such as the elderly and infirm or patients presenting after wide excision and reconstruction) as well as in patients who had a positive sentinel lymph node biopsy but did not undergo a completion regional lymphadenectomy or nodal irradiation. After the first two years, these regional nodal basin ultrasounds are performed less frequently.

The value of 'early detection' of asymptomatic metastatic Merkel cell carcinoma is much less clear-cut. There is no consensus on whether and how often to employ full body imaging in the form of PET/CT or other modalities, but we frequently use PET/CT to follow patients at high risk for distant relapse, such as those with clinically positive nodal involvement and those with distant metastases in complete remission following chemotherapy or other therapies.

9.9 Conclusion

Recommendations for imaging of Merkel cell carcinoma, for example as provided in the 2008 Guidelines of the National Comprehensive Cancer Network (NCCN), are vague at best: 'as clinically indicated.'[1] The rarity and clinical variability of Merkel cell carcinoma has so far prevented the completion of meaningful randomized trials that might provide data-driven preferences for one imaging modality over another in specific situations. This uncertainty applies both to staging and surveillance phases of management. At H. Lee Moffitt Cancer Center, we have come to rely on using lymphoscintigraphy and sentinel lymph node biopsy to stage those patients that have clinically negative nodal basins. We are judicious with our use of ultrasound of regional nodal basins at regular intervals for those patients at high risk for regional recurrence. We employ whole body cross-sectional imaging in the form of contrast-enhanced CT scans and/or ^{18}F-fluorodeoxyglucose PET/CT as imaging modalities of choice for staging those patients who are at high risk for distant disease, such as those with large primary tumors and those with known regional nodal disease. In addition, we are liberal with our whole body imaging modalities in those patients who are symptomatic or undergoing systemic therapy, to evaluate response to therapy. The low incidence of CNS metastases in our experience has led us to reserve imaging of the brain with MRI for patients with suggestive symptoms.

References

1. Miller S.J., Alam M., Andersen J., *et al.* (2009). Merkel cell carcinoma. *J Natl Compr Canc Netw* 7: 322–332.
2. Messina J.L., Reintgen D.S., Cruse C.W., *et al.* (1997). Selective lymphadenectomy in patients with Merkel cell (cutaneous neuroendocrine) carcinoma. *Ann Surg Oncol* 4: 389–395.

3. Ortin-Perez J., van Rijk M.C., Valdes-Olmos R.A., *et al.* (2007). Lymphatic mapping and sentinel node biopsy in Merkel's cell carcinoma. *Eur J Surg Oncol* 33: 119–122.
4. Maza S., Trefzer U., Hoffman M., *et al.* (2006). Impact of sentinel lymph node biopsy in patients with Merkel cell carcinoma: results of a prospective study and review of the literature. *Eur J Nucl Med Mol Imaging* 33: 433–440.
5. Warner R.E., Quinn M.J., Hruby G., *et al.* (2008). Management of Merkel cell carcinoma: the roles of lymphoscintigraphy, sentinel lymph node biopsy and adjuvant radiotherapy. *Ann Surg Oncol* 15: 2509–2518.
6. Gupta S.G., Wang L.C., Penas P.F., *et al.* (2006). Sentinel lymph node biopsy for evaluation and treatment of patients with Merkel cell carcinoma. The Dana-Farber experience and meta-analysis of the literature. *Arch Dermatol* 142: 685–690.
7. Stadelmann W.K., Cobbins L., Lentsch E.J. (2004). Incidence of nonlocalization of sentinel lymph nodes using preoperative lymphoscintigraphy in 74 consecutive head and neck melanoma and Merkel cell carcinoma patients. *Ann Plast Surg* 52: 546–550.
8. Willis A.I., Ridge J.A. (2007). Discordant lymphatic drainage patterns revealed by serial lymphoscintigraphy in cutaneous head and neck malignancies. *Head Neck* 29: 979–985.
9. Jansen L., Koops H.S., Nieweg O.E., *et al.* (2000). Sentinel node biopsy for melanoma in the head and neck region. *Head Neck* 22: 27–33.
10. Doting E.H., de Vries M., Plukker J.T., *et al.* (2006). Does sentinel lymph node biopsy in cutaneous head and neck melanoma alter disease outcome? *J Surg Oncol* 93: 564–570.
11. Lam T.K., Uren R.F., Scolyer R.A., *et al.* (2009). False-negative sentinel node biopsy because of obstruction of lymphatics by metastatic melanoma: the value of ultrasound in conjunction with preoperative lymphoscintigraphy. *Melanoma Res* 19: 94–99.
12. Mar M.V., Miller S.A., Kim E.E., Macapinlac H.A. (2007). Evaluation and localization of lymphatic drainage and sentinel lymph nodes in patients with head and neck melanomas by hybrid SPECT/CT lymphoscintigraphic imaging. *J Nuc Med Technol* 35: 10–16.
13. Voit C., Kron M., Schäfer G., *et al.* (2006). Ultrasound-guided fine needle aspiration cytology prior to sentinel lymph node biopsy in melanoma patients. *Ann Surg Oncol* 13: 1682–1689.

14. Blum A., Schmid-Wendtner M.H., Mauss-Kiefer V., *et al.* (2006). Ultrasound mapping of lymph node and subcutaneous metastases in patients with cutaneous melanoma: results of a prospective multicenter study. *Dermatology* 212: 47–52.
15. Davis J.T., Brill Y.M., Simmons S., *et al.* (2006). Ultrasound-guided fine-needle aspiration of clinically negative lymph nodes versus sentinel node mapping in patients at high risk for axillary metastasis. *Ann Surg Oncol* 13: 1545–1552.
16. Eggermont A.M. (2005). Reducing the need for sentinel node procedures by ultrasound examination of regional lymph nodes. *Ann Surg Oncol* 12: 3–5.
17. van Rijk M.C., Teertstra H.J., Peterse J.L., *et al.* (2006). Ultrasonography and fine-needle aspiration cytology in the preoperative evaluation of melanoma patients eligible for sentinel node biopsy. *Ann Surg Oncol* 13: 1511–1516.
18. Starritt E.C., Uren R.F., Scolyer R.A., *et al.* (2005). Ultrasound examination of sentinel nodes in the initial assessment of patients with primary cutaneous melanoma. *Ann Surg Oncol* 12: 18–23.
19. Rossi C.R., Pasquali S., Mocellin S. (2008). Actual false-negative rate prompts the routine use of ultrasound scan before and after sentinel node biopsy in melanoma. *Ann Surg Oncol* 15: 2976–2977.
20. Golan H., Volkov O., Linchinsky O., Melloul M. (2005). FDG-PET imaging in Merkel cell carcinoma — value of head-to-toe scan. *Nucl Med Rev Cent East Eur* 8: 135–136.
21. Yamamoto Y., Kameyama R., Murota M., *et al.* (2009). Early assessment of therapeutic response using FDG PET in small cell lung cancer. *Mol Imaging Biol* 11: 467–472.
22. Belhocine T., Pierard G., Frühling J., *et al.* (2006). Clinical added-value of 18FDG PET in neuroendocrine-Merkel cell carcinoma. *Oncol Rep* 16: 347–352.
23. Gollub M.J., Gruen D.R., Dershaw D.D. (1996). Merkel cell carcinoma: CT findings in 12 patients. *AJR Am J Roentgenol* 167: 617–620.
24. Scanga D.R., Martin W.H., Delbeke D. (2004). Value of FDG PET imaging in the management of patients with thyroid, neuroendocrine, and neural crest tumors. *Clin Nucl Med* 29: 86–90.
25. Peloschek P., Novotny C., Mueller-Mang C., *et al.* (2010). Diagnostic imaging in Merkel cell carcinoma: lessons to learn from 16 cases with correlation of sonography, CT, MRI and PET. *Eur J Radiol* 73: 317–323.

26. Iagaru A., Quon A., McDougall I.R., Gambhir S.S. (2006). Merkel cell carcinoma: is there a role for 2-deoxy-2-[f-18]fluoro-D-glucose-positron emission tomography/computed tomography? *Mol Imaging Biol* 8: 212–217.
27. Yao M., Smith R.B., Hoffman H.T., *et al.* (2005). Merkel cell carcinoma: two case reports focusing on the role of fluorodeoxyglucose positron emission tomography imaging in staging and surveillance. *Am J Clin Oncol* 28: 205–210.
28. Garneski K.M., Nghiem P. (2007). Merkel cell carcinoma adjuvant therapy: current data support radiation but not chemotherapy. *J Am Acad Dermatol* 57: 166–169.
29. Watanabe N., Shimizu M., Kageyama M., *et al.* (1998). ^{123}I-MIBG SPECT of Merkel cell carcinoma. *Br J Radiol* 71: 886–887.
30. Kwekkeboom D.J., Hoff A.M., Lamberts S.W., *et al.* (1992). Somatostatin analogue scintigraphy. A simple and sensitive method for the in vivo visualization of Merkel cell tumors and their metastases. *Arch Dermatol* 128: 818–821.
31. Guitera-Rovel P., Lumbroso J., Gautier-Gougis M.S., *et al.* (2001). Indium-111 octreotide scintigraphy of Merkel cell carcinomas and their metastases. *Ann Oncol* 12: 807–811.
32. Durani B.K., Klein A., Henze M., *et al.* (2003). Somatostatin analogue scintigraphy in Merkel cell tumours. *Br J Dermatol* 148: 1135–1140.
33. Ikawa F., Kiya K., Uozumi T., *et al.* (1999). Brain metastasis from Merkel cell carcinoma: case report and review of the literature. *Neurosurg Rev* 22: 54–57.
34. Medina-Franco H., Urist M.M., Fiveash J., *et al.* (2001). Multimodality treatment of Merkel cell carcinoma: case series and literature review of 1024 cases. *Ann Surg Oncol* 8: 204–208.
35. Cheuk W., Kwan M.Y., Suster S., Chan J.K. (2001). Immunostaining for thyroid transcription factor 1 and cytokeratin 20 aids the distinction of small cell carcinoma from Merkel cell carcinoma, but not pulmonary from extrapulmonary small cell carcinomas. *Arch Pathol Lab Med* 125: 228–231.
36. Bajetta E., Celio L., Platania M., *et al.* (2009) Single-institution series of early-stage Merkel cell carcinoma: long-term outcomes in 95 patients managed with surgery alone. *Ann Surg Oncol* 16: 2985–2993.
37. National Comprehensive Cancer Network, Inc. (2008). *Practice Guidelines in Oncology*. Version 12008. 01/03/08. www.nccn.org

Chapter 10

Surgical Management of Merkel Cell Carcinoma

Melanie D. Prince, C. Wayne Cruse, Vernon K. Sondak and Jonathan S. Zager

Merkel cell carcinoma is an aggressive neuroendocrine tumor of the skin. Although a variety of treatment methods are described in the literature, it is widely agreed that surgical excision is the treatment of choice for both primary Merkel cell carcinoma and regional metastasis. However, a multimodality approach to treatment including radiation and systemic chemotherapy may improve survival and should be considered when evaluating patients with Merkel cell carcinoma and discussing treatment options, especially those with regional or distant metastases. In an ideal situation, the management of Merkel cell carcinoma patients should be discussed at a tumor board including surgeons, radiation oncologists, medical oncologists and pathologists to collectively determine an appropriate multidisciplinary treatment regimen (see Chapter 18). In this chapter we will discuss the role of surgery in the management of primary, regional and distant metastatic Merkel cell carcinoma.

10.1 Primary Tumor Excision

Surgical excision is the gold standard initial treatment of the primary tumor in Merkel cell carcinoma. The goal of excision is the complete removal of the tumor with histologically negative margins around the periphery and deep to the tumor. A few unresolved issues that need to be studied further are (1) the optimal width of excision and (2) the indications for use of adjuvant radiation to the primary site and its influence on local recurrence.

Since Merkel cell carcinoma is rare, a randomized prospective trial comparing narrow versus wide margins of excision has never been performed. The National Comprehensive Cancer Network (NCCN) recommends excision with at least a 1–2 cm margin around the clinically obvious tumor.[1] It has been reported in individual institutional series that 1 to 2 cm margins are associated with acceptably low local recurrence rates.[2–5]

The optimal margin of excision is controversial in the literature. Bichakjian *et al.* performed an extensive review of the literature regarding treatment of Merkel cell carcinoma. Although the authors did not specifically provide evidence in favor of 1 cm versus wider margins, they concluded based on the available evidence (including some studies using Mohs surgery) that margins of 1 cm did not lead to increased local recurrence rates and that 2 cm margins should be 'reserved for larger lesions that measure greater than 2 cm in greatest dimension when feasible.'[4]

Allen *et al.* reported patient-, tumor- and treatment-related factors and their relationship on local recurrence and overall survival.[2] This large retrospective review of 251 patients treated at a single institution resulted in the following conclusions: after a median wide excision margin of 1.1 cm, local recurrence rates were 8% in those with histologically negative excision margins but 18% in those with microscopically positive margins. Although this difference was not statistically significant, the authors still recommended margin-negative resection as the standard treatment. Margin widths of more than 1 cm were also not associated with a statistically significant decrease in local recurrence in their series. Other studies have also found no clear correlation between margin width and local recurrence rates.[4,6–10] The influence of tumor diameter on local recurrence was not reported in this series, but larger tumors (≥2 cm) were more likely to be treated with adjuvant radiation to the surgical bed in their series; 23% received radiation compared to 10% for those with tumors smaller than 2 cm.

Overall, Allen *et al.* found that the use of adjuvant radiation was not associated with a decreased rate of local recurrence (8% without radiation vs. 10% with radiation). In particular, there was no evidence that the addition of radiation in those with histologically negative margins reduced local recurrence rates.

Another article in favor of surgery alone as primary treatment was recently published by Bajetta *et al.* where the authors analyzed 95 consecutive patients with Merkel cell carcinoma managed with wide excision of the primary tumor.[11] The regional nodal basins at risk were managed by either observation ($n = 42$), sentinel node biopsy ($n = 21$) or a complete node dissection for clinically involved lymph nodes ($n = 32$). With a median follow-up of 65 months, the authors reported a 5% local recurrence rate in the entire cohort, with most of those recurrences seen in patients with head and neck tumors (19%) and very few with extremity and truncal tumors (2%). They also reported no regional recurrences in patients if there were no involved nodes or 1 to 2 involved lymph nodes, compared to 39% if there were 3 or more lymph nodes involved ($p < 0.0004$).[11] It is important to note that none of the patients in this series were treated with adjuvant radiation to either the primary tumor site or regional nodal basin. Therefore, the results of this study suggest a more limited role for the addition of radiation after surgery, potentially focusing on local control of head and neck primary tumors and on regional control for patients with multiple involved lymph nodes.

Medina-Franco *et al.* published a small retrospective series and a literature review in 2001 describing patient, tumor and treatment variables that influenced survival and recurrence (local, regional and distant).[5] Their review summarized the findings of 11 single-institution reviews, including 441 patients, where local recurrence rates were reported and compared between those who received excision alone and those who received excision plus adjuvant radiation to the surgical bed. Of the 11 studies, 5 reported a significantly lower rate of local recurrence for patients who received adjuvant radiation. Although more than half of the series showed no significant improvement in local control with adjuvant radiation, when the data from all 441 patients were analyzed in aggregate, the local recurrence rate with radiation was significantly lower: 10.5% (range 0–33%) vs. 52.6% (range 6–100%) without radiation ($p < 0.00001$). Obviously many factors may play a role in these results such as width of excision, depth of excision and location of the primary tumor.[5]

Subsequently, other authors have found a significant role for radiation in increasing local control, and possibly improving survival, after wide excision. Jabbour *et al.* reported on a series of 82 patients treated with wide excision with or without radiation to the primary site and/or regional nodal basin. In this series, the median width of excision was 3 cm. The authors concluded that the addition of radiation to the surgical bed resulted in increased time to first recurrence (24.2 vs. 11.8 months) as well as increased survival (53.9 vs. 45.7 months). Neither of these differences was statistically significant. On multivariate analysis, however, *any* radiation (to the primary site and/or the regional basin) was associated with a significantly prolonged time to first recurrence (hazard ratio 0.39, 95% confidence interval 0.20–0.75; $p = 0.004$) and significantly improved survival (hazard ratio 0.39, 95% confidence interval 0.18–0.82; $p = 0.013$). A significant limitation of this study is that it is difficult if not impossible to sort out the contribution of radiation to the primary site from radiation to the nodal basin, but this series does provide one of the strongest arguments to date in favor of routine postoperative radiation.[12]

Warner *et al.* recently published results from a small series from the same institution. All patients underwent preoperative lymphoscintigraphy to identify the location of the sentinel node; some then had sentinel node biopsy and/or nodal irradiation. The median excision width for the primary tumor was 1.5 cm (range 6 mm to 3 cm). Nine of these patients had postoperative radiation to the primary site while eight did not. No local recurrences were noted during follow-up (median of 16 months) in either group, and there was one in-transit recurrence in each group. Despite these results, the authors conclude that their 'study strongly supports the use of radiation to both the primary site and the regional lymph node field for optimal loco-regional control.'[13]

Because of the rarity of this tumor, there have been no randomized trials conducted to determine the most appropriate margins of excision or the use of adjuvant radiation to the surgical bed after an excision. In our experience, postoperative radiation clearly has a role to play but is not required routinely. In the rare case of Merkel cell carcinoma of the digits treated with amputation, postoperative radiation is not utilized if a histologically negative margin has been achieved. In the more common situation of Merkel cell carcinoma treated with a 1 or 2 cm wide excision (wider margins are not routinely utilized at our institution), postoperative radiation is utilized whenever a negative margin is not achievable or when the excision width is compromised in any way (as commonly occurs in the head and neck region). Although some authors have focused on larger tumor diameter as an indicator for postoperative radiation, in our practice we are more likely to consider histologic factors: patients with deep Merkel cell tumors (>4 mm) and those with angiolymphatic invasion are more likely to be referred for adjuvant radiotherapy.

10.2 Surgical Management of Head and Neck Merkel Cell Carcinoma

Merkel cell carcinoma is commonly found on the head and neck. The margins of resection in this region are often modified to maximize the aesthetic and functional result. Although aesthetic and functional concerns must be considered, the primary oncological goal of complete surgical excision remains paramount. Special considerations for Merkel cell carcinoma of the head and neck are covered in Chapter 11.

Mohs micrographic surgery has been proposed and used by some surgeons where tissue conservation is important.[3] It has been shown to have very good results in terms of local recurrence, especially in the head and neck.[3] Mohs micrographic surgery has been shown to compare favorably with wide local excision.[3,4,14] The role and rationale of Mohs surgery in the management of Merkel cell carcinoma is discussed in Chapter 12.

10.3 Reconstruction of the Excision Defect

The surgical treatment of the primary tumor includes planning the excision and reconstruction simultaneously. Methods of reconstruction should be considered before the primary tumor excision because the extent and configuration of the excision will influence the reconstructive method used. The method of reconstruction needed will depend upon the size, depth and location of the defect created by the primary tumor excision. Reconstructive options must also consider the patient's overall medical condition, aesthetic and functional requirements of the patient, the need for sentinel lymph node biopsy and the potential need for adjuvant radiation. In most cases, a 1 to 2 cm margin can be achieved and a primary linear closure can be performed. Generally, when there are larger defects that cannot be closed primarily, reconstructive options include split thickness skin grafts, full thickness skin grafts, local advancement flaps, regional rotational flaps and free flaps. The following will discuss the method of reconstruction by the tumor location. Head and neck reconstruction is covered in detail in Chapter 11.

10.3.1 *Trunk*

Defects on the trunk are frequently closed primarily. If the defect is too large for primary closure, skin grafts or local flaps may be used. The most common reconstruction method used in our institution is skin grafting, using either full or split thickness skin grafts. Other options include local advancement, rotational and transpositional flaps. A double rhomboid flap is a good choice in many locations on the trunk because it leaves a minimal contour deformity.

10.3.2 *Hand and upper extremity*

For Merkel cell carcinomas on the distal aspects of the digits (hand or foot), amputation with 1 to 2 cm margins proximal to the tumor is the surgical procedure of choice. This is usually carried out through the next proximal interphalangeal joint, as is done in melanoma of the digits. In considering reconstructive options of the hand and upper extremity, functional outcome is the most important consideration. Skin grafts are a good choice because they are thin and conform to the hand. When prevention of contracture is important, full thickness skin grafts should be used instead of split thickness skin grafts. If there is exposed tendon without paratenon or bone without periosteum, skin grafting should not be performed as the grafts are likely to fail because of lack of blood supply from underlying tissues. Critical structures such as nerves and blood vessels require more coverage than skin grafting alone can provide. In these situations we recommend that advancement, rotational, or transpositional flaps be used to cover the aforementioned critical structures. For larger defects a radial forearm flap, reverse radial forearm flap or posterior interosseus flap could be considered. Free flaps are used for complicated and extensive defects.

10.3.3 *Lower extremity*

Defects of the thigh can be closed primarily if free of tension. Local flaps may also be used with a good cosmetic result. The abundant muscle mass in the thigh allows for many reconstructive options. Fasciocutaneous flaps include the posterior thigh flap, anterior lateral thigh flap and tensor fascia lata flap. Local muscle flaps include the gracilis, rectus femoris and vastus lateralis. Distant flaps or free flaps are rarely indicated.

A lower leg defect may be skin grafted with good results. We reported on the sentinel node biopsy incision site as the donor site for full thickness skin grafts, but use this approach sparingly in Merkel cell carcinoma because of the frequent use of postoperative radiation.[15] Local flaps, such as the keystone flap,[16] are also a good choice for smaller defects. If muscle coverage is required, the optimal flap depends upon the location and size of the defect. Defects in the proximal third of the leg may be covered with a gastrocnemius flap. The medial head of the muscle may be stretched farther than the lateral head, but either can be used. Middle leg defects may be covered with a proximally based soleus flap. Defects of the distal third of the leg may be covered using a reverse sural artery flap, dorsalis pedis flap or a distally based soleus flap. Free tissue transfer is routinely used for defects of the distal third of the leg.

10.3.4 *Foot*

Split thickness skin grafting may be used on the dorsal and plantar surface of the foot with good results. This allows thin coverage so a shoe can be easily worn. It may be necessary to perform a local rotational flap. Free flaps may be used for complicated defects.

10.3.5 *Delayed reconstruction*

Immediate reconstruction or simple linear closure may be performed for most uncomplicated Merkel cell carcinoma excisions. If the tumor is located near an aesthetically or functionally sensitive area, a significant defect will likely require a more complicated type of reconstruction. In addition, if there is any doubt about the adequacy of excision (possible microscopically involved margins), it may be preferred to delay reconstruction and use a temporary wound closure until the final margin status has been evaluated by the pathologist. This allows detailed pathological evaluation of the peripheral and deep margins with definitive reconstruction being preformed in a subsequent operation. Human allograft skin or a VAC dressing directly on the surgical bed are ideal methods of temporary wound closure that prevent desiccation of the underlying tissue while the pathologist has time to adequately assess the surgical margins. Allografts provide an epidermal closure that becomes vascularized and can remain in place for two to three weeks or more in some cases.

10.4 Surgical Treatment of Regional Merkel Cell Carcinoma

Merkel cell carcinoma has a propensity to spread to the regional lymph nodes, and the status of the regional nodes is a consistent predictor of survival.[4,17,18] Regional nodal metastases have been reported (either occult or clinically positive) in up to 30–40% of patients, including those undergoing sentinel lymph node biopsy in clinically node-negative regional basins and those who present with clinically involved regional nodal metastases.[10,13,17–20] Patients present with palpable clinical nodal disease 12–30% of the time. Nodal involvement typically precedes the development of distant metastasis.[14,15] Therefore, adequate assessment and treatment of lymph node involvement is critical for staging, individualizing treatment and providing an accurate prognosis.[18] The five-year survival rates have been described as up to 88% in those patients without regional nodal spread versus close to 50% in those patients with positive nodes.[18]

10.4.1 *The role of sentinel lymph node biopsy in Merkel cell carcinoma*

Sentinel lymph node biopsy involves the identification of the first lymph node(s) draining the primary tumor site by using lymphoscintigraphy and intraoperative mapping of the lymphatic channels with blue dye. The sentinel lymph node is the most likely place to find metastasis if the tumor has spread. The histology of the sentinel lymph node(s) has been shown to be representative of the rest of the lymph nodes in the basin.[20,21]

Preoperative lymphoscintigraphy is the nuclear medicine imaging technique used for predicting lymphatic drainage. This has been shown to be more reliable in identifying the lymph node basin at risk for metastasis than standard anatomical guidelines ('Sappey's lines').[20] A radiolabeled tracer, ^{99m}technetium-sulfur colloid, is injected around the tumor. This is taken up into the draining lymphatic channels and becomes concentrated in the sentinel lymph nodes. The tracer is then visualized with a gamma camera, guiding the surgeon to the correct lymph node basin draining the primary Merkel cell carcinoma site. Intraoperative lymphatic mapping with blue dye is also used in conjunction with lymphoscintigraphy. This is performed by injecting 0.5 to 1 ml of 1% isosulfan blue dye around the primary tumor. The lymphatic channels and sentinel nodes are stained blue. This allows for visualization of the sentinel nodes in the regional nodal basins as well as confirmation of their radioactivity via a handheld gamma probe. The sentinel node biopsy imaging technique is detailed in Chapter 9.

Sentinel lymph node biopsy provides accurate staging of Merkel cell carcinoma patients without the morbidity associated with an elective lymph node dissection. The status of the sentinel node has been shown to have both prognostic and therapeutic significance.[22] We currently offer sentinel node biopsy to most patients who present with clinically negative lymph nodes and are good surgical candidates, at the time of their wide excision. Patients without evidence of disease in the sentinel lymph node are spared further treatment of the regional basin.

The accuracy of sentinel node biopsy performed after definitive wide excision of the primary Merkel cell carcinoma site is unknown. A previous excision could possibly change the pattern of drainage through the lymphatic channels, ultimately leading the surgeon to an incorrect sentinel lymph node and/or lymph node basin. This could lead to a false negative sentinel lymph node biopsy result. However, there is data from the melanoma literature that argues a previous excision is not an absolute contraindication for sentinel node biopsy.[23] These reports indicate that the true sentinel lymph node can often be identified, although significantly more lymph nodes, sometimes in additional regional nodal basins, may be identified and removed.

The incidence of sentinel node metastases in Merkel cell carcinoma has been reported in numerous small series. These series have reported incidence rates of anywhere between 11% and 47%. One meta-analysis conducted by Mehrany *et al.* in 2002 reported a 33% incidence; rates have been described as low as 11–16% and as high as 47% in a series of 23 patients reported by Mazá *et al.*[18,20,24,25]

In those patients who are not good surgical candidates due to pre-existing medical morbidities or other specific patient-related situations, regional nodal basins may be followed clinically. Based on our experience with melanoma, we have begun to include serial ultrasound examinations of the nodal basins in following these patients, but its precise value remains to be established.

10.4.2 *Negative sentinel lymph node biopsy*

A patient with a negative sentinel node biopsy will be spared the morbidity of having a lymph node dissection. The expectation is that recurrence in the sentinel node-negative basin should be an infrequent occurrence. However, there are some investigators that recommend adjuvant radiation to the regional nodal basin even in those patients with negative sentinel node biopsies. Warner *et al.* reported on a series of 17 patients, 11 of whom had sentinel node biopsies at the time of wide excision of the primary tumor. Of these, eight patients (63%) had negative sentinel nodes, and five of the six patients with negative sentinel nodes who did not receive postoperative radiation to the nodal basin had a regional nodal (four) or in-transit (one) recurrence. The other two patients with negative sentinel nodes received postoperative radiation, and one developed an in-transit recurrence but neither failed in the nodal basin.[13] These results suggest a much higher rate of false negative sentinel node biopsies than has been reported in other series with Merkel cell carcinoma or in melanoma.[26,27]

This experience is contrasted with the meta-analysis by Mehrany *et al.* where 39 of 40 patients with a negative sentinel node biopsy, with relatively short follow-up (median of 7.3 months), did not recur despite the fact that 35 of the 40 did not receive additional treatment (either surgical or radiation) to their regional nodal basin.[18] Further evidence that not all sentinel node-negative patients are destined to recur regionally comes from Hill *et al.* who reported no evidence of regional recurrence after a negative sentinel node biopsy and no additional nodal or systemic therapy in 16 patients (again with a short median follow-up of only 7 months).[25] Allen *et al.* reported that, for all patients who had undergone pathologic nodal staging (by elective lymph node dissection or sentinel lymph node biopsy), the nodal recurrence rate was 11%, but they did not provide a specific rate of recurrence in the unirradiated sentinel node-negative basin.[2] Messina *et al.* reported their regional nodal basin recurrence rate to be two of 12 patients with negative sentinel nodes (median follow-up 10.5 months, maximum 26 months).[20]

The authors of this chapter have now accumulated a very large series of sentinel node biopsies for Merkel cell carcinoma, with post-operative radiation virtually never used to the nodal basin, and do not see nodal basin recurrences with an increased frequency compared to what would be expected from a similar population of melanoma patients. It is worth considering, however, why 'false negative' sentinel node biopsies might be more frequent in Merkel cell carcinoma compared to melanoma.

- The baseline rate of occult nodal involvement is probably higher for Merkel cell carcinoma patients than for melanoma patients, and it may be the case that multinode involvement is also more common. If so, even if the percentage of false negative procedures is the same for both Merkel cell carcinoma and melanoma patients, Merkel cell carcinoma patients would be more likely to manifest failure in the remaining nodes.
- The head and neck region is recognized as an area where sentinel node biopsy has a higher risk of false negative results due to the rich network of lymphatics and multiplicity of lymph nodes throughout the region. Since a greater percentage of Merkel cell carcinomas arise on the head and neck compared to melanoma, it is predictable that the overall false-negative rate might be somewhat higher for Merkel cell carcinoma.

- Older age has recently been recognized as a factor in lymphatic dysfunction,[28] and was also associated with an increased risk of false negative results in melanoma patients enrolled on the Sunbelt Melanoma Trial.[29] Since the average age of Merkel cell carcinoma patients is older than melanoma patients, it is predictable that the overall false-negative rate might be somewhat higher for Merkel cell carcinoma.
- Dermal and subcutaneous lymphatics likely drain to different nodes, sometimes even different basins entirely. Most melanomas are entirely confined to the dermis, whereas invasion into the subcutaneous tissue is more frequent in Merkel cell carcinoma. This could potentially lead to an increased risk of false-negative results if only the dermal lymphatics are mapped by lymphoscintigraphy and intraoperative blue dye injection.
- Merkel cell carcinoma cells in the sentinel lymph node may be more difficult to distinguish from surrounding lymphocytes than are melanoma cells, at least when routine hematoxylin and eosin staining is used. In our experience, however, immunohistochemistry using antibodies to cytokeratins clearly highlights even small deposits or isolated tumor cells in Merkel cell carcinoma. Some of the reported variation in false-negative rates after sentinel node biopsy for Merkel cell carcinoma could therefore potentially be accounted for by variations in the use of immunohistochemistry.

Even considering these potential factors that contribute to a higher risk of regional failure after a negative sentinel node biopsy, we continue to feel that sentinel node biopsy plays an important role in the staging of Merkel cell carcinoma, and we do not treat the sentinel node-negative basin in our patients.

10.4.3 *Positive sentinel lymph node biopsy*

When metastases of Merkel cell carcinoma are found within the sentinel lymph node, the incidence of which can be as high as 40%,[2,4,14,17,18,24,30–33] patients appear to be at significantly higher risk of distant metastasis and death from Merkel cell carcinoma.[2,4,17,29] There are numerous reports of the natural history after a positive sentinel node biopsy. Mehrany *et al.* report in their meta-analysis a 66% disease-free survival rate after a positive sentinel node biopsy. Over a median follow-up period of 10.5 months, the odds of recurrence were 19-fold greater in patients with a positive biopsy than in patients with a negative sentinel node biopsy (odds ratio 18.9, $p = 0.005$). Allen *et al.* reported on 251 patients and broke down nodal status to four groups: (1) those who were clinically staged as node-negative; (2) those who were pathologically staged as node-negative (either by sentinel node biopsy or elective node dissection); (3) those who were clinically node-negative but pathologically node-positive, again either by sentinel node biopsy or elective node dissection; and (4) those who were clinically node-positive. Their results demonstrated that node-negative patients had a better five-year survival rate than node-positive patients, and furthermore that those who were clinically node-negative but pathologically node-positive fared better than those who were clinically node-positive. Clinically and pathologically node-negative patients in their series had a five-year survival rate of 97%, while only 62% of clinically node-negative but pathologically node-positive patients were alive at five years. Patients with clinical evidence of disease in the regional nodal basin on presentation had a five-year survival rate of 49%.[2] Gupta *et al.* reported a three-fold increase in recurrence (60% vs. 20%) in those with a positive versus a negative sentinel node. Patients in this series had a relapse-free survival at three years of 80% if they had a negative sentinel node, which was significantly better than the 40% three-year relapse-free survival of patients with a positive sentinel node ($p = 0.03$).[30]

The management of the sentinel node-positive regional nodal basin is aimed at achieving regional control with acceptable morbidity. Management options include follow-up of the basin without additional treatment, completion lymph node dissection, definitive nodal radiation, or completion dissection followed by adjuvant postoperative radiation. Routinely employing both node dissection and postoperative radiation would be expected to lead to significantly more lymphedema than either approach alone, and we believe this combination should be used only when there is a high risk for regional recurrence.[4] Currently, the definition of 'high risk' after a positive sentinel node biopsy has not been established, but we use the presence of extracapsular invasion of tumor and/or multiple positive lymph nodes (four or more in the neck or axilla and ten or more in the groin) as strong relative indications for combined therapy.

Completion node dissection has the advantage of allowing quantitation of the number of histologically positive nodes in the entire basin, whereas definitive radiation avoids the risks and discomfort of a full node dissection. In our experience, either node dissection or nodal irradiation provide good regional control in microscopic disease that is not 'high risk' as defined above, with the caveat that we do not always have complete pathologic staging information when the sentinel node positive basin is definitively treated with radiation. However, particularly when dealing with isolated tumor cells or other 'micrometastatic' tumor deposits visualized only on immunohistochemistry, definitive radiation appears to control the regional basin quite adequately. In these cases, the management of the primary site can influence the management of the regional basin as well; if the primary site is going to undergo irradiation because of a close margin or histologic evidence of a high risk of recurrence (or because routine postoperative radiation is employed at a given center), then definitive nodal irradiation can be added with relatively little additional inconvenience, and radiation to the primary can commence sooner than would be the case if the patient had to first recover from a completion node dissection. Conversely, if the primary site has been adequately treated with surgery, then a completion node dissection may be a preferable approach. Currently, the National Comprehensive Cancer Network guidelines recommend that patients with a positive sentinel lymph node biopsy undergo a completion lymph node dissection, if the procedure can be safely performed.[1] Regardless of the strategy chosen, an informed patient and a multidisciplinary approach are key components for an optimal outcome.

10.5 Clinically Positive Lymph Node Involvement

It has been the authors' practice to evaluate patients with palpable nodes and a history of Merkel cell carcinoma in the past, or those who present with a primary tumor and synchronous palpable adenopathy, in a fashion that closely parallels the recommendations of the NCCN.[1] Patients first undergo a percutancous fine needle aspiration cytology or needle core biopsy of the suspect nodes, which can be image-guided using ultrasound or CT if needed. If the aspiration cytology does not demonstrate Merkel cell carcinoma but also fails to establish an alternative definitive diagnosis for the lymphadenopathy, an open biopsy should be considered as a next step. If the evaluation documents metastatic Merkel cell carcinoma, the patient should be evaluated for distant metastases by cross-sectional imaging (see Chapter 9). In the absence of distant metastasis, a therapeutic lymph node dissection is indicated for regional control. Unfortunately, despite these efforts, over half of the patients with clinical evidence of Merkel cell carcinoma metastatic to the lymph nodes who undergo lymphadenectomy will die from distant metastasis.[31] The potential role for adjuvant chemotherapy in node-positive Merkel cell carcinoma is discussed in Chapter 15.

Patients whose lymph node metastasis is deemed inoperable secondary to size, location or the fixed nature of the involved lymph nodes may be treated with neoadjuvant radiation and/or chemotherapy prior to undergoing an attempt at lymphadenectomy.[31] Patients with significant medical comorbidities and those who are unwilling to accept the potential risks and the morbidities of a complete node dissection may also be considered for radiation to the regional nodal basin as definitive therapy.[4]

The optimal approach to regional lymph node metastases in the presence of concomitant distant metastases has not been defined, but generally systemic chemotherapy along with definitive radiation to the regional nodal basin (especially if the patient is symptomatic in the nodal basin) is preferred to surgery directed at the lymph node basin, which would delay the initiation of systemic treatment. A possible exception is an ulcerated or bleeding matted mass of nodal disease, where lymphadenectomy and reconstruction of the attendant defect may be necessary before systemic chemotherapy can be instituted. Preoperative or definitive radiation to the nodal basin may be an alternative in that situation, depending on the magnitude of the distant metastatic disease and the patient's overall performance status.

10.6 Merkel Cell Carcinoma from an Unknown Primary

Merkel cell carcinoma is a rare entity in and of itself, and a diagnosis of metastatic Merkel cell carcinoma from an unknown primary source is exceedingly rare. Unknown primary neuroendocrine tumors can theoretically have spread from any of the following locations: lung, bronchus, islet cell tumors of the pancreas, Merkel cell carcinoma, neuroblastoma or carcinoid tumors amongst other sources.[34] When a patient presents with regional or distant metastases and the histologic and immunochemical picture is consistent with Merkel cell carcinoma but no primary is known, the evaluation should include a full history and physical examination including a thorough skin examination. We routinely ask the patient if they have ever had any skin or subcutaneous lesions removed at any time in their life, with particular attention to areas draining an involved nodal basin. Full body cross-sectional imaging should be performed in order to look for the primary source, but equally or more importantly to exclude further metastatic disease. The role of other investigations, such as upper and lower endoscopies and bronchoscopy as well as other special radiological tests, is as yet undefined and we do not routinely employ them. In the absence of definite evidence of distant metastatic disease, we follow the treatment guidelines for clinically palpable Merkel cell carcinoma from a known primary, which generally means radical lymphadenectomy plus postoperative radiation, with or without adjuvant chemotherapy.

10.7 Surgical/Regional Therapy for In-Transit Metastatic Merkel Cell Carcinoma

Like melanoma, Merkel cell carcinoma can present or recur with in-transit metastases, defined as cutaneous, dermal or subcutaneous metastases occurring between the primary site and regional nodal basin. In cases with one or a few in-transit nodules, excision of all the in-transit metastases with consideration of postoperative radiation therapy offers the best chance for disease control. Some patients who develop multiple in-transit metastases are sufficiently symptomatic from one or a few dominant lesions to merit resection and/or radiation for palliation of pain, ulceration or bleeding. There are case reports in the literature suggesting that melphalan-based hyperthermic isolated limb perfusion and more recently isolated limb infusion (both originally developed to treat in-transit melanoma) are viable options for treating in-transit metastatic Merkel cell carcinoma confined to the extremity, with durable regional response rates as high as 100%.[35–37] We have experience in treating a small number of patients with in-transit Merkel cell carcinoma via isolated limb infusion with a 100% response rate and a 66% complete response rate. The responses are durable with ongoing complete responses over four years since treatment (data not published).

10.8 Surgical Treatment of Metastatic Merkel Cell Carcinoma

Distant metastatic Merkel cell carcinoma has a very poor prognosis. The role of surgery in the treatment of distant metastatic Merkel cell carcinoma is limited, and is mainly used as a method for palliation of symptoms.[4] The presence of distant metastasis generally indicates the need for systemic therapy and limits the role for the localized control that surgery can provide. Surgery should be considered when it can be performed with limited morbidity for palliation of symptoms such as bleeding, pain, intestinal obstruction or perforation of intestinal metastases. In the rare cases of patients with oligometastatic disease confirmed by imaging, an attempt at resection may be considered if it will render the patient free of all known disease.

References

1. National Comprehensive Cancer Network. *NCCN Clinical Practice Guidelines in Oncology*, Vol. 1, 2008.
2. Allen P.J., Bowne W.B., Jacques D.P., *et al.* (2005). Merkel cell carcinoma: prognosis and treatment of patients from a single institution. *J Clin Oncol* 23: 2300–2309.
3. Boyer J.D., Zitelli J.A., Brodland D.G., D'Angelo G. (2002). Local control of primary Merkel cell carcinoma: review of 45 cases treated with Mohs micrographic surgery with and without adjuvant radiation. *J Am Acad Dermatol* 47: 885–892.
4. Bichakjian C.K., Lowe L., Loa C.D., *et al.* (2007). Merkel cell carcinoma: critical review with guidelines for multidisciplinary management. *Cancer* 110: 1–12.

5. Medina-Franco H., Urist M.M., Fiveash J., *et al.* (2001). Multimodality treatment of Merkel cell carcinoma: case series and literature review of 1024 cases. *Ann Surg Oncol* 8: 204–208.
6. Allen P.J., Zhang Z.F., Coit D.G. (1999). Surgical management of Merkel cell carcinoma. *Ann Surg* 229: 97–105.
7. Eng T.Y., Boersma M.G., Fuller C.D., *et al.* (2007). A comprehensive review of the treatment of Merkel cell carcinoma. *Am J Clin Oncol* 30: 624–636.
8. Gillenwater A.M., Hessel A.C., Morrison W.H., *et al.* (2001). Merkel cell carcinoma of the head and neck: effect of surgical excision and radiation on recurrence and survival. *Arch Otolaryngol Head Neck Surg* 127: 149–154.
9. Eng T.Y., Naguib M., Fuller C.D., *et al.* (2004). Treatment of recurrent Merkel cell carcinoma: an analysis of 46 cases. *Am J Clin Oncol* 27: 576–583.
10. Stokes J.B., Graw K.S., Dengel L.T., *et al.* (2009). Patients with Merkel cell carcinoma tumors ≤1.0 cm in diameter are unlikely to harbor regional lymph node metastasis. *J Clin Oncol* 27: 3772–3777.
11. Bajetta E., Celio L., Platania M., *et al.* (2009). Single-institution series of early-stage Merkel cell carcinoma: long-term outcomes in 95 patients managed with surgery alone. *Ann Surg Oncol* 16: 2985–2993.
12. Jabbour J., Cumming R., Scolyer R.A., *et al.* (2007). Merkel cell carcinoma: assessing the effect of wide local excision, lymph node dissection, and radiotherapy on recurrence and survival in early-stage disease — results from a review of 82 consecutive cases diagnosed between 1992 and 2004. *Ann Surg Oncol* 14: 1943–1952.
13. Warner R.E., Quinn M.J., Hruby G., *et al.* (2008). Management of Merkel cell carcinoma: the roles of lymphoscintigraphy, sentinel lymph node biopsy and adjuvant radiotherapy. *Ann Surg Oncol* 15: 2509–2518.
14. Senchenkov A., Barnes S.A., Moran S.L. (2007). Predictors of survival and recurrence in the surgical treatment of Merkel cell carcinoma of the extremities. *J Surg Oncol* 95: 229–234.
15. Lewis J.M., Zager J.S., Yu D., *et al.* (2008). Full-thickness grafts procured from skin overlying the sentinel lymph node basin; reconstruction of primary cutaneous malignancy excision defects. *Ann Surg Oncol* 15: 1733–1740.
16. Moncrieff M.D., Bowen F., Thompson J.F., *et al.* (2008). Keystone flap reconstruction of primary melanoma excision defects of the leg — the end of the skin graft? *Ann Surg Oncol* 15: 2867–2873.

17. Schmalbach C.E., Lowe L., Teknos T.N., *et al.* (2005). Reliability of sentinel lymph node biopsy for regional staging of head and neck Merkel cell carcinoma. *Arch Otolaryngol Head Neck Surg* 131: 610–614.
18. Mehrany K., Otley C.C., Weenig R.H., *et al.* (2002). A meta-analysis of the prognostic significance of sentinel lymph node status in Merkel cell carcinoma. *Dermatol Surg* 28: 113–117.
19. McAfee W.J., Morris C.G., Mendenhall C.M., *et al.* (2005). Merkel cell carcinoma: treatment and outcomes. *Cancer* 104: 1761–1764.
20. Messina J.L., Reintgen D.S., Cruse C.W., *et al.* (1997). Selective lymphadenectomy in patients with Merkel cell (cutaneous neuroendocrine) carcinoma. *Ann Surg Oncol* 4: 389–395.
21. Goessling W., McKee P.H., Mayer R.J. (2002). Merkel cell carcinoma. *J Clin Oncol* 20: 588–598.
22. Henness S., Vereecken P. (2008). Management of Merkel cell tumours: an evidence-based review. *Curr Opin Oncol* 20: 280–286.
23. Gannon C.J., Rousseau D.L., Ross M.I., *et al.* (2006). Accuracy of lymphatic mapping and sentinel lymph node biopsy after previous wide local excision in patients with primary melanoma. *Cancer* 107: 2647–2652.
24. Maza S., Trefzer U., Hofmann M., *et al.* (2006). Impact of sentinel lymph node biopsy in patients with Merkel cell carcinoma: results of a prospective study and review of the literature. *Eur J Nucl Med Mol Imaging* 33: 433–440.
25. Hill A.D., Brady M.S., Coit D.G. (1999). Intraoperative lymphatic mapping and sentinel lymph node biopsy for Merkel cell carcinoma. *Br J Surg* 86: 518–521.
26. Morton D.L., Thompson J.F., Cochran A.J., *et al.* (2006). Sentinel-node biopsy or nodal observation in melanoma. *N Engl J Med* 355: 1307–1317.
27. McMasters K.M., Noyes R.D., Reintgen D.S., *et al.* (2004). Lessons learned from the Sunbelt Melanoma Trial. *J Surg Oncol* 86: 212–223.
28. Conway W.C., Faries M.B., Nicholl M.B., *et al.* (2009). Age-related lymphatic dysfunction in melanoma patients. *Ann Surg Oncol* 16: 1548–1552.
29. Scoggins C.R., Martin R.C., Ross M.I., *et al.* (2010). Factors associated with false-negative sentinel lymph node biopsy in melanoma patients. *Ann Surg Oncol* 17: 709–717.
30. Gupta S.G., Wang L.C., Penas P.F., *et al.* (2006). Sentinel lymph node biopsy for evaluation and treatment of patients with Merkel cell carcinoma: the Dana-Farber experience and meta-analysis of the literature. *Arch Dermatol* 142: 685–690.

31. Pectasides D., Pectasides M., Economopoulos T. (2006). Merkel cell cancer of the skin. *Ann Oncol* 17: 1489–1495.
32. Sandel H.D., Day T., Richardson M.S., *et al.* (2006). Merkel cell carcinoma: does tumor size or depth of invasion correlate with recurrence, metastasis, or patient survival? *Laryngoscope* 116: 791–795.
33. Wagner J.D., Evdokimow D.Z., Weisberger E., *et al.* (2004). Sentinel node biopsy for high-risk nonmelanoma cutaneous malignancy. *Arch Dermatol* 140: 75–79.
34. Spigel D.R., Hainsworth J.D., Greco F.A. (2009). Neuroendocrine carcinoma of unknown primary site. *Semin Oncol* 36: 52–59.
35. Gupta A.S., Heinzman S., Levine E.A. (1998). Successful treatment of in-transit metastases from Merkel's cell carcinoma with isolated hyperthermic limb perfusion. *South Med J* 91: 289–292.
36. Olieman A.F., Liénard D., Eggermont A.M., *et al.* (1999). Hyperthermic isolated limb perfusion with tumor necrosis factor alpha, interferon gamma, and melphalan for locally advanced nonmelanoma skin tumors of the extremities: a multicenter study. *Arch Surg* 134: 303–307.
37. Wood B.C., Kleinpeter K.P., Levine E.A. (2007). Treatment of in-transit metastases from Merkel cell carcinoma with isolated hyperthermic limb perfusion. *Am Surg* 73: 1291–1292.

Chapter 11

Special Considerations in the Surgical Management of Merkel Cell Carcinoma in the Head and Neck

Melanie L. Aya-ay, Tapan A. Padhya and C. Wayne Cruse

Merkel cell carcinoma occurs predominantly on sun exposed areas, but especially the head and neck region (>47% of cases).[1–5] The face, scalp, neck, nose and external ear are leading sites for Merkel cell carcinoma. Surgical excision of tumors in this area can result in significant disfigurement and functional issues. Appropriate planning of incisions and reconstruction will help minimize ultimate morbidity. Numerous single institution case series have demonstrated the benefit of multimodality treatment of Merkel cell carcinoma, especially surgery followed by radiotherapy. The rich regional lymphatics of the head and neck play an integral part in staging and the overall prognosis for an individual patient. The evolving role of sentinel lymph node biopsy makes the management of Merkel cell carcinoma in the head and neck region unique and calls for special surgical considerations.

11.1 Head and Neck Anatomy

A thorough understanding of the complex anatomy of the head and neck region is essential in the management of tumors of this area. The face is comprised of aesthetic units and aesthetic lines that are of key importance when considering excision and reconstruction. Preserving function, optimizing aesthetics and avoiding complications depend in part on the surgeon's knowledge of underlying structures such as nerves and musculature. A basic overview of head and neck anatomy will be discussed in the following sections.[6]

11.1.1 *Aesthetic units*

The face can be divided into sections that represent aesthetic units and subunits (Figure 1). Anatomical boundaries and contour lines define these

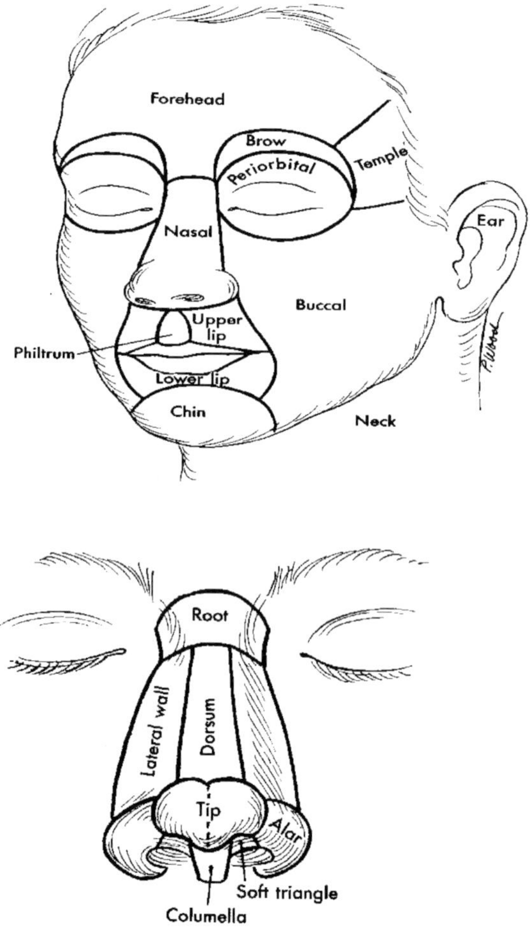

Figure 1. Major aesthetic units of the face. (Reproduced with permission from Cummings *et al.*, 1993.)[38]

units.[7] The tissue within each individual unit has similar characteristics such as skin tone, texture, and thickness. Surgical reconstruction should attempt to remain within these aesthetic units. If over 50% of an aesthetic unit is removed with excision of the Merkel cell lesion, then the decision may be made to remove and reconstruct the entire aesthetic unit.

The upper face is comprised of the forehead unit and the upper and lower eyelid units. The forehead contains the glabellar, suprabrow and temple subunits. The palpebral and orbital subunits together form the eyelid units. The orbital unit is a circular area at the periphery of the palpebral units that extends from the eyebrow to the junction of the cheek. The midface is made up of the nasal and cheek units. The nose is subdivided into the root, dorsum, lateral sidewalls, tip, ala, columella and soft triangle. The upper and lower lip units as well as the mental unit make up the lower face. The upper and lower lips extend from the mucous membrane to the vermillion border then continue as a cutaneous subunit to the nasolabial folds laterally, the nose superiorly and the labiomental crease inferiorly. At the periphery of the face lies the scalp, neck and auricular units, which can also be divided into subunits.

11.1.2 *Aesthetic lines*

There are several contour lines of the face that are important in reconstruction. These include the hairline, alar crease, nasolabial fold, vermilion border, philtrum and labiomental crease. Incisional scars are often more discrete when placed along these naturally occurring lines. As a note, these lines can be very difficult to reconstruct when a tumor excision involves these areas.

11.1.3 *Relaxed skin tension lines*

The naturally occurring lines in the skin are called the relaxed skin tension lines (Figure 2).[8] These lines are created by the muscle forces beneath the skin. The lines run perpendicular to the underlying muscle fibers. These lines can be made more evident by asking the patient to contract the facial muscles with an exaggerated smile or by pinching the skin. Incisions should be placed parallel to these relaxed skin tension lines in order to provide the best cosmetic outcome.

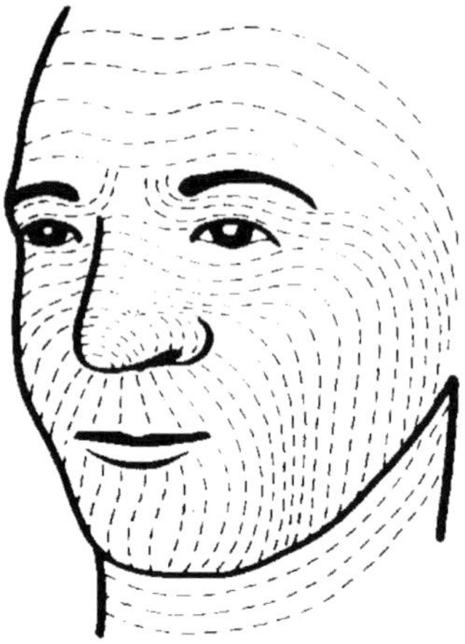

Figure 2. Relaxed skin tension lines. (Reproduced with permission from Larrabee Jr., 1989.)[39]

11.1.4 *Vasculature*

Knowledge of the arterial and venous blood supply is critical for flap reconstruction of the head and neck region. Most structures of the face, neck and scalp are supplied by branches of the external carotid artery. The majority of the scalp is supplied by the occipital, posterior auricular, supraorbital and the parietal and frontal branches of the superficial temporal artery. The supraorbital, supratrochlear and frontal branches of the superficial temporal arteries supply the forehead while the supraorbital and infraorbital arteries supply the periorbital and cheek areas. The facial, internal maxillary and lingual arteries provide blood flow to the remaining areas of the face. The venous drainage of the head and neck region mirrors the arterial system.

11.1.5 *Innervation*

The trigeminal nerve (cranial nerve V) provides sensation to the face and motor function to the muscles of mastication. The trigeminal nerve is divided into three major branches (V1, V2 and V3) which supply the upper, mid and lower face respectively. The facial nerve (cranial nerve VII) provides motor function to the muscles of facial expression. The main branches of the facial nerve are the temporal, zygomatic, buccal, mandibular and cervical. Injuries to the facial nerve may result in significant muscle weakness leading to asymmetries of the face. Oral incompetence with resulting drooling can be a distressing complication of facial nerve injury. The inability to completely close the eyelids after injury to the facial nerve branches supplying the orbicularis oculi can also be very problematic for the patient. The patient may develop chronic dry eyes or excessive tearing and have a high risk of corneal abrasion and/or ulceration.

11.1.6 *Lymphatic drainage*

The lymphatic drainage system of the head and neck also mirrors the vasculature (Figure 3). The preauricular nodes and parotid gland should be thoroughly evaluated when a malignant tumor of the face or scalp is present. The neck region is divided into six major groups of lymph nodes

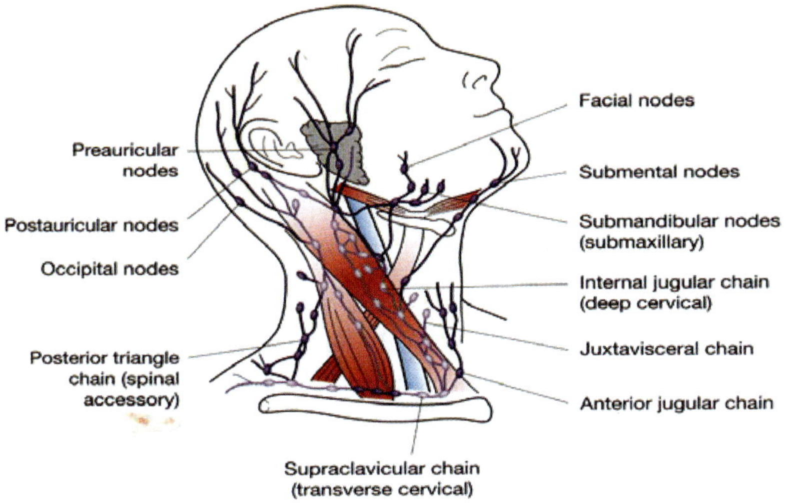

Figure 3. Cervical nodal groups as described by their anatomic location. (Reproduced with permission from Gluckman and Johnson, 2003.)[6]

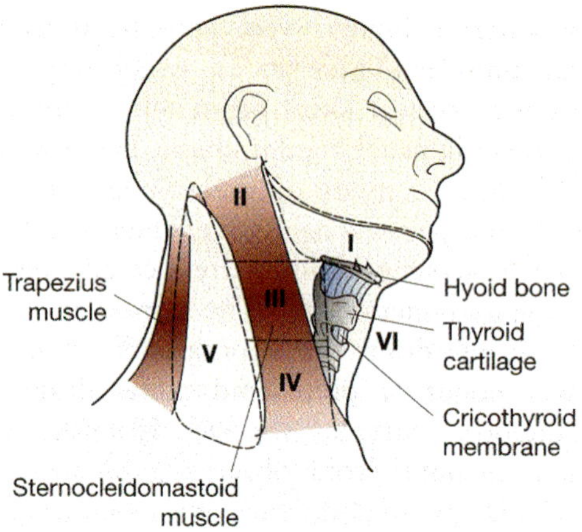

Figure 4. Classification of lymph nodes according to level. (Reproduced with permission from Gluckman and Johnson, 2003.)[6]

(levels I–VI, Figure 4).[9] Level I contains the submental and submandibular nodes. Levels II, III and IV lie deep to the sternocleidomastoid muscle with level II being located from the skull base to the level of the hyoid. Level III would be group of nodes between the hyoid and cricoid and finally level IV being located between the cricoid and the clavicle. The lymphatics in the posterior triangle formed by the sternocleidomastoid, trapezius muscle and clavicle comprise level V. Level VI includes paratracheal nodes located between the carotid sheaths.

11.2 Clinical Diagnosis

The examination of the head and neck should be undertaken in a systematic approach to assure a complete examination in each patient. A recent study by Heath *et al.* suggests increasing suspicion for Merkel cell carcinoma using the *AEIOU* acronym (see Chapter 6).[10] Examination should also note potential satellite lesions, other primary lesions or adjacent basal or squamous cell carcinomas. Mobility versus adherence of the Merkel cell tumor to the underlying structures must be assessed. The skin and soft tissue quality and turgor as well as laxity and significant rhytids should be noted. The assessment of the skin surrounding the lesion will aide in planning the reconstruction.

Preoperative assessment of facial sensation and motor function is helpful to identify any pre-existing neurologic deficits. Merkel cell tumors in the orbital region may require an eye examination, including documentation of orbital range of motion, visual fields and visual acuity. An examination of the intranasal and intraoral areas will determine mucosal involvement of overlying lesions. Physical examination of the lymphatic system of the head and neck involves thorough palpation of all potentially draining nodal basins. The parotid gland should be palpated for firm areas or potentially discrete masses. The neck examination should include all nodal levels, I–VI.

11.3 Surgical Excision

Resection and reconstruction of Merkel cell carcinoma of the head and neck requires detailed preoperative planning. Photographs of the patient taken preoperatively can assist with this planning (Figure 5). The excision and reconstruction are usually completed simultaneously, but staged reconstruction may be necessary to ensure negative margins prior to committing to an extensive reconstruction. When planning the surgery, consideration should be given to aesthetic units and lines. *Incisions should be placed parallel to the relaxed skin tension lines.* The location of the incisions should consider the possibility of future surgery such as a neck dissection. Many single institution case series have been reported stating surgery as the first modality of treatment for head and neck Merkel cell carcinoma.[11–17] Surgical margins of at least 2 cm have been suggested.[18–20] When operating in the head and neck region, margins may need to be decreased in order to improve aesthetic and functional outcomes. The depth of excision should be to deep fat and/or fascia in the face and neck, and include the galea in the scalp whenever possible.

Stage-appropriate treatment of head and neck Merkel cell carcinoma is paramount for achieving good outcomes. Stage I and II disease is treated typically with wide excision of the primary lesion, and sentinel lymph node biopsy is also recommended. Regional node dissection is performed if positive nodes are identified preoperatively or after sentinel

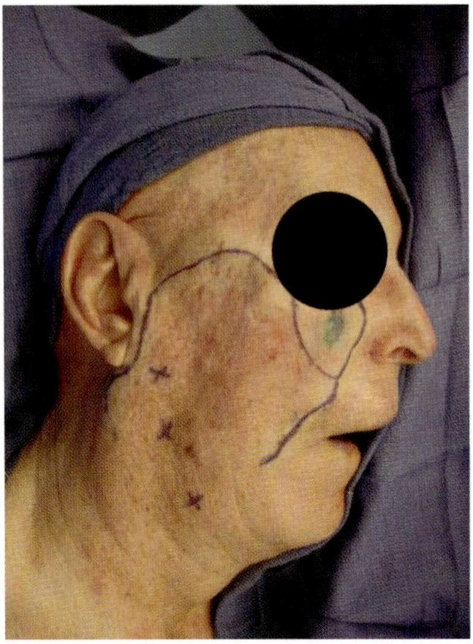

Figure 5. Merkel cell carcinoma of the medial cheek region. Wide excision with sentinel lymph node biopsy and immediate flap reconstruction is planned. The patient has undergone preoperative lymphoscintigraphy (see Figure 6); the Xs mark the site of the sentinel nodes.

node biopsy. Stage III disease is treated with wide excision of the primary and regional node dissection. Postoperative radiation and/or chemotherapy are frequently utilized (see Chapters 13 and 15). For stage IV disease, an individualized multidisciplinary plan must be initiated, which usually emphasizes chemotherapy and/or radiation as the situation warrants.

Mohs surgery has been utilized in the treatment of head and neck Merkel cell carcinoma, and is described further in Chapter 12.[21–23] With the need for concurrent sentinel node mapping and/or neck dissection, surgical excision of the primary tumor at the same setting may be a better choice.

11.4 Lymphatic Mapping and Sentinel Node Biopsy

Lymphoscintigraphy with sentinel node biopsy has become the standard of care for identifying occult regional metastases in localized Merkel cell carcinoma of the head and neck.[24–34] The technique for lymphatic mapping

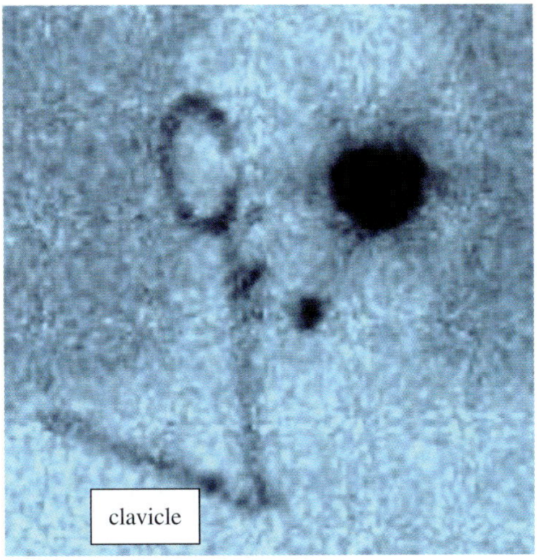

Figure 6. Lymphoscintigram of the medial cheek Merkel cell carcinoma shown in Figure 5. Obtained following the injection of ^{99m}Tc-labeled sulfur colloid, it demonstrates drainage to nodes in the parotid region and just below the inferior edge of the mandible. The ear, sternocleidomastoid muscle and clavicle have been outlined for orientation.

and sentinel node biopsy in head and neck Merkel cell carcinoma is similar to that used for most cutaneous melanoma nodal mapping. A pre-operative lymphoscintigram (see Chapter 9) is obtained and is beneficial to determine the approximate number and location of the sentinel lymph nodes (Figure 6). Lymphatic mapping may be more difficult when the primary lesion is in the neck or parotid region because the tumor may overlie the nodal basin. Thus the sentinel node may be more difficult to visualize with standard mapping techniques. Isosulfan blue dye is also used; in the head and neck, the surgeon should use less than 0.5 ml. Using larger amounts of dye will increase dermal spread which could result in long-term blue discoloration of the skin. With tumors of the face or scalp, it is important to evaluate both sides of the neck for sentinel nodes. Frozen sections are not routinely obtained on sentinel lymph nodes because the pathologist prefers permanent sections to thoroughly review each node and perform the necessary immunohistochemical stains. Therefore, patients are not usually prepared for a neck dissection at the same time as the sentinel node biopsy. Although it has been suggested that smaller

Merkel cell carcinomas may not require sentinel node biopsy,[35] as yet we have not defined a threshold tumor size or thickness below which sentinel node biopsy is unwarranted.

11.5 Neck Dissection

A neck dissection is recommended for microscopic disease detected in lymph nodes biopsied during nodal mapping, although in some cases treatment with definitive radiation may be used instead. A comprehensive neck dissection is indicated when dealing with macroscopic nodal disease detected by physical exam or by imaging.[36] Neck dissections are not performed prophylactically for N0 disease. The standard technique for cervical lymphadenectomy is also used with Merkel cell carcinoma. Because of the high risk of occult involved nodes, a neck dissection should accompany parotidectomy for positive parotid disease. Lesions of the upper neck, face and scalp anterior to the ear includes a dissection of the parotid and levels I–IV of the neck. Lesions of the upper neck and scalp posterior to the ear call for dissection of levels II–V of the neck. A dissection of levels III–V is performed with lesions of the inferior neck. Lesions of the ear and of the scalp and neck at the level of the ear drain to all areas of the neck, which dictates a parotidectomy and complete (level I–V) neck dissection.

11.6 Considerations in Reconstruction

The basic reconstructive ladder is used to determine the best technique for reconstruction of a defect following excision of Merkel cell carcinoma. The reconstructive plan and alternate or back-up options should be determined preoperatively. Attention to aesthetic units, aesthetic lines, relaxed skin tension lines and incision placement during surgical excision will aid in achieving more ideal results with reconstruction. The reconstructive options are determined in part by the size and location of the lesion. The aesthetic requirements and comorbidities of the patient will also impact the options for reconstruction. Techniques for reconstruction will be discussed for each aesthetic unit.

11.6.1 *Scalp*

Merkel cell lesions of the scalp are usually resected with at least 2 cm margins. Small defects may occasionally be able to be closed primarily with adequate undermining of the surrounding tissues. Larger defects can be closed using a split thickness skin graft if the periosteum is intact. This results in an area with non-hair bearing skin and can be somewhat fragile. Scalp rotational flaps are also a good option for coverage of scalp defects. Rotational flaps may be used for coverage of cranium if devoid of periosteum. A split thickness skin graft is typically needed for coverage of the flap donor site. For situations with very large scalp defects with deficiency of surrounding scalp skin for coverage, local pedicled flaps or free tissue transfer may be used.

11.6.2 *Forehead*

Small lesions of the forehead can occasionally be closed primarily following excision. Both split thickness and full thickness skin grafts can provide wound closure. Full thickness skin from a donor site with similar skin characteristics as the recipient site will result in a better cosmetic result. The skin of the brachiocephalic groove is frequently used as a donor site secondary to the laxity of skin in this area and good color match for the head and neck region. When using a split thickness graft, the ideal donor site is from an area of color match such as the arm. There are multiple local flaps that can be utilized for forehead reconstruction, including but not limited to rotational flaps such as the bilobed flap or rhomboid flap, advancement flaps such as the H flap or V-Y advancement flap, or the frontalis muscle myocutaneous flap. When the area of excision involves the majority of the forehead, the entire forehead may be excised and reconstructed as a total aesthetic unit.

11.6.3 *Eyelids*

Merkel cell carcinoma involving the eyelid can be very difficult to reconstruct. The complex anatomy of the orbital region, as well as the need to preserve function, contributes to this difficulty. Numerous options for reconstruction of this area are based on the characteristics of the deficit. Full thickness skin grafts, local flaps such as the cheek advancement flap, pedicled flaps such as the temporoparietal fascial flap, or free tissue transfer are all potential options. The excisional and reconstructive techniques are determined by the depth of the lesion (partial vs. full thickness), the location (upper or lower eyelid) and the involvement of the eyelid margin. Following reconstruction of the eyelid, complications such as ectropion, entropion, dacrocystitis and dry or watery eyes may be encountered.

11.6.3.1 *Partial thickness eyelid defects*

When excising a partial thickness lesion of the eyelid, incisions oriented transversely are better concealed than vertical incisions. Partial thickness defects can usually be closed primarily if they involve $<50\%$ of the eyelid surface. Partial defects $\geq 50\%$ will require at least a full thickness skin graft for reconstruction. Full thickness skin grafts can be harvested from the ipsilateral or contralateral eyelid for an excellent donor skin match. The posterior auricular skin may also be a good choice as a donor site. The resulting scar from both of these donor sites is typically well concealed.

11.6.3.2 *Full thickness eyelid defects*

Full thickness eyelid defects can be closed primarily if $<25\%$ of the eyelid margin is involved. Full thickness deficits of 25–75% require graft and flap reconstruction. Reconstruction includes an inner mucosal layer, a structural support layer and a well vascularized outer layer. Nasal septal cartilage and mucosa can be used as a composite graft to reconstruct the inner mucosal layer and structural support layer. Ear cartilage is also often used for the support layer, while palatal or buccal mucosa can be used as the mucosal graft. A local flap may then be used to provide the vascularized outer layer. Eyelid defects $>75\%$ will require a composite graft as well as multiple local flaps such as the cheek advancement flap and the lower-lid switch flap or free tissue reconstruction.

11.6.4 *Nasal*

There are several options for reconstruction of a nasal defect following surgical excision of tumors on the nose. The patient's aesthetic requirements as well as the size of the defect and subunits involved will guide the reconstructive effort. Primary closure is often not a good option in that it may result in distortion of the nasal anatomy. Skin grafts may be used with full thickness skin achieving the better cosmetic result. Bilobed flaps are a good option for small defects (<2 cm) of the nasal sidewall or nasal dorsum. A dorsal nasal flap works well for tip lesions. Nasolabial flaps can help to rebuild the nasal ala. The paramedian forehead flap is an excellent option for larger defects. With deep or full thickness tumor involvement, there may be a need for cartilage and mucosal grafts.

11.6.5 *Cheek*

The cheek is often an area with significant redundancy, especially in elderly patients. Many of these wounds may be amenable to primary closure. Care should be taken to avoid excess tension on adjacent facial features, which can result in significant distortion of the face. Larger wounds may require skin grafting or local advancement/rotation flaps (Figure 7). The V-Y advancement flap works well to reconstruct a medial cheek lesion as the incision can hide within the nasolabial fold. The bilobed flap, banner flap and rhomboid flap are all transposition flaps that can be used as well. The cheek advancement or cervicofacial flaps are excellent options for larger defects. Regional flaps such as the deltopectoral flap, pectoralis major flap or the trapezius flap are potential candidates for larger defects. Occasionally, free tissue transfer will be needed to reconstruct large or full thickness cheek defects.

11.6.6 *Lips*

The vermilion tissue of the lip presents a significant challenge in lip reconstruction. No tissue in the body has the same characteristics as the vermilion. Therefore, lip defects are best reconstructed with adjacent lip tissue. Reapproximation of the orbicularis oris is necessary for normal

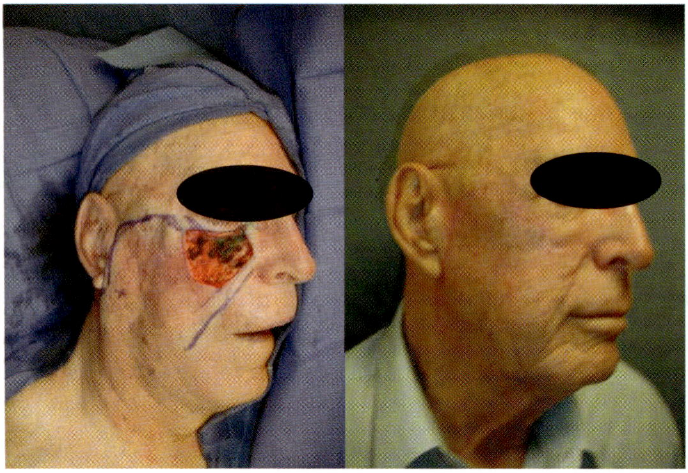

Figure 7. **(Left)** Excision of Merkel cell cancer of cheek and cervicofacial rotation advancement flap closure (same patient as in Figure 5). **(Right)** The result is shown at four months postoperatively.

lip motion. Maintaining oral competence while achieving the best aesthetic outcome is the primary goal of lip reconstruction.

11.6.6.1 *Upper lip*

Superficial defects of the skin of the upper lip can be closed primarily or covered with a full thickness graft.[37] A hair-bearing skin graft may be used in men in this location to better conceal the scar or defect. Full thickness defects of the upper lip can be closed primarily or with a wedge excision if they involve one-third or less of the length of the lip. A vermilion advancement flap can aid in this closure. Larger deficits should be reconstructed using lower lip tissue, such as with the Abbe flap. The Abbe flap borrows tissue from the lower lip but maintains the original commissure. These flaps produce a satisfactory aesthetic and functional result but do require a second stage operation. Cheek advancement and medialization can aid in obtaining closure of these defects. It is important to attempt to conceal incisions along normal anatomical lines if possible. Total or near total upper lip deficits will require more extensive reconstruction with free tissue such as the radial forearm free flap.

11.6.6.2 *Lower lip*

Many partial thickness and full thickness lower lip defects can be closed primarily or with wedge excision. For more extensive defects, the presence or absence of the commissure and size of the defect will help to determine the appropriate reconstruction.[37] The Schuchardt procedure rotates and advances the cheek and remaining lip along an incision of the labiomental fold. This flap maintains the original commissures. The reverse Abbe flap can also be used when the commissures are intact. The Estlander and Karapandzic flaps are sliding lower lip flaps that are used for reconstruction of larger lower lip defects. These flaps move the original commissure resulting in microstomia, rounding of the commissure and misplacement of the modiolus. For total or near total defects of the lower lip, the Webster-Bernard operation involves medial cheek advancement with a bipedicled mucosal sliding flap. The radial forearm free flap may be used as well. These larger reconstructions may require a palmaris longus sling for suspension of the lower lip.

11.6.7 *Ear*

The reconstructive options for an ear defect are based on the size of the lesion and the location in the upper, middle or lower third of the ear. Partial thickness defects with intact perichondrium may be skin grafted with a good result. Small full thickness defects can be closed with wedge excision. Burow's triangles may need to be excised in the conchal bowl to allow for better contour and reapproximation. Removal of a small amount of cartilage will also aide with the reapproximation. Full thickness defects are typically best reconstructed with the chondrocutaneous (Antia-Buch) flap. This flap often provides the best aesthetic result. The patient still must be aware that there will be a size discrepancy between their ears, which may or may not be obvious.

11.6.8 *Neck*

Merkel cell lesions of the neck are most often reconstructed with primary closure or local flaps. A skin graft is another option. When excising and reconstructing a primary Merkel cell carcinoma of the neck, the location and orientation of the incisions should anticipate the potential future need for a neck dissection.

In conclusion, although the surgical treatment of head and neck Merkel cell carcinoma requires knowledge of the anatomy of the region and familiarity with a wide variety of reconstructive options, treatment principles defined for Merkel cell carcinoma at other sites can and should be followed for head and neck tumors. An appropriately aggressive, multidisciplinary and multimodality approach provides the best chance for a successful oncologic, cosmetic and functional outcome for tumors in these difficult locations.

References

1. Akhtar S., Oza K.K., Wright J. (2000). Merkel cell carcinoma: report of 10 cases and review of the literature. *J Am Acad Dermatol* 43(5 Pt 1): 755–767.
2. Medina-Franco H., Urist M.M., Fiveash J., *et al.* (2001). Multimodality treatment of Merkel cell carcinoma: case series and literature review of 1024 cases. *Ann Surg Oncol* 8: 204–208.
3. Agelli M., Clegg L.X. (2003). Epidemiology of primary Merkel cell carcinoma in the United States. *J Am Acad Dermatol* 49: 832–841.
4. Hodgson N.C. (2008). Merkel cell carcinoma: changing incidence trends. *J Surg Oncol* 89: 1–4.
5. Tai P. (2008). Merkel cell cancer: update on biology and treatment. *Curr Opin Oncol* 20: 196–200.
6. Padhya T.A., Gluckman J.L. (2003). Surgical anatomy. In: Gluckman J.L. and Johnson J.T. (eds.). *Surgical Management of Neck Metastases*, pp. 1–23, Martin Dunitz, London, UK.
7. Burget G.C., Menick F.J. (1985). The subunit principle in nasal reconstruction. *Plast Reconst Surg* 76: 239–247.
8. Borges A.F. (1984). Relaxed skin tension lines (RSTL) versus other skin lines. *Plast Reconst Surg* 73: 144–150.
9. American Joint Committee on Cancer. *AJCC Cancer Staging Manual*, 6th Ed. Springer, New York, 2002.

10. Heath M., Jaimes N., Lemos B., *et al.* (2008). Clinical characteristics of Merkel cell carcinoma at diagnosis in 195 patients: the AEIOU features. *J Am Acad Dermatol* 58: 375–381.
11. Goepfert H., Remmler D., Silva E., Wheeler B. (1984). Merkel cell carcinoma (endocrine carcinoma of the skin) of the head and neck. *Arch Otolaryngol* 110: 707–712.
12. Bielamowicz S., Smith D., Abemayor E. (1994). Merkel cell carcinoma: an aggressive skin neoplasm. *Laryngoscope* 104(5 Pt 1): 528–532.
13. Azizi L., Marsot-Dupuch K., Bigel P., *et al.* (2001). Merkel cell carcinoma: a rare cause of hypervascular nasal tumor. *Am J Neuroradiol* 22: 1389–1393.
14. Brissett A.E., Olsen K.D., Kasperbauer J.L., *et al.* (2002). Merkel cell carcinoma of the head and neck: a retrospective case series. *Head Neck* 24: 982–988.
15. Karapantzos I., Tsaroucha A., Polychronidis A., *et al.* (2003). Merkel cell carcinoma: report of seven cases. *ORL J Otorhinolaryngol Relat Spec* 65: 370–374.
16. Suarez C., Rodrigo J.P., Ferlito A., *et al.* (2004). Merkel cell carcinoma of the head and neck. *Oral Oncol* 40: 773–779.
17. Veness M.J., Palme C.E., Morgan G.J. (2008). Merkel cell carcinoma: a review of management. *Curr Opin Otolaryngol Head Neck Surg* 16: 170–174.
18. Gillenwater A.M., Hessel A.C., Morrison W.H., *et al.* (2001). Merkel cell carcinoma of the head and neck: effect of surgical excision and radiation on recurrence and survival. *Arch Otolaryngol Head Neck Surg* 127: 149–154.
19. Lawenda B.D., Thiringer J.K., Foss R.D., Johnstone P.A. (2001). Merkel cell carcinoma arising in the head and neck: optimizing therapy. *Am J Clin Oncol* 24: 35–42.
20. Dancey A.L., Rayatt S.S., Soon C., *et al.* (2006). Merkel cell carcinoma: a report of 34 cases and literature review. *J Plast Reconstr Aesthet Surg* 59: 1294–1299.
21. Boyer J.D., Zitelli J.A., Brodland D.G., D'Angelo G. (2004). Local control of primary Merkel cell carcinoma: review of 45 cases treated with Mohs micrographic surgery with and without adjuvant radiation. *J Am Acad Dermatol* 47: 885–892.
22. Gollard R., Weber R., Kosty M.P., *et al.* (2000). Merkel cell carcinoma: review of 22 cases with surgical, pathologic, and therapeutic considerations. *Cancer* 88: 1842–1851.

23. O'Connor W.J., Roenigk R.K., Brodland D.G. (1997). Merkel cell carcinoma: comparison of Mohs micrographic surgery and wide excision in eighty-six patients. *Dermatol Surg* 23: 929–933.
24. Messina J.L., Reintgen D.S., Cruse C.W., *et al.* (1997). Selective lymphadenectomy in patients with Merkel cell (cutaneous neuroendocrine) carcinoma. *Ann Surg Oncol* 4: 389–395.
25. Ames S.E., Krag D.N., Brady M.S. (1998). Radiolocalization of the sentinel lymph node in Merkel cell carcinoma: a clinical analysis of seven cases. *J Surg Oncol* 67: 251–254.
26. Wasserberg N., Schachter J., Fenig E., *et al.* (2000). Applicability of the sentinel node technique to Merkel cell carcinoma. *Dermatol Surg* 26: 138–141.
27. Allen P.J., Busam K., Hill A.D., *et al.* (2001). Immunohistochemical analysis of sentinel lymph nodes from patients with Merkel cell carcinoma. *Cancer* 92: 1650–1655.
28. Mehrany K., Otley C.C., Weenig R.H., *et al.* (2002). A meta-analysis of the prognostic significance of sentinel lymph node status in Merkel cell carcinoma. *Dermatol Surg* 28: 113–117.
29. Su L.D., Lowe L., Bradford C.R., *et al.* (2002). Immunostaining for cytokeratin 20 improves detection of micrometastatic Merkel cell carcinoma in sentinel lymph nodes. *J Am Acad Dermatol* 46: 661–666.
30. Hill A.D., Brady M.D., Coit D.G. (1999). Intraoperative lymphatic mapping and sentinel lymph node biopsy for Merkel cell carcinoma. *Br J Surg* 86: 518–521.
31. Wagner J.D., Evdokimow D.Z., Weisberger E., *et al.* (2004). Sentinel node biopsy for high-risk nonmelanoma cutaneous malignancy. *Arch Dermatol* 140: 75–79.
32. Schmalbach C.E., Lowe L., Teknos T.N., *et al.* (2005). Reliability of sentinel lymph node biopsy for regional staging of head and neck Merkel cell carcinoma. *Arch Otolaryngol Head Neck Surg* 131: 610–614.
33. Gupta S.G., Wang L.S., Penas P.F., *et al.* (2006). Sentinel lymph node biopsy for evaluation and treatment of patients with Merkel cell carcinoma: the Dana-Farber experience and meta-analysis of the literature. *Arch Dermatol* 142: 685–690.
34. Warner R.E., Quinn M.J., Hruby G., *et al.* (2008). Management of Merkel cell carcinoma: the roles of lymphoscintigraphy, sentinel lymph node biopsy and adjuvant radiotherapy. *Ann Surg Oncol* 15: 2509–2518.

35. Stokes J.B., Graw K.S., Dengel L.T., *et al.* (2009). Patients with Merkel cell carcinoma tumors ≤1.0 cm in diameter are unlikely to harbor regional lymph node metastases. *J Clin Oncol* 27: 3772–3777.
36. Robbins K.T., Shaha A.R., Medina J.E., *et al.* (2008). Consensus statement on the classification and terminology of neck dissection. *Arch Otolaryngol Head Neck Surg* 134: 536–538.
37. McCarn K.E., Park S.S. (2007). Lip reconstruction. *Otolaryngol Clin North Am* 40: 361–380.
38. Cummings C.W., Haughey B., Thomas J.R., *et al.* (1993). *Otolaryngology — Head and Neck Surgery*, 2nd Ed., Mosby Publisher.
39. Larrabee W.F. Jr. (1989). Immediate repair of facial defects. *Dermatol Clin* 7: 661–676.

Chapter 12

The Role of Mohs Micrographic Surgery in Merkel Cell Carcinoma

Basil S. Cherpelis

12.1 Introduction

Surgical treatment of Merkel cell carcinoma is associated with a high rate of treatment failure,[1] but nonetheless, the primary treatment of Merkel cell carcinoma generally involves surgical excision unless precluded by health status.[2] Achieving clear surgical margins during initial resection is the best hope for cure.[3] Simple excision is associated with a high rate of local recurrence.[4] Wide surgical margins have been suggested in order to improve cure rates. Even so, wide excision has reported local recurrence rates that range from 26% to 44%.[5] Wide excision with a margin of 2 to 3 cm may result in considerable morbidity, and still sometimes fail to obtain clear margins, particularly on head and neck lesions.[2] Merkel cell carcinoma located on the head and neck accounts for 50–55% of Merkel cell carcinoma tumors.[6] For these tumors, tissue sparing is important and has led to the suggestion of Mohs micrographic surgery as a possible treatment.[7] Mohs surgery is superior to conventional excision in the treatment of basal cell and squamous cell carcinoma. It offers complete histologic evaluation and tissue sparing capability, making it attractive in the treatment of Merkel cell carcinoma.

Mohs micrographic surgery is a specialized surgical and pathologic technique used to treat a variety of cutaneous neoplasms, first described by Frederic Mohs in 1941.[8] Its design integrates the role of surgeon and pathologist and is unique in providing assessment of 100% of surgical margins intraoperatively,[9] in contrast to a significantly lower percentage

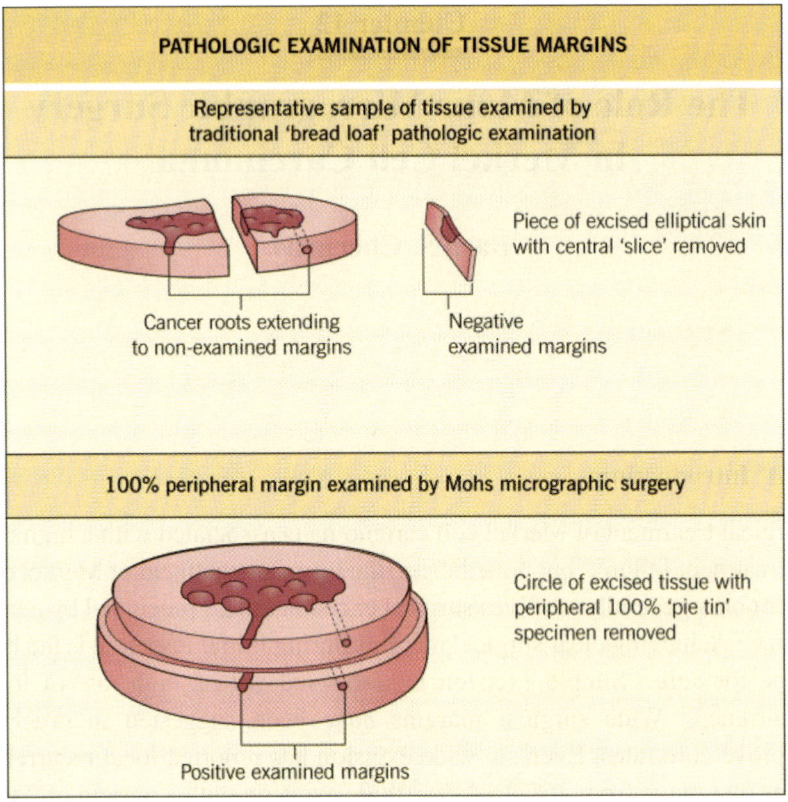

Figure 1. Pathologic examination of tissue margins. Comparison of traditional 'bread loaf' sections (<1% of total margin examined) vs. Mohs micrographic surgery (100% of total margins examined). Reproduced with permission from Otley and Roenigk, 2008.[19]

of assessed margins, typically 0.1% to 5%, by standard specimen analysis ('bread loaf' analysis, Figure 1).

In Mohs surgery, excision generally takes place under local anesthesia. The surgical site is prepared and draped in the usual manner. The surgeon marks the tumor's clinical extent and appropriate margins are drawn around the tumor (Figure 2). Margins vary depending on the surgeon performing the technique and the clinical scenario. Reference marks are placed by making small nicks overlapping the tumor and perilesional skin at 12, 3, 6 and 9 o'clock. A debulking layer is performed that removes

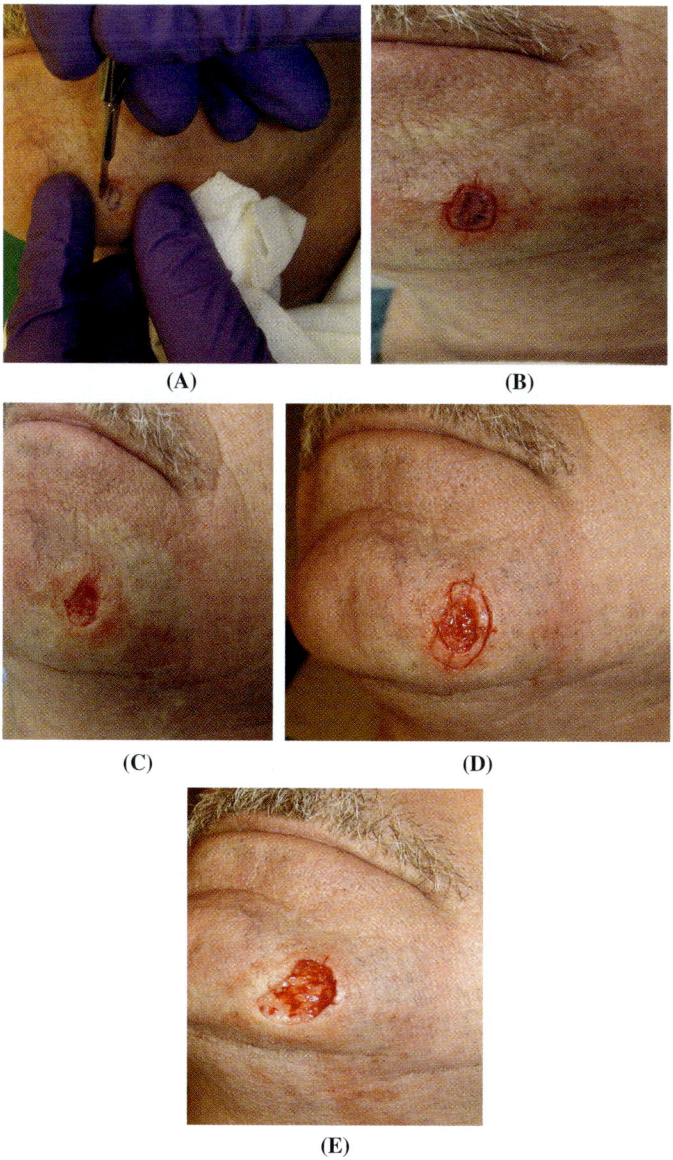

Figure 2. **(A)** Beveled excision (with scalpel at a 45° angle) of all clinically evident tumor plus a small margin of normal-appearing skin. **(B)** Placement of hash marks at 3, 6, 9 and 12 o'clock positions in adjacent surrounding tissue. **(C)** Defect after first layer of tissue is removed. **(D)** An additional margin of tissue is excised in areas of residual tumor identified by histopathologic examination. **(E)** Postoperative tumor-free defect.

the clinically visible tumor. A small 1 mm strip of tissue is taken from this debulking layer to serve as a positive control during examination of the histopathology slides. The first Mohs layer is then ready to be taken. The initial peripheral incision of each Mohs layer is beveled inward at approximately 45 degrees, until reaching the depth at which the specimen will be undercut. The remainder of the deep portion of the specimen is then excised horizontally or parallel to the tissue surface. The purpose of the angled incision is to create a bevel that allows the peripheral and deep margins to be in the same plane for processing. A detailed map of the excised tissue with reference marks is made and care is taken to preserve the orientation of the tissue. The edges are inked and the specimen is embedded top-down on the cryostat chuck. In this manner, a horizontal tissue layer will contain all of the true surgical margins, including the entire circumference of epidermis and deep tissue. Tissue staining with hematoxylin and eosin is performed. The surgeon analyzes the prepared histopathology specimens and marks any areas positive for tumor on the map. Additional stages of excision are performed as necessary with processing in the same manner as above.[10] When all margins are free of tumor, the defect is repaired. Shriner *et al.*[11] provide a detailed description of Mohs surgery.

12.2 Efficacy in Merkel Cell Carcinoma

The efficacy of Mohs micrographic surgery in the treatment of Merkel cell carcinoma has been studied in a number of retrospective studies of varying sizes. O'Conner *et al.*[12] reported that wide excision for local disease was associated with a local recurrence rate of 31.7% out of 86 patients treated. Mean follow-up was 60 months. In contrast, only one out of 12 patients (8.3%) treated with Mohs surgery had a local recurrence. This one patient underwent a second Mohs excision to treat the recurrence and has remained disease-free for 84 months. Mean follow-up for patients treated by Mohs surgery was 36 months. Regional metastasis was reported in 48.8% patients treated by wide excision and in 33.3% of Mohs patients who were not treated with postoperative radiotherapy. None of the patients treated with postoperative radiation therapy after Mohs surgery developed regional metastases. They concluded that Mohs micrographic surgery compares favorably with standard surgical excision and that radiotherapy after Mohs micrographic surgery may further reduce regional metastases.

In contrast, Boyer *et al.*[1] reported that adjuvant radiation therapy appears non-essential to secure local control of primary Merkel cell carcinoma lesions completely excised with Mohs micrographic surgery. Their retrospective study consisted of 45 patients with stage I Merkel cell carcinoma who were histologically and clinically free of disease after Mohs excision. Twenty patients subsequently received postoperative radiation to the primary site and 25 did not. In the Mohs surgery alone group, there was 4% local recurrence and three in-transit metastases were observed. No local or regional metastases were reported in the Mohs surgery plus postoperative radiation therapy. Overall and relapse-free survival were not significantly different between the treatment groups. Among the patients treated with Mohs surgery alone, Boyer reported a 79% five-year survival rate with 16% of patients developing regional recurrence and 8% developing distant metastases. These values are not statistically different from the group that received Mohs micrographic surgery and adjuvant radiation therapy, and compare favorably with results of wide excision with or without radiation. The mean overall Mohs surgical margin of clinically normal skin excised to achieve tumor-free margins in this series was 1.67 cm. However, 25% of Merkel cell carcinoma tumors in this series would have been inadequately excised if 2.0 cm margins were obtained. Similarly, 12% of Merkel cell carcinoma tumors would have been inadequately excised if 3.0 cm margins were obtained. Conversely, in 48% of the tumors, tumor-free margins were obtained with margins less than 1.0 cm. Margins of 1 cm frequently will be negative for lesions that measure under 2 cm in diameter.[13,14]

Senchenkov *et al.*[15] reported on six patients with Merkel cell carcinoma of the extremities who were treated with Mohs micrographic surgery. Three patients had recurrences; one was a local recurrence and two had regional recurrences. Adjuvant radiotherapy significantly increased the proportion of patients free from recurrence compared to surgery (wide excision or Mohs) alone (75.2% vs. 52.9%). Brissett *et al.*[16] reported a series of 33 patients; six had Mohs micrographic surgery, eight had wide excision only, and eight had wide excision and regional lymph node dissection. The survival rate at two years showed a trend toward improvement for the patients that had wide excision of the primary tumor and dissection of the lymphatic drainage basin (100%) or wide excision alone (72.9%) compared with patients who had Mohs (33.3%). Pathai *et al.*[6] reported on the use of Mohs micrographic surgery in a single patient with a Merkel cell carcinoma of the left upper eyelid. Histologically clear margins were able to be obtained and the patient was disease-free at two years postoperatively.

12.3 Conclusion

Tissue conservation is a clear benefit of Mohs micrographic surgery. The acceptably low rates of local recurrence in published retrospective series suggest that selected patients may be good candidates for Mohs. Although there are no prospective studies to allow a direct comparison with wide excision or to evaluate the role of postoperative radiation after Mohs surgery, there is reason to believe that arbitrary excision widths based on the clinical extent of tumor may be unreliable because Merkel cell carcinoma rarely has epidermal involvement and most tumors have infiltrating margins.[17] Additionally, tumors may be incompletely excised if standard 'bread-loafing' is used because typically less than 1% of the margins are examined.[18]

Merkel cell carcinoma is a rare tumor and there are few studies upon which to base firm conclusions. The data that is available supports the use of Mohs micrographic surgery in the treatment of selected patients with Merkel cell carcinoma, especially in cases that involve anatomically important areas where tissue conservation is paramount. However, Merkel cell carcinoma frequently involves regional lymph nodes. As most patients require nodal staging, Mohs micrographic surgery ideally should be performed in conjunction with sentinel lymph node biopsy, although this is often impractical in most clinical settings. Furthermore, we frequently recommend postoperative radiation to the primary site. As with other approaches to the management of primary Merkel cell carcinoma, we believe that Mohs micrographic surgery is best used as part of a multidisciplinary approach that matches the right treatment to the right patient.

References

1. Boyer J.D., Zitelli J.A., Brodland D.G., *et al.* (2002). Local control of primary Merkel cell carcinoma: review of 45 cases treated with Mohs micrographic surgery with and without adjuvant radiation. *J Am Acad Dermatol* 47: 885–892.
2. Eng T.Y., Boersma M.G., Fuller C.D., *et al.* (2007). A comprehensive review of the treatment of Merkel cell carcinoma. *Am J Clin Onc* 30: 624–636.
3. Henness S., Vereecken P. (2008). Management of Merkel tumors: an evidence-based review. *Curr Opin Oncol* 20: 280–286.
4. Kokosuka E.R., Kokoska M.S., Collins B.T., *et al.* (1997). Early aggressive treatment for Merkel cell carcinoma improves outcome. *Am J Surg* 174: 688–693.
5. Shaw J.H., Rumball E. (1991). Merkel cell tumor: clinical behavior and treatment. *Br J Surg* 78: 138–142.
6. Pathai S., Barlow R., Williams G., *et al.* (2005). Mohs' micrographic surgery for Merkel cell carcinoma of the eyelid. *Orbit* 24: 273–275.
7. The NCCN Merkel Cell Carcinoma Practice Guidelines in Oncology (version1.2008). National Comprehensive Cancer Network, Inc. http://www.nccn.org/professionals/physician_gls/ [Accessed 20 Oct 2008].
8. Mohs F.E. (1941). Chemosurgery: a microscopically controlled method of cancer excision. *Arch Surg* 42: 279–295.
9. Zitell J.A., Brown C., Hanusa B.H. (1997). Mohs micrographic surgery for the treatment of primary cutaneous melanoma. *J Am Acad Dermatol* 37(2, pt 1): 236–245.
10. Clark G.S., Pappas-Plitis E.C., Cherpelis B.S., *et al.* (2008). Surgical management of melanoma in situ on chronically sun-damaged skin. *Cancer Control* 15: 216–224.
11. Shriner D.L., McCoy D.K., Goldberg D.G., *et al.* (1998). Mohs micrographic surgery. *J Am Acad Dermatol* 39: 79–97
12. O'Conner W.J., Roenigk R.K., Brodland D.G. (1997). Merkel cell carcinoma. Comparison of Mohs micrographic surgery and wide excision in eighty-six patients. *Dermatol Surg* 23: 929–933.
13. Allen P.J., Zhang Z.F., Coit D.G. (1999). Surgical management of Merkel cell carcinoma. *Ann Surg* 229: 97–105.

14. Tai P. (2008). Merkel cell cancer: update on biology and treatment. *Curr Opin Oncol* 20: 196–200.
15. Senchenkov A., Barnes S.A., Moran S.L. (2007). Predictors of survival and recurrence in the surgical treatment of Merkel cell carcinoma of the extremities. *J Surg Oncol* 95: 229–234.
16. Brissett A.E., Olsen K.D., Kasperbauer J.L., *et al.* (2002). Merkel cell carcinoma of the head and neck: a retrospective case series. *Head Neck* 24: 982–988.
17. Wilder R.B., Harari P.M., Graham A.R., *et al.* (1991). Merkel cell carcinoma: improved locoregional control with postoperative radiation therapy. *Cancer* 68: 1004–1008.
18. Abide J.M., Nahai F., Bennett R.G. (1984). The meaning of surgical margins. *Plastic Reconstr Surg* 73: 492–496.
19. Otley C.C., Roenigk R.K. (2008). Mohs surgery. *Dermatology* 2: 2269–2279.

Chapter 13

Radiation in the Management of Primary and Regional Merkel Cell Carcinoma

George Hruby and John F. Thompson

13.1 Introduction

Merkel cell carcinoma is an exquisitely radiosensitive neuroendocrine tumor that is thought to arise from a primitive pluripotent epidermal cell.[1] Based on its radiosensitivity, the role of radiation treatment of Merkel cell carcinoma may be adjuvant (i.e. following surgery — the most common indication), definitive, elective (when nodal disease is a possibility but has not been proven histologically) or palliative. This chapter will focus on the roles of radiation (and chemoradiation) in potentially curative scenarios, i.e. as definitive, adjuvant or elective treatment.

13.2 Definitive Radiation Treatment

Several reported series document the use of radiation therapy alone to treat primary Merkel cell carcinoma, with durable levels of local control. Doses used in the definitive setting have varied from 45 to 60 Gray (Gy) in varying fractionation schedules.[2–5]

In the most recent of these reports, Mortier and colleagues compared nine patients with inoperable Merkel cell carcinoma treated by definitive radiation (group one) to 17 patients treated by surgery and adjuvant radiation (group two). All patients had stage I disease based on clinical examination, chest X-ray and ultrasound evaluation of the draining lymphatics. The mean tumor diameter was 3.7 cm in group one and 2.1 cm in group two. Tumor size was comparable between the groups with the exception of two patients in group one who had 7 and 8 cm primaries respectively. A median dose of 60 Gy (range 50–78 Gy) was delivered in daily 2 Gy fractions. Twenty-one of 26 patients also received elective radiation to the draining lymph nodes. With a median follow-up of three years for group one and 4.6 years for group two, only two patients recurred, both from group two. The first failure was a skin relapse: the recurrence was managed with definitive radiation and the patient was alive and well five years later. The second failure was both local and distant, with the patient dead of disease five months after recurrence. This small but provocative study certainly demonstrates the possibility of treating inoperable Merkel cell carcinoma with definitive radiation.

Figure 1 demonstrates the rapid response of a large Merkel cell carcinoma on the finger of a 100 year old nursing home resident treated definitively by the authors in 2008.

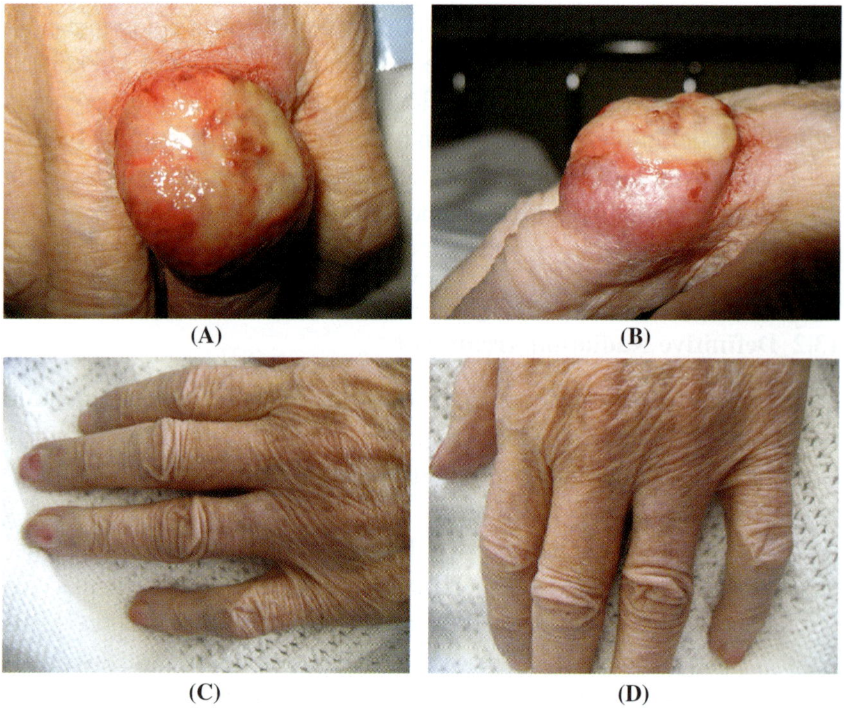

Figure 1. (**A** and **B**) Large Merkel cell carcinoma on the finger of a 100 year old nursing home resident treated definitively by radiation with rapid and complete resolution of disease (**C** and **D**).

13.3 Adjuvant Radiation Treatment

Adjuvant postoperative treatment to the primary site and/or regional lymph nodes is currently the principal role for radiotherapy in Merkel cell carcinoma. The evidence for its efficacy is retrospective, and most series demonstrate improvements in both locoregional control and disease free survival when compared to series managing this disease with surgery alone.[6–11] Medina-Franco *et al.* reported their experience with Merkel cell carcinoma at the University of Alabama and reviewed the existing literature which, at that time, included 20 series with a total of 1024 cases. Of these, 11 series comprising 441 patients reported local recurrence rates with and without adjuvant radiation.[6,7,12–19] The local recurrence rate of 10.5% (range 0–33%) following adjuvant radiation was significantly lower than the rate of 52.6% (range 6–100%) without adjuvant radiation.

These results, however, probably overstate the case for radiation due to patient selection bias, the heterogeneous nature of surgery within the surgery only group, and the possible inclusion of both local and locoregional recurrences as local relapses. Furthermore, some studies compared excision of the primary site alone with resection of the primary followed by adjuvant local and elective regional radiation; or with resection of the primary site and clinical lymph node dissection followed by adjuvant radiation treatment to both sites.[7,8,20]

Along the same lines, the majority of those advocating the use of surgery alone in this disease have included adjuvant radiation in a subset of patients. Although not reaching statistical significance (no doubt due to small patient numbers, as only 17% received adjuvant radiation), there was still a halving in nodal relapse rates from 26% to 13% with the use of adjuvant radiation.[21]

More recently, a series of 82 patients from Sydney[20] as well as an analysis of over 1600 patients in the SEER (Surveillance, Epidemiology and End Results) database[22] have demonstrated statistically significant improvements in survival with the use of postoperative radiation treatment. Again, these were retrospective series and may be subject to inherent selection bias, however in the Sydney cohort all consecutive cases were included, and the surgical margins were clearly documented. The majority of patients (60 of 73) had the primary Merkel cell carcinoma excised with clear margins, despite which, those patients who received any adjuvant radiation treatment were much less likely to recur (hazard ratio 0.39). These data challenge the notion that radiation treatment is unnecessary in the presence of clear margins.

The study by Mojica and colleagues analyzed 1665 cases of Merkel cell carcinoma found on the SEER database between 1973 and 2002. Information was available on the type of surgery performed at the primary site and lymph nodes, the use of adjuvant radiation, but not on the use of chemotherapy or of sentinel node biopsy. Surgical intervention was a component of management in 1487 cases (89%). The whole cohort had a median survival of 49 months, with a median follow-up of 40 months. Adjuvant radiation was a part of treatment in 40% of the surgical cases; in these patients the median survival was 63 months compared to 45 months for patients not receiving adjuvant radiation ($p = 0.0002$). When stratified by size of the primary tumor, adjuvant radiation was associated with an improved median survival in patients with tumors <1 cm (from 48 to 93 months, $p = 0.0447$), in patients with tumors from 1 to 2 cm (from 52 to 86 months, $p = 0.0126$) and in patients with tumors greater than 2 cm (from 21 to 50 months, $p = 0.0003$). Thus, the use of adjuvant radiation was associated with improved survival in all age groups, and for all tumor sizes.

The weight of evidence therefore supports the use of adjuvant radiation treatment after surgery. Furthermore, the extent of surgical margins, or the need for re-resection or disfiguring surgery for Merkel cell carcinoma (which occurs predominantly in exposed and often cosmetically challenging areas) becomes less important if adjuvant radiation is delivered. What remains controversial, however, is the most appropriate integration of surgery and radiation treatment.[23] Therefore, surgeons and radiation oncologists should manage these patients together in a team approach. Barriers to timely radiation treatment such as long waiting times need to be overcome. These delays may also come from failure to recognize this quixotic disease, as well as lack of knowledge regarding the role of radiation, particularly among clinicians practicing outside a multidisciplinary setting.

There are data suggesting that delayed commencement of radiation treatment is associated with worse outcomes. An unacceptably high risk of progression (41%) was seen in patients who waited a median of 24 days for radiation treatment.[24] Patients who progressed while awaiting radiation had a median wait of ten days longer than those who did not progress (median 30 vs. 20 days). Consequently, some radiation oncology departments will prioritize patients with Merkel cell carcinoma for early treatment.

In addition to its role as adjuvant therapy following surgery, radiation treatment may be used electively, particularly at sites such as the head and neck where the draining node field is usually in close proximity to the primary lesion. Pragmatically, this may in some cases obviate the need for sentinel lymph node biopsy, as radiation can be given as adjuvant therapy to the primary site and electively to the nodal basin, in continuity.

The role of sentinel node biopsy in this disease remains controversial. In a recent series from the Sydney Melanoma Unit,[25] eight patients had negative sentinel nodes. Despite the negative biopsy results, two of these patients received elective radiation treatment to the node field and did not recur; however five of the six remaining patients recurred in the node field. The sentinel node specimens were all re-reviewed by a pathologist subspecialized in melanoma and Merkel cell carcinoma, with no changes to the original reports. At the Sydney Melanoma Unit, the failure rate for melanoma detection after a negative sentinel node biopsy was only 2.7% in over 1000 patients treated.[25] The expertise of the two author surgeons dealing with Merkel cell carcinoma is not in doubt, and if this experience is substantiated it would appear that Merkel cell carcinoma may behave in a very different fashion than melanoma. Treating this disease using standard melanoma or non-melanoma skin cancer paradigms is flawed and inappropriate. However, it seems likely that preoperative lymphoscintigraphy to identify the location of sentinel lymph nodes and draining node fields may be of value in rational radiotherapy field planning.[9]

Studies reporting the use of sentinel node biopsy for Merkel cell carcinoma were summarized recently by Warner *et al.*[25] It is apparent that in various series recurrence rates range from 5% to 33%.[21,26–29] Again, consistent with our experience, in many cases these are unacceptably high.

13.4 The Role of Chemoradiation in the Treatment of Merkel Cell Carcinoma

Chemotherapy may sensitize Merkel cell carcinoma to the effects of radiation treatment and therefore enhance the local cell kill from radiotherapy.

It may also act further afield to eliminate micrometastatic disease, particularly in a chemosensitive disease with a propensity to disseminate. These two mechanisms of action at distinct sites are known as 'spatial cooperation.'

The Australia and New Zealand Trans-Tasman Radiation Oncology Group (TROG) has conducted two prospective trials utilizing adjuvant chemoradiotherapy in high risk Merkel cell carcinoma. The trials are important not only because they are among the only prospective trials reported in the literature, but also because they are testament to several important management principles that can only be coordinated in the multi-disciplinary care setting. Given that adjuvant (chemo) radiotherapy was to be delivered to the primary tumor site and nodes in all cases, excision with clear margins was not required, nor was resection of nodal disease or sentinel node biopsy mandated.

The first of these TROG trials was trial 96.07,[30] which included 53 patients with high risk Merkel cell carcinoma. To be eligible for the study, patients had to have a cutaneous primary with no evidence of spread beyond the regional lymph nodes. High risk was defined as meeting at least one of the following criteria: primary tumor size >1 cm, involved lymph nodes, recurrence after initial surgery, or gross residual disease after surgery. From 1997 to 2001, 53 patients were treated with radiation to the primary site and nodes using a dose of 50 Gy in 25 fractions over five weeks to clinically involved areas. Concomitant carboplatin (area under the curve (AUC) 4.5 given intravenously on day 1) and etoposide (80 mg per m^2 intravenously on days 1–3) were administered on weeks 1 and 4. Two further cycles followed the initial combination chemoradiotherapy during weeks 7 and 10. The radiation treatment was delivered to the primary site with a 3–5 cm margin, and to draining lymph nodes — which were treated in the same field as the primary if the basin was within 20 cm of the primary. Clinically uninvolved areas were treated to 46 Gy in 23 fractions over five weeks, and if volumes were thought to be too large, fields could be shrunk after 46 Gy. Despite the high-risk status of the group, overall survival and locoregional control were excellent, with three-year overall and relapse-free survival rates of 76% and 65% respectively. However, grade 3 or more neutropenia occurred in 57% of the patients, with febrile neutropenia in 35%. It has been postulated that the marrow suppression coincides with the acute skin radiation reaction, which provides a portal for colonization.

In order to reduce the toxicity seen in trial 96.07, TROG investigators have piloted the use of weekly carboplatin (AUC 2) synchronous with the radiation treatment.[31] This is then followed by three cycles of adjuvant carboplatin (AUC 4.5) and etoposide (instead of the two cycles given with, and two cycles after, radiation treatment in TROG 96.07). Again, as with TROG 96.07, wide surgical clearance and sentinel node biopsy were not mandated, nor was it a prerequisite for positive margins to be re-excised. Four patients with high risk stage I and 14 with high risk stage II disease were recruited. Only one patient did not complete weekly carboplatin (due to myelosuppression after three infusions). All three cycles of adjuvant chemotherapy were delivered in 15 of 18 patients. Skin toxicity was greatest during the last week of radiation (week 5). It was gratifying to note that neutropenia peaked during the second cycle of combination chemotherapy, by which time the skin was healing. Compared to trial 96.07, grade 3 skin toxicity was much lower (23% vs 65%), as was grade 3 and 4 neutropenia (25% and 6% respectively). Given the advanced age of most patients with Merkel cell carcinoma, a better tolerated treatment regimen is important, and this pilot chemoradiotherapy schedule is being used in ongoing trials.

As yet, chemoradiotherapy cannot be regarded as standard treatment for Merkel cell carcinoma.[32] Our approach at present is to utilize it in the clinical trial setting only, using the regime described above.

References

1. Toker C. (1972). Trabecular carcinoma of the skin. *Arch Dermatol* 105: 107–110.
2. Mortier L., Mirabel X., Fournier C., *et al.* (2003). Radiotherapy alone for primary Merkel cell carcinoma. *Arch Dermatol* 139: 1587–1590.
3. Ashby M.A., Jones D.H., Tasker A.D., *et al.* (1989). Primary cutaneous neuroendocrine (Merkel cell or trabecular carcinoma) tumour of the skin: a radioresponsive tumour. *Clin Radiol* 40: 85–87.
4. Pacella J., Ashby M., Ainslie J., *et al.* (1988). The role of radiotherapy in the management of primary cutaneous neuroendocrine tumors (Merkel cell or trabecular carcinoma): experience at the Peter MacCallum Cancer Institute (Melbourne, Australia). *Int J Radiat Oncol Biol Phys* 14: 1077–1084.

5. Suntharalingam M., Rudoltz M.S., Mendenhall W.M., *et al.* (1995). Radiotherapy for Merkel cell carcinoma of the skin of the head and neck. *Head Neck* 17: 96–101.
6. Medina-Franco H., Urist M.M., Fiveash J., *et al.* (2001). Multimodality treatment of Merkel cell carcinoma: case series and literature review of 1024 cases. *Ann Surg Oncol* 8: 204–208.
7. Meeuwissen J.A., Bourne R.G., Kearsley J.H. (1995). The importance of postoperative radiation therapy in the treatment of Merkel cell carcinoma. *Int J Radiat Oncol Biol Phys* 31: 325–331.
8. Veness M.J., Perera L., McCourt J., *et al.* (2005). Merkel cell carcinoma: improved outcome with adjuvant radiotherapy. *ANZ J Surg* 75: 275–281.
9. Eng T.Y., Boersma M.G., Fuller C.D., *et al.* (2004). Treatment of Merkel cell carcinoma. *Am J Clin Oncol* 27: 510–515.
10. Gillenwater A.M., Hessel A.C., Morrison W.H., *et al.* (2001). Merkel cell carcinoma of the head and neck: effect of surgical excision and radiation on recurrence and survival. *Arch Otolaryngol Head Neck Surg* 127: 149–154.
11. Lawenda B.D., Arnold M.G., Tokarz V.A., *et al.* (2008). Analysis of radiation therapy for the control of Merkel cell carcinoma of the head and neck based on 36 cases and a literature review. *Ear Nose Throat J* 87: 634–643.
12. Allen P.J., Zhang Z.F., Coit D.G. (1999). Surgical management of Merkel cell carcinoma. *Ann Surg* 229: 97–105.
13. Boyle F., Pendlebury S., Bell D. (1995). Further insights into the natural history and management of primary cutaneous neuroendocrine (Merkel cell) carcinoma. *Int J Radiat Oncol Biol Phys* 31: 315–323.
14. Kokoska E.R., Kokoska M.S., Collins B.T., *et al.* (1997). Early aggressive treatment for Merkel cell carcinoma improves outcome. *Am J Surg* 174: 688–693.
15. O'Connor W.J., Roenigk R.K., Brodland D.G. (1998). Merkel cell carcinoma. Comparison of Mohs micrographic surgery and wide excision in eighty-six patients. *Dermatol Surg* 23: 929–933.
16. Ott M.J., Tanabe K.K., Gadd M.A., *et al.* (1999). Multimodality management of Merkel cell carcinoma. *Arch Surg* 134: 388–392.
17. Perez J.A., Poblete M.T., Castillo P., *et al.* (1998). Merkel cell carcinoma. Report of 4 cases. *Rev Med Chil* 126: 553–558.
18. Pergolizzi J. Jr., Sardi A., Pelczar M., *et al.* (1997). Merkel cell carcinoma: an aggressive malignancy. *Am Surg* 63: 450–454.

19. Wong K.C., Zuletta F., Clarke S.J., *et al.* (1998). Clinical management and treatment outcomes of Merkel cell carcinoma. *Aust N Z J Surg* 68: 354–358.
20. Jabbour J., Cumming R., Scolyer R.A., *et al.* (2007). Merkel cell carcinoma: assessing the effect of wide local excision, lymph node dissection, and radiotherapy on recurrence and survival in early-stage disease — results from a review of 82 consecutive cases diagnosed between 1992 and 2004. *Ann Surg Oncol* 14: 1943–1952.
21. Allen P.J., Bowne W.B., Jaques D.P., *et al.* (2005). Merkel cell carcinoma: prognosis and treatment of patients from a single institution. *J Clin Oncol* 23: 2300–2309.
22. Mojica P., Smith D., Ellenhorn J.D. (2007). Adjuvant radiation therapy is associated with improved survival in Merkel cell carcinoma of the skin. *J Clin Oncol* 25: 1043–1047.
23. Poulsen M., Harvey J. (2002). Is there a diminishing role for surgery for Merkel cell carcinoma of the skin? A review of current management. *ANZ J Surg* 72: 142–146.
24. Tsang G., O'Brien P., Robertson R., *et al.* (2004). All delays before radiotherapy risk progression of Merkel cell carcinoma. *Australas Radiol* 48: 371–375.
25. Warner R.E., Quinn M.J., Hruby G., *et al.* (2008). Management of Merkel cell carcinoma: the roles of lymphoscintigraphy, sentinel lymph node biopsy and adjuvant radiotherapy. *Ann Surg Oncol* 15: 2509–2518.
26. Maza S., Trefzer U., Hofmann M., *et al.* (2006). Impact of sentinel lymph node biopsy in patients with Merkel cell carcinoma: results of a prospective study and review of the literature. *Eur J Nucl Med Mol Imaging* 33: 433–440.
27. Pan D., Narayan D., Ariyan S. (2002). Merkel cell carcinoma: five case reports using sentinel lymph node biopsy and a review of 110 new cases. *Plast Reconstr Surg* 110: 1259–1265.
28. Rodrigues L.K., Leong S.P., Kashani-Sabet M., *et al.* (2001). Early experience with sentinel lymph node mapping for Merkel cell carcinoma. *J Am Acad Dermatol* 45: 303–308.
29. Schmalbach C.E., Lowe L., Teknos T.N., *et al.* (2005) Reliability of sentinel lymph node biopsy for regional staging of head and neck Merkel cell carcinoma. *Arch Otolaryngol Head Neck Surg* 131: 610–614.
30. Poulsen M., Rischin D., Walpole E., *et al.* (2003) High-risk Merkel cell carcinoma of the skin treated with synchronous carboplatin/etoposide and

radiation: a Trans-Tasman Radiation Oncology Group Study — TROG 96:07. *J Clin Oncol* 21: 4371–4376.

31. Poulsen M., Walpole E., Harvey J., *et al.* (2008) Weekly carboplatin reduces toxicity during synchronous chemoradiotherapy for Merkel cell carcinoma of skin. *Int J Radiat Oncol Biol Phys* 72: 1070–1074.
32. Poulsen M.G., Rischin D., Porter I., *et al.* (2006) Does chemotherapy improve survival in high-risk stage I and II Merkel cell carcinoma of the skin? *Int J Radiat Oncol Biol Phys* 64: 114–119.

Chapter 14

Management of Recurrent and Metastatic Merkel Cell Carcinoma

Ronald C. DeConti

Merkel cell carcinoma may be the most deadly of the skin malignancies and its rise in incidence is likely to make it more problematic in the future, justifying increased attention and new efforts to improve therapy and prognosis. The Surveillance, Epidemiology and End Results (SEER) program of the National Cancer Institute reported an observed five-year survival rate of 45% with a five-year relative survival of 62%. Survival after the onset of systemic metastasis is poor, with median survival in the range of eight to 12 months; the SEER Program reported a five-year relative survival of 25%.[1] Few patients present with distant metastatic disease; early reviews described 1–2% but recent individual institutions and a large SEER database report 6–8% of patients presenting with metastatic disease.[2–5] The difference is likely related to improved evaluation techniques.[1]

Clinically, most patients have localized disease at presentation; at least 20–30% of these will be upstaged with micrometastatic nodal disease found at sentinel node evaluation. While the prognostic value of age, sex, size, depth and location have each been debated (see Chapters 7 and 8), the risk for systemic relapse has been most convincingly related to regional lymph node involvement.[6,7] Distant nodal disease is often the first site of systemic relapse, but rapid spread to multiple sites is common including soft tissue, lung, liver, bone and eventually brain. More unusual foci include testis,[8–10] pancreas,[11] heart,[12] bone marrow[13] and meninges.[14]

Merkel cell carcinoma, a neuroendocrine tumor, has been likened to both small cell lung cancer and malignant melanoma because of its histologic features as well as some clinical similarities. However, there are many very distinct differences from both. Like small cell lung cancer, Merkel cell carcinoma shares some neuroendocrine features, is likely to spread widely to soft tissue, nodes, lung, liver, bone and brain, and has been shown to frequently respond to combination chemotherapy and to radiation. Unlike small cell lung cancer, it is commonly a localized skin neoplasm at presentation, and usually progresses with nodal involvement first and dissemination later. These latter features are more reminiscent of melanoma, though the prognostic value of primary tumor thickness is uncertain in Merkel cell carcinoma and the chronology of relapse is quite different. More than 90% of metastases have been reported to develop within two years of diagnosis in Merkel cell carcinoma, whereas melanoma recurrences continue for well beyond ten years.[15,16] It must be acknowledged, however, that long term outcome studies in Merkel cell carcinoma are rare, and in fact the relapse pattern of 'typical' Merkel cell carcinoma is really quite similar to that of thick primary cutaneous melanoma.

The appreciation that many Merkel cell patients at high risk (e.g. node positive patients) will demonstrate relapse within months permits close clinical follow-up and periodic radiographic evaluations to detect asymptomatic disease, and calls attention to the need for prompt evaluation of new symptoms during this period.

14.1 Local and In-Transit Recurrences

The management of these recurrences relates to their location, extent and any previous therapy. As described in Chapters 10 and 13, the primary lesion may have been subjected to prior wide resection and/or radiation therapy. A review in 2000 by Medina *et al.* of 11 collected series reported the effect of radiation therapy on reducing local recurrence.[17] Evaluating 441 patients in these non-randomized reports, the local recurrence rate without radiation was 52% compared to 10% with radiation. More recently, in a meta-analysis of 1254 patients, Lewis *et al.* found a similar impact of radiation therapy upon local recurrence rates. Patients with negative margins recurred more often after surgery alone than after surgery plus postoperative radiation therapy (39% vs. 12%, $p < 0.001$).[18] This collected adjuvant radiation data is in marked contrast to the single-institution Memorial Sloan-Kettering experience.[4] Their relatively low recurrence rate with surgery alone (11%) was not substantially affected by the addition of radiation therapy (8%), and radiation has not been recommended by them as standard practice. Only 25 of their 185 patients (13.5%) with margin-negative excisions received adjuvant radiotherapy. Some guidelines suggest that radiation therapy is unnecessary for small lesions with adequate margins,[19] though an analysis of SEER data showed a survival benefit associated with radiotherapy for tumors of all sizes.[20]

When possible, local recurrences are managed with additional resection and radiation therapy, as determined by the location and extent of the recurrence and prior radiation dose. Unless combined with more extensive regional soft tissue disease, chemotherapy is not routinely indicated for the management of locally recurrent Merkel cell carcinoma.

Isolated in-transit recurrences, generally defined as dermal or subcutaneous metastases located 2 cm or more from the primary excision site but between that site and the regional nodal basin, are commonly also resected and treated with postoperative radiation therapy. In-transit recurrences occur more frequently in Merkel cell carcinoma than in melanoma (although again adjustments for tumor thickness or other risk factors to truly compare the incidence is not currently possible), and these recurrences may be quite extensive and bulky. In many reports, they are included together with local recurrences and nodal relapses under the category of 'local-regional recurrence.' Widely different recurrence rates in the literature may in part be accounted for by the inability to separate local, regional soft tissue and regional nodal involvement. The role of chemotherapy in management of locoregional recurrences has not been defined, but we have occasionally encountered such extensive soft tissue recurrence as to preclude surgery and for which radiation and concurrent chemotherapy may be appropriate. When chemotherapy is used, locoregional disease is reported to respond more often than disseminated metastases. Cytotoxic chemotherapy may also improve response rates when administered concomitant with radiation,[21] but clear evidence of an effect on survival has not been demonstrated.

A few cases of extensive, usually multifocal, recurrence confined solely to one extremity have been successfully treated with isolated limb perfusion utilizing melphalan alone as well as a combination of TNF, interferon and melphalan,[22,23] and more recently with isolated limb infusion using melphalan and dactinomycin. Grandpeix *et al.* described two cases achieving complete response after isolated limb perfusion with melphalan, lasting more than 18 months and 66 months, respectively.[24]

14.1.1 *Case illustration — management of in-transit metastasis*

An 89 year old woman was found to have a 1.5 cm diameter, 4.6 mm thick Merkel cell carcinoma of her right forearm, with satellite metastases evident within 2 cm of the main tumor nodule. At presentation to Moffitt less than three weeks later, two additional satellite nodules were noted. She underwent a wide excision of the primary site and surrounding satellite nodules; postoperatively she received 2500 cGy in eight fractions to the surgical site. Four months after the completion of radiation, multiple new dermal and subcutaneous nodules proximal to the primary site and outside the radiation field were noted (Figure 1A and B). Biopsy was positive for recurrent Merkel cell carcinoma. Isolated limb infusion was performed and ultimately resulted in the complete regression of all tumor nodules (Figure 1C and D). She remains free of disease 13 months post-treatment.

14.2 Nodal Recurrence

Initial management of the clinically negative nodal basin is outlined in Chapter 10, and can include observation, sentinel lymph node biopsy or primary nodal irradiation. Regional nodal recurrence is frequent in patients undergoing resection of the primary tumor without treatment of the nodal basin. Such regional (or even distant nodal) recurrences in the absence of previous treatment are treated in a manner analogous to patients presenting with clinically evident nodal involvement: generally with radical node dissection and postoperative radiation therapy. Selected patients may be considered for adjuvant chemotherapy (see Chapter 15).[3] The rate of nodal relapse after primary irradiation of the clinically

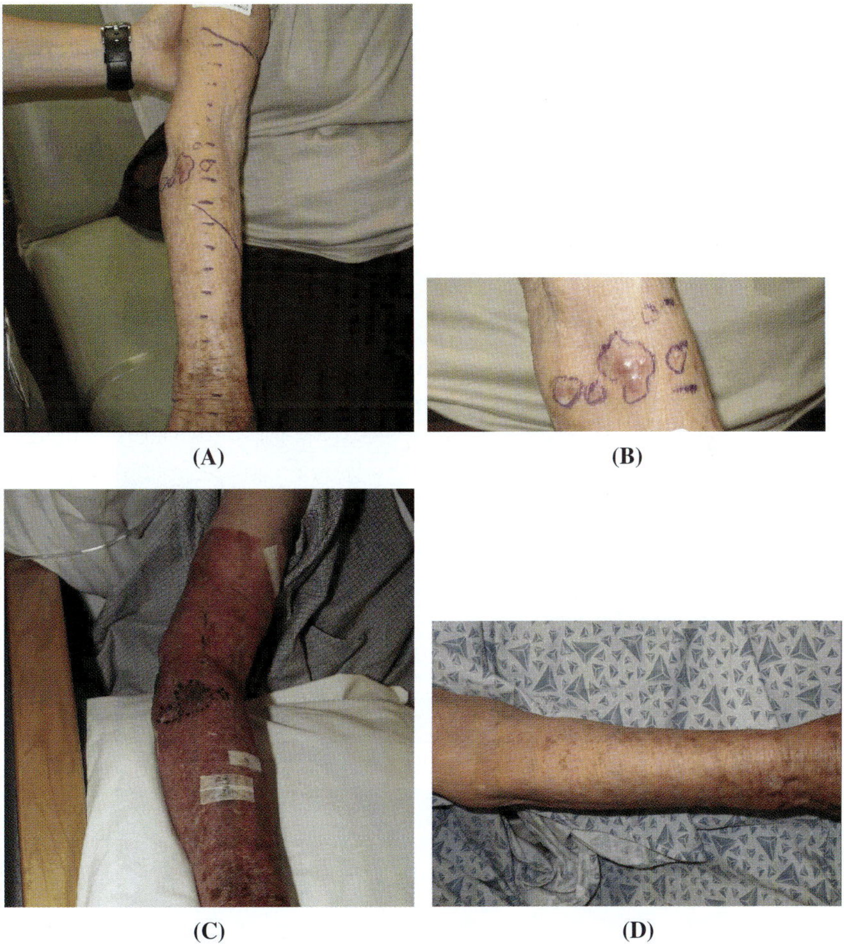

Figure 1. (**A** and **B**) Multifocal in-transit recurrence confined to the upper extremity of an 89 year old woman, developing four months after wide excision and radiation of a Merkel cell carcinoma of the forearm. **(C)** The patient underwent an isolated limb infusion with melphalan and dactinomycin, and demonstrates the characteristic inflammatory reaction 24 hours later. **(D)** Six weeks after the infusion, all visible and palpable evidence of tumor has resolved.

negative nodal basin is not well defined. Nodal recurrences after radiation therapy should be evaluated for additional surgery with possible chemotherapy thereafter, or if too extensive (with evidence of vascular or nerve compromise), be considered for upfront chemotherapy. Nodal

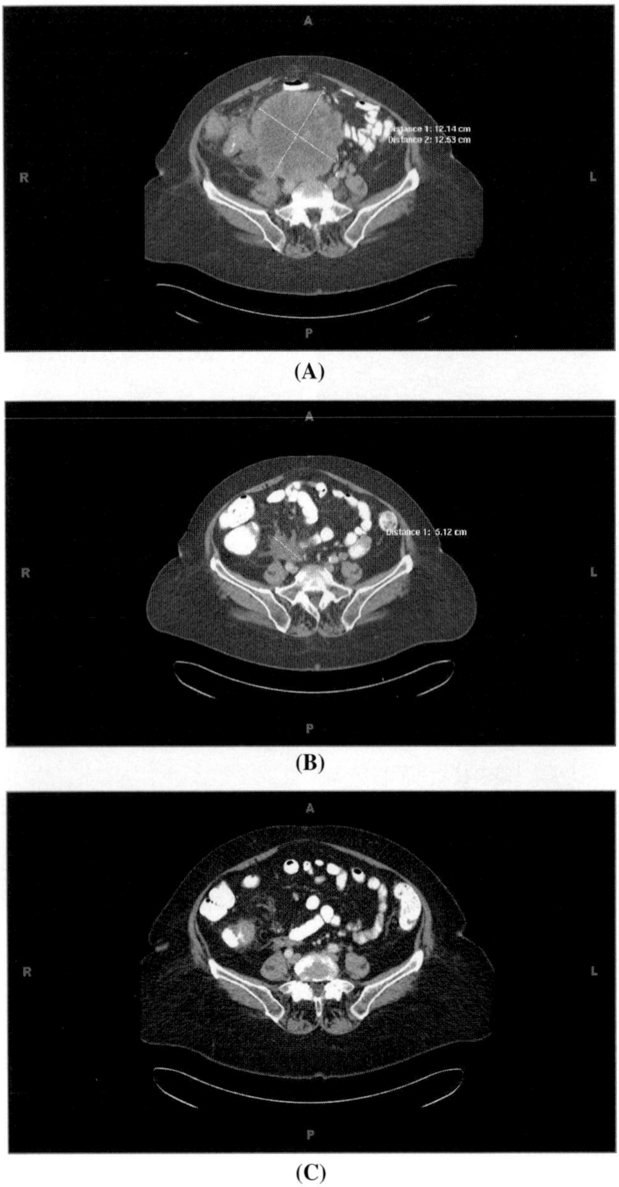

Figure 2. Serial abdominal CT scans demonstrating sustained regression of advanced intraabdominal disease. **(A)** Large intraabdominal mass pretreatment. **(B)** Less than three months after the initiation of systemic chemotherapy, the tumor was dramatically smaller, and the patient remains in sustained complete remission nearly four years after therapy **(C)**.

disease may also be the first site of distant metastasis; if isolated, management as for regional metastasis is warranted. The collected reviews of both Voog *et al.*[25] and Tai *et al.*[26] as well as individual reports[27,28] suggest higher response rates with more frequent longer lasting complete responses for chemotherapy of regional and distant nodes than achieved in non-nodal metastatic disease. Details of the regimens, doses and number of cycles of therapy to achieve these responses are usually lacking. Most appear to be given as concomitants to radiation therapy. Small numbers of patients with nodal recurrence have been treated with chemotherapy initially, using radiation therapy thereafter to consolidate remission.[21,29–31]

14.3 Nodal Disease with Unknown Primary

As is the case for melanoma, a small number of Merkel cell carcinoma patients present with nodal disease without a known primary site, with estimated frequencies ranging from 3–20%.[32,33] Explanations for this phenomenon include prior removal or ablation of an unrecognized primary, a concealed non-cutaneous primary or spontaneous regression of the primary. The workup of unknown primary Merkel cell carcinoma includes a history and physical examination aimed at identifying skin or subcutaneous lesions that may have been removed or have regressed, as well as routine staging to define the extent of disease, but extensive efforts to identify the primary site are not of value. Radical node dissection, postoperative radiation therapy and consideration of chemotherapy form the mainstays of treatment, just as for clinically evident nodal involvement from a known primary.

14.4 Distant Metastatic Disease

In a disease process well known for distant lymphatic, lung, liver, intraabdominal, bone and brain metastases, current radiologic evaluation techniques have made possible an improved appreciation of the extent of disease and are frequently used to discover asymptomatic disease and to characterize symptomatic tumors (see Chapter 9). Radiation therapy is used to relieve symptoms and prevent progression of metastases in critical sites, e.g. painful bone metastases or asymptomatic metastases in weight-bearing bones, and to treat symptomatic or asymptomatic spinal cord and brain metastases. The sensitivity of Merkel cell carcinoma to radiation therapy has made it an effective palliative tool in managing symptomatic metastatic disease either alone or in conjunction with chemotherapy (see Chapter 13). Multifocal areas of metastasis without a single major symptom-producing focus may be better managed with chemotherapy.

14.4.1 *Chemotherapy for metastatic disease*

Our understanding of the value of cytotoxic agents in the management of metastatic Merkel cell carcinoma derives largely from multiple small, frequently retrospective assessments of the results of their empiric use collected over several decades. Because of histologic similarities to small cell lung cancer, agents useful in that entity were usually selected for use; the rarity of Merkel cell carcinoma effectively prevented any large-scale prospective studies of individual agents, dose, schedule or combination of drugs. The latter were essentially extrapolated from experience with the management of other malignancies. No comparative data are available, yet despite these weaknesses, some generalities have emerged.

1. Merkel cell carcinoma is a chemotherapy-responsive malignancy, but is rarely curable with chemotherapy alone.
2. A significant number of complete responses can be achieved and at least some of them are long lasting (Figure 2).
3. Partial responses are generally short-lived, in the range of several months.
4. As with other malignancies, higher response rates and more frequent complete responses are seen with therapy of limited rather than extensive metastatic disease. Patients with non-visceral disease and good performance status respond better.
5. Greater toxicity and fewer responses are seen in the elderly, the immunocompromised and those with significant comorbidity limiting therapy.

These conclusions largely derive from two sources. In 1999, Voog *et al.* reviewed the literature regarding chemotherapy of locally advanced and metastatic Merkel cell carcinoma from 1980 to 1995 and collected 101 cases from 37 publications, adding six cases of their own.[25] No publication included more than 13 patients. Eighty-seven percent of patients received multi-agent chemotherapy utilizing some combination of an anthracycline, an alkylating agent, 5-fluorouracil, cisplatin and/or etoposide. Overall, an objective response was reported in 60%, with 39% said to achieve complete remission. The objective response rate for distant metastatic disease was 57% (41 of 72), compared with 69% for locally advanced disease, but this difference did not reach statistical significance ($p = 0.37$).

Cyclophosphamide, doxorubicin (Adriamycin) and vincristine (CAV) was the most frequently used combination, with a response rate of 61%. Etoposide/cisplatin (EP) achieved a 47% response rate. The median duration of response was eight months, and was shorter for partial responses (approximately three months) but more than 20 months for complete responders. Thirty-three evaluable patients received second line therapy; 15 (45%) achieved an objective response. Limited survival data revealed a median survival of nine months for patients with metastatic disease and 24 months for those with locally advanced disease. Nine treatment-related deaths were described, five due to neutropenia with septic shock. Treatment-related death appeared related to age; seven of 43 patients over 65 years old died (16%) as compared to two of 57 of younger patients (3%).[25]

In 2000, Tai *et al.* expanded the above review to include 204 cases collected between 1966–1998, and added 25 patients from the London Regional Cancer Center.[26] Cyclophosphamide, doxorubicin or epirubicin, and vincristine, with or without prednisone were used in 47 cases, with a reported 70% objective response rate (35% complete responses). Etoposide with either cisplatin or carboplatin was used in 27 cases, achieving a 36% complete and 24% partial response rate. Among the 204 cases, there were seven toxic deaths (3.4%). Incomplete reporting and fragmented data prevent a more comprehensive analysis of these regimens.

Only handfuls of patients have been reported who were treated with other agents including methotrexate, 5-fluorouracil, dacarbazine, ifosfamide, streptozotocin and bleomycin, usually in some combination.

A few reports detail patients who received single agent oral chemotherapy using cyclophosphamide, chlorambucil or etoposide.[27] Fenig *et al.* demonstrated that oral etoposide could induce remission in three patients previously treated with intravenous etoposide.[34] Wobser *et al.* used single agent liposomal doxorubicin intravenously along with radiation therapy.[35]

A few other reports of chemotherapy for Merkel cell carcinoma are worthy of mention. Pectasides *et al.* achieved lasting complete responses in two of five patients treated with second line cisplatin, ifosfamide and epirubicin.[31] Fenig *et al.* used cyclophosphamide/methotrexate/5-fluorouracil in five patients, achieving complete responses in four. Radiation therapy was used for consolidation. Three patients were reported alive and well without disease five, 12 and 37 months from initiation of chemotherapy.[30] Bajetta *et al.* evaluated a combination of 5-fluorouracil, dacarbazine and epirubicin in multiple neuroendocrine tumors. The single patient with Merkel cell carcinoma achieved a complete response lasting more than 21 months.[36] Hainesworth *et al.*, in reporting the results of a phase II trial of paclitaxel, carboplatin and etoposide in advanced neuroendocrine carcinomas, described complete remissions of 36+ and 66+ months in two of four patients with Merkel cell carcinoma.[37] After four cycles of the combination, responders were treated with 24 weeks of single agent paclitaxel.

The last ten years have seen little innovation, development or application of new agents that might improve the management of this malignancy. Topical dinitrochlorobenzol,[38] intratumoral injection of tumor necrosis factor[39,40] and interferon,[41] as well as autologous stem cell transplantation[42] have shown isolated responses. More recently, taxanes and topoisomerase inhibitors have emerged but remain largely unstudied. Advances in molecular biology and the recognition of potential molecular targets may only now be beginning to stimulate clinical investigations to test new hypotheses. Based on the recognition that Merkel cell carcinomas have a high incidence of over-expression of the tyrosine kinase c-KIT, imatimib was evaluated in a phase II trial by the Southwest Oncology Group (SWOG). Unfortunately, only one partial response was observed despite the fact that all tumors were c-KIT positive by immunohistochemistry.[43] The details of this trial are reviewed in Chapter 16.

14.5 Toxicity and Patient Selection Factors

Merkel cell carcinoma is largely a disease of the elderly and the immunocompromised and these populations require special attention to minimize morbidity and drug-related mortality. Almost 50% of patients with Merkel cell carcinoma are 75 or older; 14% are immunosuppressed.[1] Significant comorbid conditions are common. Many older individuals may have difficulties with communication, transportation and social support systems, compromising their ability to receive adequate treatment. Table 1 lists the clinical parameters that help guide the choice of therapy for an individual patient.

The drug combinations CAV or cisplatin/etoposide are the most widely used treatment regimens, although the ideal dose and schedule for a geriatric population remains uncertain. No phase II studies of dose or schedule effectiveness have been conducted. Voog *et al.* were unable to detect response differences by drug doses, i.e. doxorubicin <50 mg/m^2 vs. ≥ 50 mg/m^2 per course, cisplatin <75 mg/m^2 vs. ≥ 75 mg/m^2 per course, or cyclophosphamide <500 mg/m^2 vs. ≥ 500 mg/m^2 per course.[25] Table 2 describes several drug combinations and schedules used in other carcinomas that have been applied to Merkel cell carcinoma.

Each of the known active agents has its limitations and cautions. Major side effects of doxorubicin include tissue necrosis from extravasation, nausea and vomiting, mucositis, myelosuppression and cardiomyopathy.

Table 1. Patient factors influencing selection of chemotherapy.

Performance status
Geriatric assessment scale
Comorbidity factors
Presence of another concurrent malignancy
Prior chemotherapy
Prior radiation to marrow areas
Immunosuppressive drugs
Cardiac status
Hematologic values (blood counts)
Renal function
Neurologic status

Table 2. Chemotherapy regimens used in the management of Merkel cell carcinoma.

Cisplatin	20–25 mg/m^2 IV Day 1–3	Q 3 wks
Etoposide	80–100/m^2 IV Day 1–3	
Cyclophosphamide	750 mg/m^2 Day 1	Q 3 wks
Doxorubicin	50 mg/m^2 Day 1	
Vincristine	2 mg Day 1	
Carboplatin	AUC 4.5 Day 1	Q 4 wks
Etoposide	80 mg/m^2 Days 1–3	
Cyclophosphamide	600 mg/m^2	Q 4 wks
Methotrexate	40 mg/m^2 Days 1 and 8	
5-Fluorouracil	600 mg/m^2	

AUC: Area under the (concentration-time) curve.

Percutaneous indwelling central catheters and ports are commonly placed to avoid the first complication. Contemporary antiemetics are considerable improved and pretreatment cardiac evaluations are now commonly done, allowing for improved patient selection. The usefulness of granulocyte stimulating factors has not been directly studied in Merkel cell carcinoma but may ameliorate neutropenia.

The potential neuropathy, hearing loss and renal damage from cisplatin may be reduced by pretreatment creatinine clearance determinations, hydration during treatment, slow rates of infusion, more effective anti-nausea agents and close follow-up to prevent dehydration. The dose may be divided over the three days of etoposide administration. For the frail, those intolerant of a fluid load or those with neuropathy, carboplatin is an appropriate alternative.

The largest prospective toxicity assessment of carboplatin/etoposide available is that from the TROG-07 trial with concurrent radiation.[44] Grade 3–4 neutropenia occurred in 30 patients (57%). Febrile neutropenia, which was seen in 19 patients (35%), was most likely to occur at the nadir of the second cycle of chemotherapy, when the radiation skin reactions were most severe (64% grade 3–4). In a subsequent study, weekly carboplatin (AUC 2) during radiation therapy reduced the extent of grade 3–4 neutropenia and patients did not become febrile.[45]

Immunocompromised patients may require dose reductions depending on the extent or severity of the process. Patients with chronic lymphocytic leukemia are likely to experience more profound myelosuppression, especially thrombocytopenia, from carboplatin and may benefit from a 25% dose reduction even if baseline platelet values are normal. HIV-positive patients with normal CD4 counts, lower or absent viral loads and normal hematologic values may be treated with some caution. Transplant recipients on immunosuppressants likewise require special dosage considerations.

The data available suggest that CAV and EP are comparable in their ability to achieve complete responses.[25] Complete remission with either regimen may be anticipated in approximately 30–40% of patients. Barring specific patient comorbidity factors, which should be the initial therapy? Is it possible that study of these agents in small cell lung cancer will prove helpful in selecting therapies in Merkel cell carcinoma? A randomized Phase III trial in extensive small cell cancer revealed similar initial response rates; at progression, patients were treated with the alternative regimen. Twenty-three percent of patients who initially received CAV responded to subsequent EP compared to a 12% response rate to secondary CAV after EP.[46]

Clearly, these two neuroendocrine malignancies are quite different, limiting the ability to extrapolate from one disease to the other, so this intriguing question of the order of drug use remains unanswered. In other malignancies, patients who relapse after a long complete response are commonly retreated with the same agents, whereas if the response was brief or only partial, other alternatives are sought. CMF may be a reasonable third choice. NCCN guidelines suggest topotecan as a third choice; to date no published Merkel cell data supports that recommendation.[47]

14.5.1 *Case illustration — management of metastatic disease*

A 73 year old white woman underwent incisional biopsy of a scalp lesion she described as progressing over a two-month period. Pathology revealed an 8 mm thick Merkel cell carcinoma. On presentation to Moffitt, a 3.5 cm tumor with clinically negative regional nodes was noted, and she underwent wide excision, skin grafting and a sentinel node biopsy. The latter revealed a minute focus of Merkel cell carcinoma in one sentinel lymph node. A return visit just one month postoperatively revealed multiple nodular recurrences in and around the graft site; she also described vaginal bleeding and abdominal distention. CT scans demonstrated pulmonary metastases, extensive intra-abdominal disease (Figure 2A) and an enlarged inguinal node. Vaginal biopsy revealed metastatic Merkel cell carcinoma. She began cisplatin/etoposide, responded quickly and continues in clinical complete remission nearly four years after initiation of therapy, and has been off treatment for more than three years (Figures 2B and C).

14.6 The Future

Merkel cell carcinoma has been shown to be a highly responsive disease, with chemotherapy offering significant palliation to the majority of patients with advanced disease and long term disease control to some. Several regimens have demonstrated activity, although no prospective phase II or III trials have examined the relative merits of each, and many unanswered management questions remain in this relatively uncommon malignancy. As its increasing incidence brings the problems of these patients to more oncologists, interest in resolving them will increase. Meaningful advances in management can be achieved through cooperative group, consortia or working party efforts to overcome the difficulties of low single institution accruals. Both the TROG 96–07 adjuvant trial with radiation[45] and the more recent SWOG trial of imatinib in advanced disease[44] exemplify the value of cooperative group efforts. The SWOG trial, although a negative study, was able to accrue 25 patients from 13 institutions in three years. There are clearly enough patients to address some key questions in prospective studies. Similar efforts should continue as advances in molecular biology identify potential targets, newer drugs become available and the use of currently available drugs is optimized for this geriatric population.

References

1. Agelli M., Clegg L.X. (2003). Epidemiology of primary Merkel cell carcinoma in the United States. *J Am Acad Dermatol* 49: 832–841.

2. Hitchcock C.L., Bland K.I., Laney R.G. 3rd, *et al.* (1988). Neuroendocrine (Merkel cell) carcinoma of the skin. *Ann Surg* 207: 201–207.
3. Shaw J.H., Rumball E. (1991). Merkel cell tumour: clinical behaviour and treatment. *Br J Surg* 78: 138–142.
4. Allen P.J., Bowne W.B., Jaques D.P., *et al.* (2005). Merkel cell carcinoma: prognosis and treatment of patients from a single institution. *J Clin Oncol* 23: 2300–2309.
5. Eng T.Y., Boersma M.G., Fuller C.D., *et al.* (2007). A comprehensive review of the treatment of Merkel cell carcinoma. *Am J Clin Oncol* 30: 624–636.
6. Goldberg S.R., Neifeld J.P., Frable W.J. (2007). Prognostic value of tumor thickness in patients with Merkel cell carcinoma. *J Surg Oncol* 95: 618–622.
7. Sandel H.D., Day T., Richardson M.S., *et al.* (2006). Merkel cell carcinoma: does tumor size or depth of invasion correlate with recurrence, metastasis, or patient survival? *Laryngoscope* 116: 791–795.
8. Gleason J.M., Kohler T.S., Monga M. (2006). Merkel cell carcinoma metastatic to testis. *Urology* 67: 423.e13–423.e14.
9. Schwindl B., Meissner A., Giedl J., Klotz T. (2006). Merkel cell carcinoma — a rarity in the urogenital tract. *Onkologie* 29: 326–328.
10. Tummala M.K., Hausner P.F., McGuire W.P., *et al.* (2006). Testis: a sanctuary site in Merkel cell carcinoma. *J Clin Oncol* 24: 1008–1009.
11. Ouellette J.R., Woodyard L., Toth L., Termuhlen P.M. (2004). Merkel cell carcinoma metastatic to the head of pancreas. *JOP* 5: 92–96.
12. Conley M., Hawkins K., Ririe D. (2006). Complete heart block and cardiac tamponade secondary to Merkel cell carcinoma cardiac metastases. *South Med J* 99: 74–78.
13. Tam C.S., Turner P., McLean C., *et al.* (2005). Leukaemic presentation of metastatic Merkel cell carcinoma. *Br J Haematol* 129: 446.
14. Chang D.T., Mancuso A.A., Riggs C.E. Jr., Mendenhall W.M. (2005). Merkel cell carcinoma of the skin with leptomeningeal metastases. *Am J Otolaryngol* 26: 210–213.
15. Pectasides D., Pectasides M., Economopoulos T. (2006). Merkel cell cancer of the skin. *Ann Oncol* 17: 1489–1495.
16. Eng T., Naguib M., Fuller C.D., *et al.* (2004). Treatment of recurrent Merkel cell carcinoma: an analysis of 46 cases. *Am J Clin Oncol* 27: 576–583.

17. Medina-Franco H., Urist M.M., Fiveash J., *et al.* (2001). Multimodality treatment of Merkel cell carcinoma: case series and literature review of 1024 cases. *Ann Surg Oncol* 8: 204–208.
18. Lewis K.G., Weinstock M.A., Weaver A.L., Otley C.C. (2006). Adjuvant local irradiation for Merkel cell carcinoma. *Arch Dermatol* 142: 693–700.
19. Bichakjian C.K., Lowe L., Lao C.D., *et al.* (2007). Merkel cell carcinoma: critical review with guidelines for multidisciplinary management. *Cancer* 110: 1–12.
20. Mojica P., Smith D., Ellenhorn J.D. (2007). Adjuvant radiation therapy is associated with improved survival in Merkel cell carcinoma of the skin. *J Clin Oncol* 25: 1043–1047.
21. Fenig E., Brenner B., Katz A., *et al.* (1997). The role of radiation therapy and chemotherapy in the treatment of Merkel cell carcinoma. *Cancer* 80: 881–885.
22. Gupta A.S., Heinzman S., Levine E.A. (1998). Successful treatment of in-transit metastases from Merkel's cell carcinoma with isolated hyperthermic limb perfusion. *South Med J* 91: 289–292.
23. Olieman A.F., Liénard D., Eggermont A.M., *et al.* (1999). Hyperthermic isolated limb perfusion with tumor necrosis factor α, interferon gamma, and melphalan for locally advanced nonmelanoma skin tumors of the extremities. *Arch Surg* 134: 303–307.
24. Grandpeix C., Bonvalot S., Petrow P., *et al.* (2006). Continued complete remission of Merkel cell carcinoma with in-transit metastasis after treatment with isolated limb perfusion regional chemotherapy. *Ann Dermatol Venereol* 133(8–9 Pt 1): 700–703.
25. Voog E., Biron P., Martin J.P., Blay J.Y. (1999). Chemotherapy for patients with locally advanced or metastatic Merkel cell carcinoma. *Cancer* 85: 2589–2595.
26. Tai P., Yu E., Winquist E., *et al.* (2000). Chemotherapy in neuroendocrine/Merkel cell carcinoma of the skin: case series and review of 204 cases. *J Clin Oncol* 18: 2493–2499.
27. Boyle F., Pendlebury S., Bell D. (1995). Further insights into the natural history and management of primary cutaneous neuroendocrine (Merkel cell) carcinoma. *Int J Radiat Oncol Biol Phys* 31: 315–323.
28. Wynne C.J., Kearsley J.H. (1988). Merkel cell tumor: a chemosensitive skin cancer. *Cancer* 62: 28–31.

29. Davis M.P., Miller E.M., Rau R.C., *et al.* (1990). The use of VP16 and cisplatin in the treatment of Merkel cell carcinoma. *J Dermatol Surg Oncol* 16: 276–278.
30. Fenig E., Lurie H., Sulkes A. (1993). The use of cyclophosphamide, methotrexate and 5-fluorouracil in the treatment of Merkel cell carcinoma. *Am J Clin Oncol* 16: 54–57.
31. Pectasides D., Pectasides M., Psyrri A., *et al.* (2006). Cisplatin-based chemotherapy for Merkel cell carcinoma of the skin. *Cancer Invest* 24: 780–785.
32. Poulsen M. (2004). Merkel-cell carcinoma of the skin. *Lancet Oncol* 5: 593–599.
33. Yanguas I., Goday J.J., Gonzalez-Guemens M., *et al.* (1997). Spontaneous regression of Merkel cell carcinoma of the skin. *Br J Dermatol* 137: 296–298.
34. Fenig E., Brenner B., Njuguna E., *et al.* (2000). Oral etoposide for Merkel cell carcinoma in patients previously treated with intravenous etoposide. *Am J Clin Oncol* 23: 65–67.
35. Wobser M., Kurzinger N., Ugurel S., *et al.* (2009). Therapy of metastasized Merkel cell carcinoma with liposomal doxorubicin in combination with radiotherapy. *J Dtsch Dermatol Ges* 7: 521–525.
36. Bajetta E., Rimassa L., Carnaghi C., *et al.* (1998). 5-Fluorouracil, dacarbazine, and epirubicin in the treatment of patients with neuroendocrine tumors. *Cancer* 83: 372–378.
37. Hainsworth J.D., Spigel D.R., Litchy S., Greco F.A. (2006). Phase II trial of paclitaxel, carboplatin, and etoposide in advanced poorly differentiated neuroendocrine carcinoma: A Minnie Pearl Cancer Research Network Study. *J Clin Oncol* 24: 3548–3554.
38. Herrmann G., Groth W., Krieg T., Mauch C. (2004). Complete remission of Merkel cell carcinoma of the scalp with local and regional metastases after topical treatment with dinitrochlorobenzol. *J Am Acad Dermatol* 50: 965–969.
39. Hata Y., Matsuka K., Ito O., *et al.* (1997). Two cases of Merkel cell carcinoma cured by intratumoral injection of natural human tumor necrosis factor. *Plast Reconstr Surg* 99: 547–553.
40. Ito Y., Kawamura K., Miura T., *et al.* (1989). Merkel cell carcinoma: a successful treatment with tumor necrosis factor. *Arch Dermatol* 125: 1093–1095.
41. Durand J.M., Weiller C., Richard M.A., *et al.* (1991). Treatment of Merkel cell tumor with interferon-alpha-2b. *Br J Dermatol* 124: 509.

42. Waldmann V., Goldschmidt H., Jackel A., *et al.* (2000). Transient complete remission of metastasized Merkel cell carcinoma by high-dose polychemotherapy and autologous peripheral bone stem cell transplantation. *Br J Dermatol* 143: 837–839.
43. Samlowski W.E., Moon J., Tuthill R.J., *et al.* (2009). A Phase II trial of imatinib mesylate in Merkel cell carcinoma (neuroendocrine carcinoma of the skin): a Southwest Oncology Group Study (S0331). *Am J Clin Oncol* 2009 Dec 16 [Epub ahead of print].
44. Poulsen M., Rischin D., Walpole E., *et al.* (2003). High-risk Merkel cell carcinoma of the skin treated with synchronous carboplatin/etoposide and radiation: a Trans-Tasman Radiation Oncology Group Study — TROG 96: 07. *J Clin Oncol* 21: 4371–4376.
45. Poulsen M., Walpole E., Harvey J., *et al.* (2008). Weekly carboplatin reduces toxicity during synchronous chemoradiotherapy for Merkel cell carcinoma of the skin. *Int J Radiat Oncol Biol Phys* 72: 1070–1074.
46. Roth B.J., Johnson D.H., Einhorn L.H., *et al.* (1992). Randomized study of cyclophosphamide, doxorubicin, and vincristine versus etoposide and cisplatin versus alternation of these two regimens in extensive small-cell lung cancer: a phase III trial of the Southeastern Cancer Study Group. *J Clin Oncol* 10: 282–291.
47. Miller S.J., Alam M., Andersen J., *et al.* (2009). Merkel cell carcinoma. *J Natl Comp Cancer Netw* 7: 322–332.

Chapter 15

Adjuvant Chemotherapy of Merkel Cell Carcinoma

Ronald C. DeConti

To date, no body of data clearly supports the use of chemotherapy in the adjuvant setting for patients with Merkel cell carcinoma, not because of demonstrated lack of efficacy, but because of the paucity of data in a heretofore rare disease. Virtually no randomized trials have been done and no large historical database is available. While a number of authors have been optimistic,[1–4] little data has been generated to solidify that optimism to date. However, a number of anecdotal and preliminary experiences provide some suggestion of possible benefit and ideas for the future.

Historically, adjuvant chemotherapy has most readily been demonstrated to be effective in a number of clinical situations satisfying these prerequisites: (1) in a disease with a subset of individuals with a clearly defined poor prognosis, (2) with a regimen shown capable of achieving responses in a large proportion of patients with advanced measurable disease, and (3) the accrual of sufficient numbers of patients to demonstrate statistical evidence of improvements in local control, recurrence-free survival and/or overall survival. How do these criteria apply to Merkel cell carcinoma?

The current reporting systems fail to stratify patient risk well. Many reports of adjuvant therapy refer to patients with locoregional recurrence and others to nodal relapse. It is frequently unclear if the designation 'locoregional relapse' includes both nodal relapse and satellite soft tissue involvement, and these may be heterogeneous populations with variable survivals. Nodal involvement has been demonstrated to be the most reliable predictor of relapse and poor prognosis,[5–8] but even these patients also have a quite variable prognosis. Patients with microscopic foci identified by sentinel node procedures fare better than those with clinically evident gross nodal involvement.[9]

Patients with grossly positive nodal disease are estimated to have a 40–60% probability of recurrence,[6] approximately 90% of which will manifest within two years,[6,10] clearly satisfying the requirement for a defined high risk subset for future trials.

Node number may also prove to be a significant stratification factor. Allen *et al.*[9] reported a five-year survival rate of 30% for patients with more than four positive nodes, about half that of individuals with fewer nodes. Not only can this poor prognostic subset be identified at presentation but the effectiveness of therapy may be evaluated after a relatively brief follow-up period given the natural history of relapse in this disease. This contrasts markedly in some malignancies with a more indolent pattern of relapse requiring a longer period of post-treatment observation.

Two regimens have been identified as possible candidates for use as adjuvant therapy.[11,12] Both cyclophosphamide/doxorubicin/vincristine and etoposide (VP-16)/cisplatin appear similar in efficacy in advanced disease, though the doses and schedules used in the past have been variable and rarely completely described. Extent of disease, response duration and survival are frequently omitted in published reports. Despite these limitations, both regimens produce overall responses in 50–70% of patients with advanced disease; complete responses are achieved in approximately 30%. Relapse is common however; no phase II study has been done to evaluate the incidence of long term freedom from relapse. Patients with distant nodal foci without visceral involvement do best. Voog *et al.* projected a 17% three-year survival for patients with distant metastases compared with 35% for patients with unresectable or locoregional nodal disease.[1]

The greatest impediments to our understanding of the role of adjuvant chemotherapy have been lack of adequate patient numbers in single institution experiences and the absence of large multi-institutional trials which might overcome the accrual problems of a single institution. Nevertheless, a number of adjuvant strategies have been explored, none with adequate numbers or clearly stratified patients enabling clear conclusions.

Chemotherapy is used as an adjuvant to definitive interventions in several ways in a number of different neoplasms. Neoadjuvant or induction chemotherapy is administered prior to definitive therapy, thereby allowing an assessment of the responsiveness of the neoplasm before surgical intervention or radiation therapy. Effective chemotherapy may then be continued during or after definitive local/regional therapy. Concurrent adjuvant drug therapy is administered during radiation therapy. Endpoints in this situation include an evaluation of the extent of local regression achieved, as well as percent of in-field recurrences, distant failures, local and distant disease free survival times and ultimately overall survival. Post-surgical or post-radiation adjuvant therapy is given after complete surgical removal of the primary tumor and/or radiation. Efficacy is assessed by rates of both local and distant relapse and duration of relapse free and overall survival.

15.1 Neoadjuvant Chemotherapy

Small numbers of patients with nodal disease have received chemotherapy as induction treatment, achieved remission and then were given radiation as a remission consolidation.[13–16] Some of these remissions were sustained. Response rates in these multiple small experiences appear high, consistent with other chemotherapy data suggesting that responses to regional disease are superior to those with advanced disease.[1,6] Fenig *et al.* used two to four cycles of cisplatin-etoposide followed by radiation therapy to the primary site and regional nodal basin in seven patients with advanced disease. Two patients relapsed and died of metastatic disease at 12 and 36 months. The other five were followed for 25–125 months without relapse.[17] However, once again, small numbers and potential selection bias limits the interpretation of this data.

15.2 Post-Surgical Adjuvant Therapy Experiences

Eng *et al.*[6] in their review noted that the recurrence rate for patients receiving surgery and adjuvant radiation therapy was approximately the same as that of a small number of patients treated with surgery and four to six cycles of cisplatin/etoposide without other adjuvant therapies (40% [11 of 27] vs. 40% [two of five] respectively).

McFee *et al.*[2] described the University of Florida experience. Thirty-four patients were treated with radiation therapy to the primary site; 24 of 26 patients with clinically negative regional nodes received therapy to the nodal basin; eight of 11 patients with clinically positive nodes received radiation therapy to the regional node basin. Nine patients received one to four cycles of adjuvant chemotherapy. Five of these nine recurred compared to eight of 25 who did not receive drugs. Five-year cause specific survival was 38% for those with locoregional disease compared to 58% for stage I patients. Small numbers, incomplete staging and lack of detail limit interpretation of these data. The authors concluded that it is reasonable to add chemotherapy to initial management despite the lack of convincing data.

Kokoska *et al.*[4] evaluated 35 patients with Merkel cell carcinoma. Wide local excision, prophylactic node dissection and adjuvant radiation therapy significantly decreased locoregional and distant recurrence rates and improved survival. Adjuvant chemotherapy did not achieve statistical benefit, not surprisingly given the small number of treated patients. However, four of nine chemotherapy-treated patients experienced locoregional recurrence (44%) compared to 16 of 24 (67%) who did not receive chemotherapy. Three of the nine developed distant recurrence (33%) compared to 13 of 24 patients who did not receive drug therapy (54%). Rather than being regarded as negative, these very limited data are actually suggestive of benefit.

Allen *et al.*,[9] in reviewing Memorial Sloan-Kettering data, describe the node positive patients who were selected for chemotherapy as having poorer outcomes in both recurrence and survival rates. Neither the prescribed regimens nor the number of cycles given were specified. Sixty individuals presented with clinical nodal involvement and 16 additional patients were identified by sentinel node evaluation. Twenty-three individuals received chemotherapy whereas 53 did not. Thirty-two percent of patients who received adjuvant chemotherapy recurred with distant disease compared with 19% who did not. The authors also report the effect of node number on survival. Of their 76 node-positive patients, 40 patients with a single positive node had a five-year survival of 66%; 21 patients with two to four positive nodes had a 62% five-year survival while 16 individuals with more than four positive nodes had a survival of 30%. It seems most probable that the patients given adjuvant chemotherapy would have been those with the greatest nodal burden and the poorest prognosis, but this is not specified in their report. No prospective studies have yet clearly evaluated the effect of the magnitude of node burden on survival. Unfortunately, this experience is frequently cited as evidence of the lack of efficacy of adjuvant drug therapy.[18,19] A more reasonable conclusion might be that no conclusions could be drawn from this data.

15.3 Concurrent Chemoradiotherapy

Though not universally accepted, adjuvant radiation therapy is commonly used to reduce recurrence,[20] and has been shown to improve survival in at least one analysis using the SEER database.[21] The only prospective trial of chemoradiation includes individuals with both local and/or regional nodal involvement as well as some patients with residual or persistent gross disease.

TROG 96–07[7] evaluated concurrent chemoradiation in 53 patients with local and/or regional nodal involvement by Merkel cell carcinoma. Nodal involvement was present in 33 and absent in 20 patients. Treatment was adjuvant in 38 and therapeutic in 15. Fifty Gray was administered in 25 fractions over five weeks. Two cycles of carboplatin/etoposide were given during radiation (weeks 1 and 4) and two subsequent cycles thereafter (weeks 7 and 10). A cycle of therapy consisted of carboplatin (AUC 4) on day 1 and etoposide 80 mg/m^2 (days 1, 2 and 3). This study also combined concurrent chemoradiation with post-radiation adjuvant carboplatin/VP-16 chemotherapy. Two subsequent cycles were added following the completion of radiation.

The three-year overall survival, locoregional control and distant control rates were 76%, 75% and 76% respectively. These favorable results suggested that chemoradiotherapy in high risk situations warranted further investigation. The three-year survival for patients with involved nodes was 66% compared to 93% for those without. Patients treated with gross residual disease had a 45% three-year survival compared to 90% for those without. Small numbers prevented these differences from reaching statistical significance. Cox's proportional hazard modeling demonstrated a hazard ratio of 4.34 for N1 disease and 76.71 for N2 involvement.

To determine whether chemotherapy improved survival in high risk patients, Poulsen *et al.*[22] subsequently compared the patients in this trial to selected historic controls treated with radiation therapy alone. Univariate analysis revealed a statistically significant difference in overall survival between those who received chemotherapy (52% five-year survival) compared to those treated without chemotherapy (31% five-year survival). However, a multivariate analysis of this small group of patients failed to confirm a statistical advantage, though a favorable chemotherapy effect could not be excluded. The addition of chemotherapy was associated with a hazard ratio of 0.64 (95% CI 0.34–1.2, $p = 0.16$). The superior patient outcomes in this prospective trial provide the most suggestive evidence to date in support of further studies of concomitant chemoradiation.

To reduce the high incidence of febrile neutropenia noted late in the course of radiation in this study, the authors have since studied single agent weekly carboplatin (AUC 2×5 doses) in 18 patients. Though grade 3–4 neutropenia occurred in seven patients, none became febrile, demonstrating the safety of this regimen.[23] Relative efficacy has not yet been evaluated.

15.4 Future Directions

Improvement in our understanding of the value and limitations of adjuvant chemotherapy will clearly depend on a number of developments. The lack of a uniform staging system may be remedied by the development and approval of a specific staging system for Merkel cell carcinoma by the American Joint Committee on Staging of Cancer (see Chapter 7). Specifying clinical or pathologic assessment of the nodal basin, distinguishing sentinel node micrometastases from clinically evident nodal disease, and incorporating the number of positive lymph nodes will likely greatly improve stratification of prognosis and permit improved patient selection for and evaluations of therapy.

Prospective evaluation of current therapy options in phase II trials in advanced disease to determine appropriate doses and schedules suitable for a geriatric population are necessary. These may allow novel applications as induction, concomitant or post-treatment adjuvants. The TROG data has provided the most reliable basis for concurrent chemoradiation trials to date. The demonstrated value of cisplatin and/or carboplatin as a radiosensitizer in other diseases make continued study of this concurrent strategy attractive in larger trials of well-stratified patients.

Cooperative efforts to pool information, create clinical trials, test hypotheses and evaluate results are needed to overcome the difficulties of small numbers of patients treated at individual institutions, even centers with an interest in this rare disease. Whether the appropriate mechanism is a cooperative group, a consortium or a working party remains to be determined. Hopefully, growing awareness of Merkel cell carcinoma as an important neoplasm ready for advances in therapy will create interest in collaborative efforts to promote the development of trials of multiple competing strategies, and the growing body of basic and translational science will provide further impetus for new drug development and trials in Merkel cell carcinoma.

References

1. Eng T.Y., Boersma M.G., Fuller C.D., *et al.* (2007). A comprehensive review of the treatment of Merkel cell carcinoma. *Am J Clin Oncol* 30: 624–636.
2. McAfee W., Morris C.G., Mendenhall C.M., *et al.* (2005). Merkel cell carcinoma. *Cancer* 104: 1761–1764.
3. King M.M., Osswald M.B. (2005). Adjuvant chemotherapy for Merkel cell carcinoma. *Am J Clin Oncol* 28: 634.
4. Kokoska E.R., Kokoska M.S., Collins B.T., *et al.* (1997). Early aggressive treatment for Merkel cell carcinoma improves outcome. *Am J Surg* 174: 688–693.
5. Goldberg S.R., Neifeld J.P., Frable W.J. (2007). Prognostic value of tumor thickness in patients with Merkel cell carcinoma. *J Surg Oncol* 95: 618–622.
6. Eng T.Y., Boersma M.G., Fuller C.D., *et al.* (2004). Treatment of Merkel cell carcinoma. *Am J Clin Oncol* 27: 510–515.
7. Poulsen M., Rischin D., Walpole E., *et al.* (2003). High-risk Merkel cell carcinoma of the skin treated with synchronous carboplatin/etoposide and

radiation: a Trans-Tasman Radiation Oncology Group Study — TROG 96:07. *J Clin Oncol* 21: 4371–4376.
8. Morrison W.H., Peters L.J., Silva E.G., *et al.* (1990). The essential role of radiation therapy in securing locoregional control of Merkel cell carcinoma. *Int J Radiat Oncol Biol Phys* 19: 583–591.
9. Allen P.J., Bowne W.B., Jaques D.P., *et al.* (2005). Merkel cell carcinoma: prognosis and treatment of patients from a single institution. *J Clin Oncol* 23: 2300–2309.
10. Medina-Franco H., Urist M.M., Fiveash J., *et al.* (2001). Multimodality treatment of Merkel cell carcinoma: case series and literature review of 1024 cases. *Ann Surg Oncol* 8: 204–208.
11. Voog E., Biron P., Martin J.P., Blay J.Y. (1999). Chemotherapy for patients with locally advanced or metastatic Merkel cell carcinoma. *Cancer* 85: 2589–2595.
12. Tai P.T., Yu E., Winquist E., *et al.* (2000). Chemotherapy in neuroendocrine/Merkel cell carcinoma of the skin: case series and review of 204 cases. *J Clin Oncol* 18: 2493–2499.
13. Poon D., Yap S.P., Mancer K., *et al.* (2001). Induction chemotherapy followed by radiotherapy in Merkel-cell carcinoma. *Lancet Oncol* 5: 509–510.
14. Pectasides D., Pectasides M., Psyrri A., *et al.* (2006). Cisplatin-based chemotherapy for Merkel cell carcinoma of the skin. *Cancer Invest* 24: 780–785.
15. Davis M.P., Miller E.M., Rau R.C., *et al.* (1990). The use of VP16 and cisplatin in the treatment of Merkel cell carcinoma. *J Dermatol Surg Oncol* 16: 276–278.
16. Fenig E., Lurie H., Sulkes A. (1993). The use of cyclophosphamide, methotrexate and 5-fluorouracil in the treatment of Merkel cell carcinoma. *Am J Clin Oncol* 16: 54–57.
17. Fenig E., Brenner B., Katz A., *et al.* (1997). The role of radiation therapy and chemotherapy in the treatment of Merkel cell carcinoma. *Cancer* 80: 881–885.
18. Veness M.J., Perera L., McCourt J., *et al.* (2005). Merkel cell carcinoma: improved survival with adjuvant radiotherapy. *ANZ J Surg* 55: 275–281.
19. Heath M.L., Nghiem P. (2007). Merkel cell carcinoma: If no Breslow, then what? *J Surg Oncol* 95: 614–615.

20. Lewis K.G., Weinstock M.A., Weaver A.L., Otley C.C. (2006). Adjuvant local irradiation for Merkel cell carcinoma. *Arch Dermatol* 142: 693–700.
21. Mojica P., Smith D., Ellenhorn J.D. (2007). Adjuvant radiation therapy is associated with improved survival in Merkel cell carcinoma of the skin. *J Clin Oncol* 25: 1043–1044.
22. Poulsen M.G., Rischin D., Porter I., *et al.* (2006). Does chemotherapy improve survival in high-risk stage I and II Merkel cell carcinoma of the skin? *Int J Radiat Oncol Biol Phys* 64: 114–119.
23. Poulsen M., Walpole E., Harvey J., *et al.* (2008). Weekly carboplatin reduces toxicity during synchronous chemoradiotherapy for Merkel cell carcinoma of the skin. *Int J Radiat Oncol Biol Phys* 72: 1070–1074.

Chapter 16

The Potential for Targeted Therapy of Merkel Cell Carcinoma

Wolfram A. Samlowski and Jürgen C. Becker

There is a striking need for a better understanding of the molecular biology of Merkel cell carcinoma despite immense progress in our understanding of cancer pathogenesis overall. Numerous tyrosine and serine/threonine kinases, as well as growth factors, can now be targeted with small molecular inhibitors. Due to the relative rarity of Merkel cell carcinoma, these novel agents have not yet been extensively tested. The purpose of this chapter is to overview current knowledge in the field with an eye toward future opportunities for clinical investigation.

Merkel cell carcinoma was initially described as a rare neuroendocrine tumor of the skin.[1] It has subsequently been established that this tumor is one of the most aggressive forms of skin cancer with a five-year survival of less than 75%.[2–4] Merkel cell carcinoma has a high risk of both regional lymph node involvement (55%) and distant metastases (36%).[5] Typically, the tumor presents in middle-aged to elderly patients, but younger patients in their teens and early adulthood have been described, particularly in immunosuppressed individuals.[1,6,7]

The significant frequency of distant metastases in Merkel cell carcinoma (25–35%) has resulted in a series of retrospective chemotherapy reports, each describing treatment of a small numbers of patients.[8–14] These are described in more detail in Chapter 14. Selection of chemotherapy for Merkel cell carcinoma has been patterned after small cell lung cancer treatments since Kultchitzsky cells in the lung and Merkel cells in the skin appear similar by light microscopy and are probably both part of the amine precursor uptake and decarboxylation (APUD) system.[9,15]

A variety of combination chemotherapy regimens have been employed in patients with metastatic Merkel cell carcinoma, with resulting clinical responses. These regimens have included cyclophosphamide, methotrexate and 5-fluorouracil, etoposide and cisplatin, cisplatin plus doxorubicin, and cyclophosphamide, doxorubicin and vincristine.[11,12,14,16] Although most studies include only a small number of treated patients (due to the rarity of this cancer), they indicate potential responsiveness to multidrug combinations. Unfortunately, these responses tend to be of short duration. Long-term responses and complete remissions are at best anecdotal.[10] As many of the individuals that develop Merkel cell carcinoma are upwards of 70 years of age (mean age of onset is 69), multi-agent chemotherapy with anthracyclines and platinum compounds is often poorly tolerated. Identification of novel small molecule agents to treat Merkel cell carcinoma is, therefore, highly desirable.

16.1 Potential Molecular Targets in Merkel Cell Carcinoma

16.1.1 *c-KIT*

A number of studies have identified over-expression of c-KIT (CD117) following immunostaining of Merkel cell carcinoma, in contrast to a lower incidence of c-KIT expression in small cell lung carcinoma.[17–20] For example, Su *et al.* evaluated c-KIT expression in 22 biopsies of Merkel cell carcinoma.[17] These investigators showed that 21 of 22 Merkel cell carcinoma (95%) stained with an anti-CD117 antibody. Intensity of CD117 expression did not appear to correlate with aggressive behavior. While the incidence of activating mutations in c-KIT in Merkel cell carcinoma was not evaluated in this report, the pathogenic role of this oncogene in other malignant neoplasms suggested the possibility of a similar role in Merkel cell carcinoma.[20]

16.1.2 *Survivin*

Inhibition of apoptosis appears to be a critical step in tumorigenesis.[21] Survivin is an inhibitor of apoptosis that is undetectable in most terminally differentiated human tissues.[22] It is strongly expressed in embryonic and fetal organs and in many cancers.[22] Kim and McNiff recently evaluated survivin expression in Merkel cell carcinoma.[23] These investigators stained 19 samples of primary Merkel cell carcinoma. All 19 showed strong immunoreactivity with anti-survivin antibodies. Patients demonstrating strong nuclear survivin expression appeared to have a poorer prognosis. While this result will require prospective verification, there are molecular inhibitors of survivin already in clinical trials (e.g. YM 155, Astellas Pharma).[21] This class of agent seems promising for further investigation in Merkel cell carcinoma.

16.1.3 *VEGF and PDGF receptor inhibitors*

Neuroendocrine tumors frequently are highly vascular. This has been studied in Merkel cell carcinoma specifically, where 20% of cases demonstrated pericyte hyperplasia, pyogenic granuloma-like, hemangioendothelial-like, epithelioid hemangioma-like, peliosis-like, and follicular dendritic cell tumor-like morphologic patterns.[24] Vascular endothelial growth factor receptor (VEGFR)-2 expression has been seen in 91% of large primary tumors.[25] Brunner *et al.* performed staining of a tissue microarray containing 32 samples for VEGF-A and -C, VEGFR-2, and platelet-derived growth factor (PDGF)-α or -β.[26] A high percentage of these samples stained for VEGF-A and -C, VEGFR-2, and PDGF-α. Tumor samples generally lacked Her2-neu and EGFR over-expression. Swick *et al.* have identified a novel single base substitution in PDGFR-α in at least one-third of Merkel cell carcinoma patients tested.[27] When taken together, these studies suggest that combined VEGFR/PDGFR receptor inhibitors such as sunitinib may be potentially active in the treatment of Merkel cell carcinoma. Further support is provided by a case report documenting a partial response of Merkel cell carcinoma lasting six months with pazopanib therapy (a second-generation multi-targeted tyrosine kinase inhibitor that inhibits VEGFR-1, -2, and -3; PDGFR-α and -β, and c-KIT).[28] This concept will be further tested in a planned Southwest Oncology Group phase II study of sunitinib currently in development. Other angiogenic molecules, such as endostatin, may also be over-expressed in Merkel cell carcinoma, suggesting additional treatment targets.[29]

16.1.4 *Acetylcholine receptor*

Neural crest-derived tissues express muscarinic and nicotinic acetylcholine receptors.[30] These receptors appear to be critical for the migration of these cells during development. Bowers *et al.* recently published the results of immunostaining for M3 and M5 muscarinic acetylcholine receptors in 15 cases of Merkel cell carcinoma.[31] All cases stained diffusely positive. In contrast, none stained for the β2-nicotinic acetylcholine receptor. This result suggests that development of agents that block M3 or M5 acetylcholine receptors may prove fruitful.

16.1.5 *Fluoroquinolones*

With the recent identification of a polyomavirus related to SV-40 and BK virus in association with Merkel cell carcinoma (see Chapter 3),[32–34] the possibility of virally directed antibiotic therapy comes to mind. There is some data to suggest that the related BK polyomavirus can be suppressed by fluoroquinolones. Leung *et al.* treated 68 bone marrow transplant patients with a variety of antibiotic regimens. They analyzed the BK virus load and urinary ciprofloxacin levels in their patients.[35] Patients who received ciprofloxacin had a significantly lower peak BK virus load and lower incidence of viruria and hemorrhagic cystitis. One potential mechanism may be via the capacity of fluoroquinolones to inhibit viral helicase.[36] This intriguing concept may not be directly relevant to the Merkel cell polyomavirus, but it could easily be tested in clinical trials in advanced Merkel cell carcinoma with the expectation of low toxicity.

16.1.6 *Additional molecular pathways*

It should be noted that there are reports of other molecular pathways that may be targetable in Merkel cell carcinoma. These include tenascin C, p63 and matrix metalloproteinases.[37–39] In contrast, overactivity of the classic MAP kinase pathway (RAS/RAF/MEK/MAP kinases) has not been demonstrated.[40] Cox-2 also appears to be expressed at low levels in Merkel cell carcinoma.[41]

16.2 Recently Completed Clinical Trials of Signaling Inhibitors

Imatinib mesylate (Gleevec, formerly STI-571) is a small molecule that has been demonstrated to be a highly selective inhibitor of certain receptor tyrosine kinases, including Abl and the chimeric BCR-Abl fusion protein found in certain leukemias such as chronic myeloid leukemia; the platelet-derived growth factor receptor; and KIT, the product of the c-KIT proto-oncogene.[42,43] Imatinib inhibits KIT at an IC_{50} of approximately 100 nM, which is similar to that required for inhibiting the tyrosine kinase activity associated with BCR-Abl and the PDGF receptor.[44] Imatinib has been extensively tested in Philadelphia chromosome-positive leukemia patients where the main target is inhibition of the dysregulated kinase activity associated with the chimeric BCR-Abl fusion protein.[45] Additionally, single center and multicenter trials have now documented significant activity of imatinib in gastrointestinal stromal tumors (GIST), a solid tumor type that usually expresses gain-of-function somatic mutation of c-KIT.[46]

From July 2003 to July 2006, a total of 25 patients were accrued to a phase II trial of imatinib in Merkel cell carcinoma by the Southwest Oncology Group. Two patients were found to be ineligible (one whose tumor was found not to express CD117 on central pathology review, and one who did not have measurable disease). Therefore 23 patients were included in the analysis. Median age was 77 (with a range of 56 to 91 years). Seventeen patients (74%) were men, six (26%) were women and all were Caucasian.

Toxicity in this trial was typical for clinical trials of imatinib. There were three episodes of grade 4 toxicities (one each of dyspnea, hyperglycemia and vomiting). Three patients experienced grade 3 toxicities including one episode each of peripheral edema, fatigue, lymphopenia and rash. Grade 1–2 toxicities that were observed were mostly hematological and gastrointestinal, including four patients with diarrhea, six patients with nausea, 12 with anemia, four with neutropenia, and four patients with hypokalemia. It should be noted that there were three deaths on study, but all were felt attributable to cancer progression.

There were no complete responses and one confirmed partial response in the 23 evaluable patients (4% objective response rate, 95% confidence

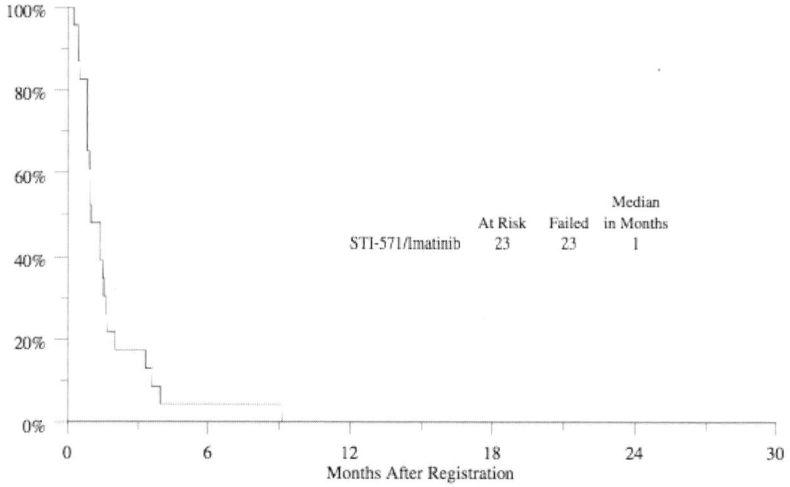

Figure 1. Progression-free survival of patients with metastatic Merkel cell carcinoma following imatinib therapy.

interval <1–22%). In addition, three patients with stable disease were observed. At the time of analysis, all evaluable patients had developed progressive disease (Figure 1). The median progression-free survival was only one month (95% confidence interval one to two months). The median overall survival was five months (95% confidence interval two to eight months). The one-year survival rate was 20%.

Our data demonstrate that cooperative oncology group clinical trials in Merkel cell carcinoma are feasible and can be completed in a timely fashion. Unfortunately, imatinib proved to have minimal activity against Merkel cell carcinoma despite apparent over-expression of c-KIT protein as assessed by CD117 staining. Subsequent laboratory studies may explain this clinical result, as despite over-expression, Merkel cell carcinoma generally does not express activating mutations in c-KIT.[47,48]

16.3 Future Directions

There is a striking need for a better understanding of the molecular biology of Merkel cell carcinoma. It is hoped that the recent identification of the Merkel cell carcinoma-associated polyoma virus[33,49–51] and elucidation of its effect on cells will provide additional therapeutic targets.[52] In general, there has been immense progress made in understanding molecular signaling pathways in cancer cells. Numerous tyrosine and serine/threonine kinases and growth factors can now be targeted with small molecular inhibitors or antibodies. Due to the relative rarity of Merkel cell carcinoma, these novel agents have not yet been extensively tested. The key to the development of successful therapy will be the development of a Merkel cell carcinoma directed research consortium and selective and thoughtful evaluation of new agents based on an improved understanding of the molecular pathogenesis of this enigmatic neoplasm.

References

1. Toker C. (1972). Trabecular carcinoma of the skin. *Arch Dermatol* 105: 107–110.
2. Shaw J.H., Rumball E. (1991). Merkel cell tumour: clinical behaviour and treatment. *Br J Surg* 78: 138–142.
3. Raaf J.H., Urmacher C., Knapper W.K., *et al.* (1986). Trabecular (Merkel cell) carcinoma of the skin. Treatment of primary, recurrent, and metastatic disease. *Cancer* 57: 178–182.
4. Yiengpruksawan A., Coit D.G., Thaler H.T., *et al.* (1991). Merkel cell carcinoma. Prognosis and management. *Arch Surg* 126: 1514–1519.
5. Hitchcock C.L., Bland K.I., Laney R.G., *et al.* (1988). Neuroendocrine (Merkel cell) carcinoma of the skin. Its natural history, diagnosis, and treatment. *Ann Surg* 207: 201–207.
6. Gould V.E., Moll R., Moll I., *et al.* (1985). Neuroendocrine (Merkel) cells of the skin: hyperplasias, dysplasias, and neoplasms. *Lab Invest* 52: 334–353.
7. Wick M.R., Goellner J.R., Scheithauer B.W., *et al.* (1983). Primary neuroendocrine carcinomas of the skin (Merkel cell tumors). A clinical, histologic, and ultrastructural study of thirteen cases. *Am J Clin Pathol* 79: 6–13.
8. Crown J., Lipzstein R., Cohen S., *et al.* (1991). Chemotherapy of metastatic Merkel cell cancer. *Cancer Invest* 9: 129–132.
9. Feun L.G., Savaraj N., Legha S.S., *et al.* (1998). Chemotherapy for metastatic Merkel cell carcinoma. Review of the M.D. Anderson Hospital's experience. Cancer 62: 683–685.

10. Fenig E., Brenner B., Njuguna E., *et al.* (2000). Oral etoposide for Merkel cell carcinoma in patients previously treated with intravenous etoposide. *Am J Clin Oncol* 23: 65–67.
11. Tai P.T., Yu E., Winquist E., *et al.* (2000). Chemotherapy in neuroendocrine/Merkel cell carcinoma of the skin: case series and review of 204 cases. *J Clin Oncol* 18: 2493–2499.
12. Voog E., Biron P., Martin J.P., *et al.* (1999). Chemotherapy for patients with locally advanced or metastatic Merkel cell carcinoma. *Cancer* 85: 2589–2595.
13. Bajetta E., Rimassa L., Carnaghi C., *et al.* (1998). 5-Fluorouracil, dacarbazine, and epirubicin in the treatment of patients with neuroendocrine tumors. *Cancer* 83: 372–378.
14. Fenig E., Lurie H., Sulkes A. (1993). The use of cyclophosphamide, methotrexate, and 5-fluorouracil in the treatment of Merkel cell carcinoma. *Am J Clin Oncol* 16: 54–57.
15. De Wolff-Peeters C., Marien K., Mebis J., *et al.* (1980). A cutaneous APUDoma or Merkel cell tumor? A morphologically recognizable tumor with a biological and histological malignant aspect in contrast with its clinical behavior. *Cancer* 46: 1810–1816.
16. Poulsen M., Rischin D., Walpole E., *et al.* (2003). High-risk Merkel cell carcinoma of the skin treated with synchronous carboplatin/etoposide and radiation: a Trans-Tasman Radiation Oncology Group Study — TROG 96:07. *J Clin Oncol* 21: 4371–4376.
17. Su L.D., Fullen D.R., Lowe L., *et al.* (2002). CD117 (KIT receptor) expression in Merkel cell carcinoma. *Am J Dermatopathol* 24: 289–293.
18. Bobos M., Hytiroglou P., Kostopoulos I., *et al.* (2006). Immunohistochemical distinction between Merkel cell carcinoma and small cell carcinoma of the lung. *Am J Dermatopathol* 28: 99–104.
19. Strong S., Shalders K., Carr R., *et al.* (2004). KIT receptor (CD117) expression in Merkel cell carcinoma. *Br J Dermatol* 150: 384–385.
20. Feinmesser M., Halpern M., Kaganovsky E., *et al.* (2004). c-Kit expression in primary and metastatic Merkel cell carcinoma. *Am J Dermatopathol* 26: 458–462.
21. Mita A.C., Mita M.M., Nawrocki S.T., *et al.* (2008). Survivin: key regulator of mitosis and apoptosis and novel target for cancer therapeutics. *Clin Cancer Res* 14: 5000–5005.

22. Ambrosini G., Adida C., Altieri D.C. (1997). A novel anti-apoptosis gene, survivin, expressed in cancer and lymphoma. *Nat Med* 3: 917–921.
23. Kim J., McNiff J.M. (2008). Nuclear expression of survivin portends a poor prognosis in Merkel cell carcinoma. *Mod Pathol* 21: 764–769.
24. Vazmitel M., Michal M., Shelekhova K.V., *et al.* (2008). Vascular changes in Merkel cell carcinoma based on a histopathological study of 92 cases. *Am J Dermatopathol* 30: 106–111.
25. Kukko H., Koljonen V., Lassus P., *et al.* (2007). Expression of vascular endothelial growth factor receptor-2 in Merkel cell carcinoma. *Anticancer Res* 27: 2587–2589.
26. Brunner M., Thurnher D., Pammer J., *et al.* (2008). Expression of VEGF-A/C, VEGF-R2, PDGF-alpha/beta, c-kit, EGFR, Her-2/Neu, Mcl-1 and Bmi-1 in Merkel cell carcinoma. *Mod Pathol* 21: 876–884.
27. Swick B.L., Ravdel L., Fitzpatrick J.E., *et al.* (2008). Platelet-derived growth factor receptor alpha mutational status and immunohistochemical expression in Merkel cell carcinoma: implications for treatment with imatinib mesylate. *J Cutan Pathol* 35: 197–202.
28. Davids M., Charlton A., Ng S.S., *et al.* (2009). Response to a novel multi-targeted tyrosine kinase inhibitor pazopanib in metastatic Merkel cell carcinoma. *J Clin Oncol* 27: e97–100.
29. Kukko H., Koljonen V., Lassus P., *et al.* (2007). Expression of endostatin in Merkel cell carcinoma. *Anticancer Res* 27: 2583–2586.
30. Kirby M.L., Aronstam R.S., Buccafusco J.J. (1985). Changes in cholinergic parameters associated with failure of conotruncal septation in embryonic chick hearts after neural crest ablation. *Circ Res* 56: 392–401.
31. Bowers J.W., Schlauder S.M., Calder K.B., *et al.* (2008). Acetylcholine receptor expression in Merkel cell carcinoma. *Am J Dermatopathol* 30: 340–343.
32. Garneski K.M., Warcola A.H., Feng Q., *et al.* (2009). Merkel cell polyomavirus is more frequently present in North American than Australian Merkel cell carcinoma tumors. *J Invest Dermatol* 129: 246–248.
33. Feng H., Shuda M., Chang Y., *et al.* (2008). Clonal integration of a polyomavirus in human Merkel cell carcinoma. *Science* 319: 1096–1100.
34. Becker J.C., Houben R., Ugurel S., *et al.* (2009). MC polyomavirus is frequently present in Merkel cell carcinoma of European patients. *J Invest Dermatol* 129: 248–250.

35. Leung A.Y., Chan M.T., Yuen K.Y., *et al.* (2005). Ciprofloxacin decreased polyoma BK virus load in patients who underwent allogeneic hematopoietic stem cell transplantation. *Clin Infect Dis* 40: 528–537.
36. Ali S.H., Chandraker A., DeCaprio J.A. (2007). Inhibition of Simian virus 40 large T antigen helicase activity by fluoroquinolones. *Antivir Ther* 12: 1–6.
37. Koljonen V., Jahkola T., Tukiainen E., *et al.* (2005). Tenascin-C in primary Merkel cell carcinoma. *J Clin Pathol* 58: 297–300.
38. Asioli S., Righi A., Volante M., *et al.* (2007). p63 expression as a new prognostic marker in Merkel cell carcinoma. *Cancer* 110: 640–647.
39. Fernandez-Figueras M.T., Puig L., Musulen E., *et al.* (2007). Expression profiles associated with aggressive behavior in Merkel cell carcinoma. *Mod Pathol* 20: 90–101.
40. Houben R., Michel B., Vetter-Kauczok C.S., *et al.* (2006). Absence of classical MAP kinase pathway signalling in Merkel cell carcinoma. *J Invest Dermatol* 126: 1135–1142.
41. Koljonen V., Lassus P., Tukiainen E., *et al.* (2005). Cyclooxygenase-2 expression in primary Merkel cell carcinoma. *J Cutan Pathol* 32: 55–58.
42. Druker B.J., Sawyers C.L., Kantarjian H., *et al.* (2001). Activity of a specific inhibitor of the BCR-ABL tyrosine kinase in the blast crisis of chronic myeloid leukemia and acute lymphoblastic leukemia with the Philadelphia chromosome. *N Engl J Med* 344: 1038–1042.
43. Savage D.G., Antman K.H. (2002). Imatinib mesylate — a new oral targeted therapy. *N Engl J Med* 346: 683–693.
44. Druker B.J., Tamura S., Buchdunger E., *et al.* (1996). Effects of a selective inhibitor of the Abl tyrosine kinase on the growth of Bcr-Abl positive cells. *Nat Med* 2: 561–566.
45. O'Brien S.G., Guilhot F., Larson R.A., *et al.* (2003). Imatinib compared with interferon and low-dose cytarabine for newly diagnosed chronic-phase chronic myeloid leukemia. *N Engl J Med* 348: 994–1004.
46. Demetri G.D., von Mehren M., Blanke C.D., *et al.* (2002). Efficacy and safety of imatinib mesylate in advanced gastrointestinal stromal tumors. *N Engl J Med* 347: 472–480.
47. Swick B.L., Ravdel L., Fitzpatrick J.E., *et al.* (2007). Merkel cell carcinoma: evaluation of KIT (CD117) expression and failure to demonstrate activating mutations in the C-KIT proto-oncogene — implications for treatment with imatinib mesylate. *J Cutan Pathol* 34: 324–329.

48. Kartha R.V., Sundram U.N. (2008). Silent mutations in KIT and PDGFRA and coexpression of receptors with SCF and PDGFA in Merkel cell carcinoma: implications for tyrosine kinase-based tumorigenesis. *Mod Pathol* 21: 96–104.
49. Kassem A., Technau K., Kurz A.K, *et al.* (2009). Merkel cell polyomavirus sequences are frequently detected in nonmelanoma skin cancer of immunosuppressed patients. *Int J Cancer* 125: 356–361.
50. zur Hausen H. (2008). A specific signature of Merkel cell polyomavirus persistence in human cancer cells. *Proc Natl Acad Sci USA* 105: 16063–16064.
51. zur Hausen H. (2008). Novel human polyomaviruses — re-emergence of a well known virus family as possible human carcinogens. *Int J Cancer* 123: 247–250.
52. Houben R., Schrama D., Becker J.C. (2009). Molecular pathogenesis of Merkel cell carcinoma. *Exp Dermatol* 18: 193–198.

Chapter 17

Potential for Immunotherapy in Merkel Cell Carcinoma

Kelly M. McLean, Ronald C. DeConti and Vernon K. Sondak

17.1 Introduction

Most patients with Merkel cell carcinoma initially present with localized disease. Merkel cell carcinoma, however, behaves aggressively with recurrence and metastases often occurring within two years.[1] Once Merkel cell carcinoma metastasizes, it is responsive to, but rarely cured by, chemotherapy and radiation. Additional therapies and new modalities are clearly needed to cure this disease.

Merkel cell carcinoma is prevalent in immunosuppressed populations including the elderly, transplant patients with CLL and HIV-positive patients. Compared with the general population, the risk of Merkel cell carcinoma is 40 times greater in immunosuppressed transplant patients and 13 times greater in HIV-positive patients.[2,3] Chronically immunosuppressed patients are more than 15 times more likely to develop Merkel cell carcinoma than age-matched controls.[4] Mortality from Merkel cell carcinoma has also been reported to be greater in immunosuppressed patients.[5] In addition, in at least some cases, reduction of immunosuppression has induced tumor regression.[6] Clearly, immunocompetence plays a role in tumor suppression.

As with melanoma, the literature contains accounts of spontaneous regression of primary Merkel cell carcinoma, as well as its metastases, particularly after biopsy (reviewed in Richetta *et al.*, 2008 and Connelly *et al.*, 2000).[7,8] In a retrospective study, Inoue *et al.* compared the levels of tumor infiltrating lymphocytes in Merkel cell carcinomas that spontaneously regressed with levels in tumors which did not spontaneously regress and found significantly higher levels in those that did regress. Uchl-1 positive T-cells combined with a high TUNEL index confirmed the importance of T-cell activation in the regression,[9] illustrating the role that activation of the immune system can play in the control of Merkel cell carcinoma. Regression has also been reported associated with therapies such as TNF,[10] IFN-alpha,[11] and dinitrochlorbenzol.[12] What is striking is that these therapies create both a local response and also a systemic effect, attacking tumor throughout the body. All of these studies suggest that when properly stimulated, the immune system can potentially fight Merkel cell carcinoma.

Cancer immunotherapy is predicated on targeting tumor antigens that identify the cancer as non-self and activate the body's natural defense mechanisms. The necessary steps to stimulate an immune response to a cancer are to mount a tumor antigen on an antigen-presenting cell, present the antigen, activate cytotoxic lymphocytes *in vivo* and inhibit autoregulatory control mechanisms. This process can be enhanced by the co-administration of immunologic adjuvants such as immune stimulatory cytokines or suppressors of immune inhibitors. Virally derived proteins, cell type-specific proteins, oncofetal proteins and cancer-testis antigens, proteins that are mutated or upregulated in tumor cells and clonal rearrangement of immunoglobulin genes are all potential immunotherapy targets (Table 1). Dendritic cells are the most powerful antigen-presenting cells. They can be cultured *ex vivo* with the desired immunogenic antigens or even whole tumor lysates and then injected intratumorally as a

Table 1. Classes of proteins that are appropriate potential targets for immunotherapy.

Appropriate targets for immunotherapy
Virally derived proteins
Cell type-specific proteins
Oncofetal proteins/cancer-testis antigens
Mutated proteins or those that are upregulated in tumor cells
Clonal rearrangement of immunoglobulin genes

vaccine to stimulate an immune response to tumor.[13] Serologic analysis of recombinant cDNA expression libraries (SEREX) has been used in multiple tumor types to identify potential tumor-specific antigens.[14]

Many advances in immunotherapy have been made over the last decade. Little is known about applying immunotherapy to Merkel cell carcinoma; however, possibilities can be extrapolated from similarities to other cancers in which it has been used.

17.2 Parallels with Neuroendocrine Tumor Therapy

Merkel cells are normal constituents of the skin that belong to the neuroendocrine/APUD system. Examining successful immunotherapy treatments for neuroendocrine cancers may provide insight on potential approaches for Merkel cell carcinoma.

Small cell lung carcinoma is the most common neuroendocrine malignancy. Because of the morphologic similarities between small cell lung carcinoma and Merkel cell carcinoma, NCCN guidelines recommend similar treatment for metastatic Merkel cell carcinoma as for small cell lung carcinoma (NCCN home page, http://www.nccn.org).[15,16] Genomic analysis demonstrated only 17 different genes between Merkel cell carcinoma and small cell lung carcinoma, further supporting the similarity between the two malignancies.[17] Although the extent of the parallels between the two tumor types has been debated, the histologic appearance, metastatic incidence, pattern of spread and sensitivity to chemotherapy and radiation of the two tumors resemble each other.[18] In addition, JC virus, a member of the same virus family responsible for Merkel cell carcinoma, has been suggested to play a role in the generation of non-adenomatous lung cancer, particularly small cell lung carcinoma.[19] The vast majority of immunotherapeutic treatments for lung carcinoma have been studied in non-small cell lung carcinoma;[13] however, a few studies have focused on small cell lung carcinoma. Improved survival in small cell lung carcinoma has been associated with auto-antibodies against tumor,[20] although results of trials have been mixed and have shown little clinical efficacy of vaccines.[21]

Antonia *et al.* investigated vaccination of extensive-stage small cell lung carcinoma with dendritic cells transduced with full length wild-type p53.[22] Studies in mice and *ex vivo* human cells showed that anti-p53 cytotoxic lymphocytes killed tumor cells and spared normal cells.[23–25] In Antonia's study, a T-cell response to vaccination was seen in 57%. This, however, translated to a clinical response in only one patient. Instead, most patients had disease progression. At first, the vaccination strategy appeared unsuccessful, until they noticed that 61.9% of the vaccinated patients responded to subsequent chemotherapy. In addition, of the patients who did not develop a p53-specific response to vaccination, only 30% responded to second line chemotherapy. In contrast, 75% of the patients who did develop a p53 cellular immune response had objective clinical responses to chemotherapy after vaccination. One year after vaccination, 38% of the patients were alive, a time period well beyond median survival rates previously shown for end-stage small cell lung carcinoma.

Merkel cell carcinoma and small cell lung carcinoma are similar in that they are held at bay by chemotherapy, but generally not cured by it. First line therapy produces a tumor response in small cell lung carcinoma approximately half of the time. Once small cell lung carcinoma recurs, however, prognosis is dismal with most patients dying from disease within a few months.[26,27] Merkel cell carcinoma also has a low survival rate for advanced disease. When a tumor is first exposed to chemotherapy the majority of cells are killed. Similar to what is seen with antibiotics, however, the process selects for tumor cells that are resistant to the chemotherapeutic agent. Any recurrent tumor is now resistant to the first line chemotherapeutic agents. Prognosis is poor and median survival time is low after recurrence. High level expression of anti-apoptotic proteins is one of the methods through which tumors manifest resistance. The same method that grants them chemotherapeutic resistance, however, may make them vulnerable to immunotherapy, thus, combining chemotherapy and immunotherapy can produce a synergistic effect.[28]

Chemotherapy may also enhance the effectiveness of immunotherapy by suppressing immune inhibitors such as regulatory T (T_{reg}) cells. Anthracyclines, widely used in chemotherapeutic treatment of Merkel cell carcinoma,[29] appear to be especially effective in eliciting an immune response secondary to translocation of calreticulin.[30] Cyclophosphamide, also an active agent against Merkel cell carcinoma,[29] has also been used to down-regulate T_{reg} cells.[31]

Evidence indicates that, as in small cell lung carcinoma, the regulation of p53 may be disturbed in Merkel cell carcinoma.[15] Expression of p63, a member of the p53 family is seen in 53% of Merkel cell carcinomas and is an indicator of poor prognosis.[32] Both p53 and p63 have been shown to be over-expressed in Merkel cell carcinoma compared to normal Merkel cells. In addition, over-expression of Ki-67 was associated with over-expression of p63, propensity to metastasize and poor prognosis, making it a prime target for adjuvant immunotherapy aimed toward preventing or treating metastatic disease.[33–35] Co-targeting biologically connected proteins may enhance the effectiveness of immunotherapy, particularly in heterogeneous tumors.[28]

Dendritic cell therapy has also been used in other chemotherapy-resistant neuroendocrine carcinomas.[36] In a case report by Schott *et al.* a dendritic cell vaccine based on whole cell tumor-derived lysate induced a strong T-cell response, lowered tumor markers and showed slight regression of a liver metastasis without progression of other disease in a patient with metastatic neuroendocrine carcinoma of the pancreas resistant to conventional chemotherapy.[37] In another series of seven patients with metastatic medullary thyroid carcinoma, dendritic cell therapy induced a clinical response which included regression of pulmonary and liver metastases in one patient. Five other patients maintained stable disease. Only one patient, who did not demonstrate a T-cell response, had progression of disease.[38] Other studies demonstrated cytotoxic T-cell activity against medullary thyroid carcinoma tumor cells both *in vitro*,[39] in animal models,[40] and in human models.[41] In addition, CD8+ T-cells that recognized tumor-associated antigens have spontaneously developed in patients with midgut carcinoid tumors.[42] Although these T-cells are anergic without exogenous stimulation, if cultured with healthy dendritic cells, they could initiate an immune response against tumor cells. Although only pilot studies, these case reports demonstrate the potential of successful immunotherapy treatment for multiple types of neuroendocrine tumors increasing the prospects that this therapy can be extended to Merkel cell carcinoma as well.

17.3 Application of Immunotherapy Techniques from Melanoma

Melanoma, like Merkel cell carcinoma, is a malignancy of the skin that has proven difficult to cure once it has metastasized. Melanoma is highly immunogenic. In incidences of spontaneous regression of melanoma, infiltration of the tumor with lymphocytes has been found.[43] Melanocyte proliferation has been associated with immunosuppression, as well as reversal with cessation of immunosuppression.[44] In addition, tumor antigen-specific antibodies present in melanoma patients and peripheral blood lymphocytes have been shown to be cytotoxic to melanoma cells *in vitro*.[43] T-lymphocytes have been shown to prevent tumor formation in both a murine and human model.[45,46] Excision of metastases may enhance the immune response to melanoma by removing inhibitors of the immune response and by increasing the number of tumor-specific antibodies and lymphocytes available for immune-mediated killing.[47] Although immunotherapy in melanoma has demonstrated efficacy against metastases in all parts of the body, the best results have been seen with skin and soft tissues metastases versus visceral metastases.[48]

Immunotherapeutic approaches to melanoma have taken three approaches: (1) non-specific stimulation of anti-tumor immune responses by stimulating endogenous effector cells or removing inhibition; (2) active immunization against melanoma; and (3) adoptive cell transfer using tumor infiltrating lymphocytes (Table 2). Non-specific therapy has included interferon therapy, IL-2, and CTLA-4 and PD-1 antagonists. Vaccines have been made from autologous or allogeneic tumor, peptide fragments from known or suspected tumor antigens, or recombinant DNA. Early trials of vaccines had shown some benefit, although more recent trials have not.[49] Dendritic cell therapy has also been used in combination with melanoma-associated antigens.[43] Even though results have not been consistent, treatment has been effective in a subset of patients with initial human trials demonstrating some delay in tumor progression.[50,51]

Table 2. Current immunotherapy strategies against melanoma from which potential approaches to treat Merkel cell carcinoma could be drawn.

Current immunotherapeutic approaches to melanoma
1. Non-specific stimulation of anti-tumor responses
2. Active immunization against melanoma
3. Adoptive cell transfer

One of the most successful immunotherapies for treating melanoma has been adoptive cell transfer using tumor-specific lymphocytes. Cytotoxic T-lymphocytes (CTL) against melanoma tumors are found in the peripheral blood, lymph nodes and in melanoma tumors, but are either too few in number or existing in an immunosuppressive environment limiting their effectiveness.[49] By isolating and proliferating these CTL *ex vivo*, large numbers of potentially more effective cells can be created. Up to 78% of melanoma tumor infiltrating lymphocytes can be tumor reactive.[52] Combined with non-myeloablative chemotherapy, objective results have been seen in 51% of patients with metastatic melanoma.[53,54] Adoptively transferred T-cells obtained from tumor-draining lymph nodes have also triggered regression of melanoma metastases in animal models.[55] When the T-cells were primed with GM-CSF, a durable clinical response in stage IV melanoma was observed.[52] Addition of highly-avid T-cell receptors increases the affinity of the tumor infiltrating lymphocytes for tumor cells. These T-cells have been shown to persist in blood for up to one year.[56] Spontaneously regressing Merkel cell tumors show high levels of tumor-infiltrating lymphocytes, as well.[9] Merkel cell carcinoma is well-known to drain to lymph nodes. Isolation and proliferation of T-cells from Merkel cell tumors or tumor-draining lymph nodes is a potential approach for immunotherapy of Merkel cell carcinoma.

17.4 Potential Viral Protein Derived Immunotherapy Targets

Studies have indicated that up to 80% of Merkel cell carcinomas show evidence of infection by the Merkel cell polyomavirus (MCPyV), a newly discovered member of the polyomavirus family[57] (see Chapter 3 for a detailed account). In short, the polyomavirus family includes five known human viruses — BKV, JCV, Karolinska Institute Virus, Washington University Virus, and MCPyV. While Merkel cell carcinoma provides the first evidence of a polyomavirus-induced malignancy in humans,[58,59] polyomavirus sequences have been detected in multiple other human tumors,[60] and other polyomaviruses can induce malignancies in animals or transform human cells in culture.[15]

Epitopes derived from oncoviral proteins serve as potential tumor antigens. Vaccination for the treatment and prevention of the human papilloma virus (HPV) induced cervical cancer illustrates this example well (reviewed in Mahdavi and Monk, 2005 and Beaudenon and Huibregtse, 2008).[61,62] Polyomaviruses and papillomavirus are closely related, previously grouped together in the same viral family — Papovaridae. Perhaps lessons learned from HPV can be applied to immunotherapy for Merkel cell carcinoma.

Virtually all cervical cancers contain the genes of HPV. Similar to MCPyV, the immune system appears to be integral in controlling oncogenic transformation with HPV. The incidence of HPV associated cancers is higher in immunocompromised patients such as transplant patients and HIV-positive patients. To develop preventative and therapeutic vaccines against human papilloma virus, two types of oncoviral proteins have been targeted — viral capsid-specific proteins and oncogenic HPV proteins.

HPV viral capsid proteins are themselves highly immunogenic and have been successful antigens for preventative vaccines against HPV. Therapeutic vaccines utilizing HPV capsid protein antigens have not been efficacious, however, because malignant cells already transformed by HPV do not express these antigens sufficiently to generate an immune response. The viral etiology of Merkel cell carcinoma lends itself to developing a preventative vaccine for polyomavirus, as has been done with the human papilloma virus. The MCPyV genome encodes for three viral capsid proteins — VP1, VP2, and VP3 — all of which are all potential antigens for preventative vaccines. As in HPV, whether or not the viral capsid proteins are expressed in the final Merkel cell tumor cell would determine the potential to use them as antigens for therapeutic vaccines. At risk populations including the elderly, people who are HIV-positive, transplant recipients and people with CLL could be vaccinated to prevent them from infection with the virus, hopefully preventing future development of Merkel cell carcinoma. The key to prevention, however, would be vaccination prior to viral exposure. Most people demonstrate evidence of exposure to other human polyomaviruses before adulthood; few studies, however, have looked at the timing of infection with MCPyV. If MCPyV infection occurs early, followed by a period of viral dormancy, focusing on therapeutic vaccinations may prove more beneficial.

An approach to therapeutic vaccination for HPV targets the viral proteins E6 and E7, which are integral to both the malignant transformation of the cell and to the maintenance of malignancy. Most HPV cancers express one of these oncoviral proteins. In preclinical studies in both animals and humans, these proteins have elicited strong antitumor immunologic responses. Since other polyomaviruses appear to express some cell tropism, it would be reasonable to suspect that MCPyV expresses itself predominantly in Merkel cells.[60] The selectivity of MCPyV for only Merkel cells would make any resulting oncoproteins ideal immunotherapy targets. The viral genome of MCPyV encodes for the large tumor (large T), small tumor, T3 and T4 antigens in the early region and for viral capsid proteins VP1, VP2, and VP3 in the late region, any of which are potential therapeutic antigens targets.

The large T antigen is mandatory for viral DNA replication, controlling the transcription of early and late genes.[60] The large T antigen interferes with the normal action of cell cycle regulatory proteins, cellular gene expression, cell survival, cellular protein turnover, chromosomal stability, and angiogenesis. Specifically, the large T antigen interferes with the retinoblastoma tumor suppressor protein and the p53 pathway. In tumor cells, the large T protein is prematurely truncated compared with viral proteins expressed in non-tumor cells.[63] Both the wild type and the truncated large T protein maintain interaction with the retinoblastoma pathway, however the DNA damage response is impaired, resulting in oncogenesis. The mutated protein preserves the cell-cycle progression activity but prevents genomic instability which would lead to cell death. In addition, the truncated protein is seen both in primary tumor cells and in metastases.[5] As mentioned before, proteins involved with anti-apoptotic pathways are preferred targets for immunotherapy because they tend to be highly expressed in tumor cells that are resistant to chemotherapy. The expression of the same truncated large T protein in metastases makes it a good immunotherapeutic target choice in both primary and metastatic disease.

17.5 Other Protein Targets

Anti-apoptotic proteins are ideal targets for immunotherapy: they are expressed in high number in all the tumor cells, they confer resistance to chemotherapy, they are not expressed in normal cells and they are

Table 3. Proteins which are potential antigenic targets in the treatment of Merkel cell carcinoma.

Viral Proteins:	Survivin	Mcl-1
VP1	MUC-1	Bmi-1
VP2	Ep-CAM	VEGF-A
VP3	Bcl-2	VEGF-C
Large T	p63	VEGF-R2
Small T	Ki-67	PDGF-α
T3	KOC	
T4		

antigenic. Merkel cell carcinomas inhibit apoptotic pathways. Survivin, MUC-1, Ep-CAM, bcl-2, p63 are all anti-apoptotic proteins which have been shown to be over-expressed in Merkel cell carcinoma and thus would make good targets for immunotherapy (Table 3). Many of these proteins are already being targeted to treat other malignancies.

Survivin is a fetal oncoprotein that is strongly expressed in many human malignancies, including Merkel cell carcinoma, while almost undetectable in normal, differentiated tissues. Survivin is an inhibitor of apoptosis as well as a regulator of mitosis. While all of the Merkel cell tumors tested expressed survivin, nuclear expression of survivin was associated with worse prognosis and increased incidence of metastases.[64] Survivin's selective expression in tumor cells makes it a great target for tumor immunotherapy. Spontaneous anti-survivin T-cell reactivity has been observed in a wide variety of cancer patients.[65] In addition, survivin-specific T-cells harvested from a patient with one type of malignancy have been shown *ex vivo* to lysis HLA-matched cells harvested from a different tumor type[66–68] without lysing normal cells.[69] In mice, lung metastases were eradicated by combined immunotherapy against survivin and angiogenesis proteins.[70] Clinical trials have begun to confirm the efficacy of a survivin-based vaccine. In one example, a patient with carcinoma of the pancreas had regression of liver metastases.[71] Clearly, immunotherapy targeting the expression of survivin holds potential for treating a wide variety of malignancies, Merkel cell carcinoma included.

Mucin 1 (MUC-1) is another protein that is expressed in a wide variety of adenocarcinomas and that has been an immunotherapeutic target in multiple epithelial malignancies.[72] MUC-1 is a highly glycosylated protein that is secreted by glandular epithelial cells. MUC-1 is an integral part of cell-cell adhesions and cellular proliferation. Although MUC-1 is found in both malignant and normal cells, variations in glycosylation patterns have allowed it to be successfully targeted by immunological therapies. Kurzen *et al.* demonstrated that MUC-1 is expressed in normal Merkel cells, in 82% of Merkel cell carcinomas, and in 66% of Merkel cell carcinoma metastases — levels that are comparable to those seen in breast carcinoma and squamous cell carcinoma. As had been seen in other tissue types, MUC-1 glycosylation patterns differed between normal Merkel cells and malignant Merkel cells.[73] Many preclinical studies in mice have demonstrated that MUC-1 can stimulate an adequate immune response which has lead to numerous human clinical trials.[74]

Kurtzen *et al.* also examined the expression of Ep-CAM in both normal and malignant Merkel cells. Similar to the expression of MUC-1, Ep-CAM was expressed in normal Merkel cells, in 70% of primary Merkel cell carcinomas, and in 70% of metastases. Ep-CAM appeared to have stronger expression in Merkel cell carcinomas that metastasized than those that did not.[73] Immunotherapy against Ep-CAM may, therefore, target the most aggressive disease, while leaving the disease less likely to metastasize for local excision. Ep-CAM is a transmembrane molecule that acts as a tumor-associated calcium signal transducer as well as a cell-cell adhesion molecule. It is one of the most immunogenic tumor-associated proteins. In human trials, edrecolomab, a monoclonal antibody against Ep-CAM has shown some efficacy in treating adenocarcinoma of the colon.[75]

Over-expression of bcl-2, another anti-apoptotic protein, has been observed in the majority of Merkel cell carcinomas.[76,77] Inhibition in an animal model demonstrated reduction in tumor size.[78] Although inhibition of bcl-2 *in vivo* has not yet been shown to be therapeutically effective,[5] bcl-2 is still a potential immunotherapy target either alone or combined with other antigenic epitopes.

Other potential targets for immunotherapy are p63, Ki-67, and K homology domain-containing protein over-expressed in cancer (KOC).

Although each of these has not been specifically investigated for immunotherapy, each one has the characteristics of a desirable antigen: over-expression in tumors, scant expression in normal tissue, higher expression in more aggressive tumors, and interaction with the apoptotic pathways. p63 is a member of the p53 family which has been shown to be important in the development of the basal cell differentiation of epithelial tissues. Expression of p63 has been shown to be increased in multiple squamous cell tumors[79] including those of the head and neck,[80] lung,[81] esophagus,[82] and cervix.[83] Its expression in neuroendocrine tumors has been proportional to the aggressiveness of the tumor. Aggressive small cell lung cancers highly expressed p63 while indolent carcinoids had a low level of expression.[81] When studied in Merkel cell carcinoma, 53.1% were found to be positive for p63. Expression of p63 was highly associated with Ki-67 expression ($p = 0.0006$). In addition, expression of p63 correlated with worse prognosis.[32]

KOC, also known as L523S and IMP-3, is an insulin-like growth factor II messenger RNA-binding protein that increases tumor cell proliferation. KOC is an oncofetal protein that is expressed in early embryonic tissues. KOC is over-expressed in high-grade neuroendocrine carcinomas[84,85] in addition to other malignancies such as pancreatic cancer,[86] melanoma[87]and ovarian cancer.[88] Pryor *et al.* showed that 90% of Merkel cell carcinomas also expressed KOC. In addition, those tumors that had the highest level of expression of KOC were the most likely to metastasize.[89] Recombinant KOC elicited an immunological response when given to patients with lung carcinoma.[90] As KOC is expressed in the placenta, gonads and intestinal mucosa,[91] patients would need to be monitored for autoimmune side-effects, particularly of the reproductive and GI tracts.

Multiple promising targets for immunotherapy are listed above. Some of these, such as survivin and MUC 1, have been successfully used to stimulate an immune response *in vivo* in other malignancies causing regression of tumor. Others targets have not been investigated to the same extent, but display promising characteristics. Brunner performed a tissue microarray of Merkel cell carcinoma to identify potential targets for immunotherapy. Immunoreactivity scores greater than 70% were seen for myeloid cell leukemia sequence-1 (Mcl-1) (88%), Bmi-1 (78%), vascular endothelial growth factor-A (VEGF-A) (91%), VEGF-C (75%),

VEGF-R2 (88%), and platelet-derived growth factor (PDGF-α) (72%). Mcl-1 is a member of the bcl-2 protein family, an anti-apoptotic protein which avoids the release of cell-damage induced mitochondrial cytochrome c. Bmi-1 is a member of the polycomb group family of proteins which is important in the immortalization of cell lines. Either would be potential immunotherapy targets.[92]

Serologic analysis of recombinant cDNA expression library (SEREX) is another option for identifying potential immunotherapy targets. SEREX analyzes lysate from a fresh tumor specimen to identify unique peptides that elicit an immunogenic response from the host. It has been integral in identifying antibody targets for tumor types including melanoma, astrocytoma, Hodgkin's lymphoma, and prostate, renal cell, esophageal, gastric, colon, lung, and breast carcinomas. IgG-specific antibodies identify epitopes that have already been targeted by the host's T-cells. Comparison of reactivity of normal serum with that of cancer patients helps to identify cancer-specific targets, minimizing autoimmune effects. Many of the antigens identified are novel. SEREX has been used to develop tumor markers such as CEA and AFP as well as identify markers for metastasis including cancer/testis antigens, over-expressed gene products, mutated cancer genes, splice variants, and cancer-related autoantigens. In addition, SEREX allows for adaptation. As tumors recur, they can be re-analyzed for new targets which may be more efficacious.[14, 93,94]

17.6 Challenges

Merkel cell carcinoma is predominantly a disease of immunosuppressed individuals. Although it may occur in patients with fully functioning immune systems, it is much more prevalent in the immunocompromised. As a result, even if presented with the ideal antigen, patients may not be able to mount an immune response sufficient to fight the tumor. Even in the absence of pre-existing immunosuppression, malignancies themselves create an immunosuppressed state. As tumors grow, their effect on immune suppression, particularly of T-cells, increases. Adjuvant therapies that address the individual etiology of each patient's immunosuppression may be required to assist immunotherapy treatments for Merkel cell carcinoma.

Merkel cell carcinoma is also predominantly a disease of the elderly. Immunosenescence in the elderly is an accumulation of alterations in both B- and T-cells, which include decreased circulating memory B-cells, decreased germinal center B-cell formation, decreased follicular dendritic cell function, decreased thymic generation of naïve T-cells, increased terminal effector cells, and increased inflammatory mediators. NK cells, which inhibit tumor growth and metastases, show decreased cytotoxity per cell in the elderly. Humoral immunity is also impaired. B-cells, in general, are less stimulated by dendritic cells resulting in decreased T-cell function. The elderly have fewer T-cells than the young, particularly secondary to thymic involution.[95] Among these T-cells, the proportion of naïve cells relative to the proportion of activated effector cells is lower in the elderly than in the young.

Merkel cell carcinoma is inherently a heterogeneous disease. No single chromosomal defect has consistently been found.[96] Based on biochemical markers and neurosecretory granule morphology, colony shape and aggregation, two types of Merkel cell carcinoma, a Classic and Variant type, have been described. Genomic analysis of the two different subtypes demonstrated 76 differentially expressed genes. The Classic cell line showed increased gene expression for neuromediators, neurotransmittors, ion-channels and proteins involved with neuronal development. In contrast, the Variant cell line showed increased expression of genes related to cell cycle control, cell proliferation and vimentin.[17] Cells in tissue culture also display distinct morphologies. Some are small, closely resembling small cell lung carcinoma, while other cells are much larger, greater than three times the size of lymphocytes with high mitotic activity and multiple nucleoli. A mixture of both morphologies may be found in one tumor. The two cell types stain distinctly for different receptors and proteins. In a microarray analysis of tissue, c-kit and PDGF-β expression was only seen in the large cell tumor group while VEGF-R2 expression trended toward higher expression in the large cell group.[92] In addition, not all Merkel cell carcinomas express the MCPyV sequence. About 75% of tumors from North American patients[57] and 85% of the tumors in European patients showed evidence of MCPyV infection.[97] In contrast, only 24% of tumors from Australian patients showed evidence of MCPyV infection.[98] As a result of the diverse etiologies of Merkel cell carcinoma, one antigen or immunotherapy approach may not work for every case.

17.7 Conclusion

Merkel cell carcinoma is a malignancy of cutaneous neuroendocrine cells which, once metastasized, is aggressive and difficult to cure. Its innate responsiveness to the immune system makes it an appropriate candidate for immunotherapeutic approaches. To date, little research has been done on immunotherapeutic treatments for Merkel cell carcinoma. Potential approaches can be derived from therapeutic analogies with other similar malignancies. Since Merkel cell carcinoma is a disease of immunocompromised patients, adjuvant strategies that strengthen patients' own immune system may need to accompany the therapies directed at Merkel cell carcinoma. In addition, the heterogeneous nature of Merkel cell carcinoma indicates that one single therapy may not work for every tumor. Multiple treatment options may need to be developed to attain adequate treatment for all.

References

1. Henness S., Vereecken P. (2008). Management of Merkel tumours: an evidence-based review. *Curr Opin Oncol* 20: 280–286.
2. Kanitakis J., Euvrard S., Chouvet B., *et al.* (2006). Merkel cell carcinoma in organ-transplant recipients: report of two cases with unusual histological features and literature review. *J Cutan Pathol* 33: 686–694.
3. Engels E.A., Frisch M., Goedert J.J., *et al.* (2002) Merkel cell carcinoma and HIV infection. *Lancet* 359(9305): 497–498.
4. Buell J.F., Trofe J., Hanaway M.J., *et al.* (2002). Immunosuppression and Merkel cell cancer. *Transplant Proc* 34: 1780–1781.
5. Becker J.C., Schrama D., Houben R. (2009) Merkel cell carcinoma. *Cell Mol Life Sci* 66: 1–8.
6. Friedlaender M.M., Rubinger D., Rosenbaum E., *et al.* (2002). Temporary regression of Merkel cell carcinoma metastases after cessation of cyclosporine. *Transplantation* 73: 1849–1850.

7. Richetta A.G., Mancini M., Torroni A., *et al.* (2008). Total spontaneous regression of advanced Merkel cell carcinoma after biopsy: review and a new case. *Dermatol Surg* 34: 815–822.
8. Connelly T.J., Cribier B., Brown T.J., Yanguas I. (2000). Complete spontaneous regression of Merkel cell carcinoma: a review of the 10 reported cases. *Dermatol Surg* 26: 853–856.
9. Inoue T., Yoneda K., Manabe M., Demitsu T. (2000). Spontaneous regression of Merkel cell carcinoma: a comparative study of TUNEL index and tumor-infiltrating lymphocytes between spontaneous regression and non-regression group. *J Dermatol Sci* 24: 203–211.
10. Hata Y., Matsuka K., Ito O., *et al.* (1997). Two cases of Merkel cell carcinoma cured by intratumor injection of natural human tumor necrosis factor. *Plast Reconstr Surgery* 99: 547–553.
11. Durand J.M., Weiller C., Richard M.A., *et al.* (1991). Treatment of Merkel cell tumor with interferon-alpha-2b. *Br J Dermatol* 124: 509.
12. Herrmann G., Groth W., Krieg T., Mauch C. (2004). Complete remission of Merkel cell carcinoma of the scalp with local and regional metastases after topical treatment with dinitrochlorbenzol. *J Am Acad Dermatol* 50: 965–969.
13. Ribas A., Butterfield L.H., Glaspy J.A., Economou J.S. (2003). Current developments in cancer vaccines and cellular immunotherapy. *J Clin Oncol* 21: 2415–2432.
14. Sittler T., Zhou J., Park J., *et al.* (2008). Concerted potent humoral immune responses to autoantigens are associated with tumor destruction and favorable clinical outcomes without autoimmunity. *Clin Cancer Res* 14: 3896–3905.
15. Becker J.C., Kauczok C.S., Ugurel S., *et al.* (2008). Merkel cell carcinoma: molecular pathogenesis, clinical features and therapy. *J Dtsch Dermatol Ges* 6: 709–719.
16. Busse P.M., Clark J.R., Muse V.V., Liu V. (2008). Case records of the Massachusetts General Hospital. Case 19–2008. A 63-year-old HIV-positive man with cutaneous Merkel-cell carcinoma. *N Engl J Med* 358: 2717–2723.
17. Van Gele M., Boyle G.M., Cook A.L., *et al.* (2004). Gene-expression profiling reveals distinct expression patterns for classic versus variant Merkel cell phenotypes and new classifier genes to distinguish Merkel cell from small-cell lung carcinoma. *Oncogene* 23: 2732–2742.

18. Lemos B.D., Yu S.S., Nghiem P. (2008). Case 19-2008: Merkel-cell carcinoma. *N Engl J Med* 359: 1629–1631.
19. Zheng H., Abdel Aziz H.O., Nakanishi Y., *et al.* (2007). Oncogenic role of JC virus in lung cancer. *J Pathol* 212: 306–315.
20. Winter S.F., Sekido Y., Minna J.D., *et al.* (1993). Antibodies against autologous tumor cell proteins in patients with small-cell lung cancer: association with improved survival. *J Natl Cancer Inst* 85: 2012–2018.
21. Bradbury P.A., Shepherd F.A. (2008). Immunotherapy for lung cancer. *J Thorac Oncol* 3(6 Suppl 2): S164–S170.
22. Antonia S.J., Mirza N., Fricke I., *et al.* (2006). Combination of p53 cancer vaccine with chemotherapy in patients with extensive stage small cell lung cancer. *Clin Cancer Res* 12: 878–887.
23. Ishida T., Chada S., Stipanov M., *et al.* (1999). Dendritic cells transduced with wild-type p53 gene elicit potent anti-tumour immune responses. *Clin Exp Immunol* 117: 244–251.
24. Mayordomo J.I., Loftus D.J., Sakamoto H., *et al.* (1996). Therapy of murine tumors with p53 wild-type and mutant sequence peptide-based vaccines. *J Exp Med* 183: 1357–1365.
25. Nikitina E.Y., Clark J.I., Van Beynen J., *et al.* (2001). Dendritic cells transduced with full-length wild-type p53 generate antitumor cytotoxic T lymphocytes from peripheral blood of cancer patients. *Clin Cancer Res* 7: 127–135.
26. Schiller J.H. (2001). Current standards of care in small-cell and non-small-cell lung cancer. *Oncology* 61(Suppl 1): 3–13.
27. Eckardt J.R. (2004). Emerging role of weekly topotecan in recurrent small cell lung cancer. *Oncologist* 9(Suppl 6): 25–32.
28. Andersen M.H., Sorensen R.B., Schrama D., *et al.* (2008). Cancer treatment: the combination of vaccination with other therapies. *Cancer Immunol Immunother* 57: 1735–1743.
29. Tai P. (2008). Merkel cell cancer: update on biology and treatment. *Curr Opin Oncol* 20: 196–200.
30. Obeid M., Tesniere A., Ghiringhelli F., *et al.* (2007). Calreticulin exposure dictates the immunogenicity of cancer cell death. *Nat Med* 13: 54–61.
31. Ghiringhelli F., Menard C., Puig P.E., *et al.* (2007). Metronomic cyclophosphamide regimen selectively depletes CD4+CD25+ regulatory T cells and

restores T and NK effector functions in end stage cancer patients. *Cancer Immunol Immunother* 56: 641–648.
32. Asioli S., Righi A., Volante M., *et al.* (2007). p63 expression as a new prognostic marker in Merkel cell carcinoma. *Cancer* 110: 640–647.
33. Koljonen V., Tukiainen E., Haglund C., Bohling T. (2006). Proliferative activity detected by Ki67 correlates with poor outcome in Merkel cell carcinoma. *Histopathology* 49: 551–553.
34. Llombart B., Monteagudo C., Lopez-Guerrero J.A., *et al.* (2005). Clinicopathological and immunohistochemical analysis of 20 cases of Merkel cell carcinoma in search of prognostic markers. *Histopathology* 46: 622–634.
35. Fernandez-Figueras M.T., Puig L., Musulen E., *et al.* (2005). Prognostic significance of p27Kip1, p45Skp2 and Ki67 expression profiles in Merkel cell carcinoma, extracutaneous small cell carcinoma, and cutaneous squamous cell carcinoma. *Histopathology* 46: 614–621.
36. Schott M., Seissler J. (2003). Dendritic cell vaccination: new hope for the treatment of metastasized endocrine malignancies. *Trends Endocrinol Metab* 14: 156–162.
37. Schott M., Feldkamp J., Lettmann M., *et al.* (2001). Dendritic cell immunotherapy in a neuroendocrine pancreas carcinoma. *Clin Endocrinol* 55: 271–277.
38. Schott M., Seissler J., Lettmann M., *et al.* (2001). Immunotherapy for medullary thyroid carcinoma by dendritic cell vaccination. *J Clin Endocrinol Metab* 86: 4965–4969.
39. Schott M., Feldkamp J., Klucken M., *et al.* (2002). Calcitonin-specific antitumor immunity in medullary thyroid carcinoma following dendritic cell vaccination. *Cancer Immunol Immunother* 51: 663–668.
40. Papewalis C., Wuttke M., Seissler J., *et al.* (2008). Dendritic cell vaccination with xenogenic polypeptide hormone induces tumor rejection in neuroendocrine cancer. *Clin Cancer Res* 14: 4298–4305.
41. Bachleitner-Hofmann T., Stift A., Friedl J., *et al.* (2002). Stimulation of autologous antitumor T-cell responses against medullary thyroid carcinoma using tumor lysate-pulsed dendritic cells. *J Clin Endocrinol Metab* 87: 1098–1104.
42. Vikman S., Giandomenico V., Sommaggio R., *et al.* (2008). CD8+ T cells against multiple tumor-associated antigens in peripheral blood of midgut carcinoid patients. *Cancer Immunol Immunother* 57: 399–409.

43. Jack A., Boyes C., Aydin N., *et al.* (2006). The treatment of melanoma with an emphasis on immunotherapeutic strategies. *Surg Oncol* 15: 13–24.
44. Zattra E., Fortina A.B., Bordignon M., *et al.* (2009). Immunosuppression and melanocyte proliferation. *Melanoma Res* 19: 63–68.
45. Shankaran V., Ikeda H., Bruce A.T., *et al.* (2001). IFN gamma and lymphocytes prevent primary tumour development and shape tumour immunogenicity. *Nature* 410: 1107–1111.
46. Chiao E.Y., Krown S.E. (2003). Update on non-acquired immunodeficiency syndrome-defining malignancies. *Curr Opin Oncol* 15: 389–397.
47. Hsueh E.C., Gupta R.K., Yee R., *et al.* (2000). Does endogenous immune response determine the outcome of surgical therapy for metastatic melanoma? *Ann Surg Oncol* 7: 232–238.
48. Demierre M.F., Sabel M.S., Margolin K.A., *et al.* (2008). State of the science 60th anniversary review: 60 years of advances in cutaneous melanoma epidemiology, diagnosis, and treatment, as reported in the journal Cancer. *Cancer* 113(7 Suppl): 1728–1743.
49. Fang L., Lonsdorf A.S., Hwang S.T. (2008). Immunotherapy for advanced melanoma. *J Invest Dermatol* 128: 2596–2605.
50. Engell-Noerregaard L., Hansen T.H., Andersen M.H., *et al.* (2009). Review of clinical studies on dendritic cell-based vaccination of patients with malignant melanoma: assessment of correlation between clinical response and vaccine parameters. *Cancer Immunol Immunother* 58: 1–14.
51. Nestle F.O., Alijagic S., Gilliet M., *et al.* (1998). Vaccination of melanoma patients with peptide- or tumor lysate-pulsed dendritic cells. *Nat Med* 4: 328–332.
52. Tsai S., Chang A.E. (2008). Adoptive T cell immunotherapy. In: Agarwala, S.S. and Sondak, V.K. (eds.). *Melanoma: Translational Research and Emerging Therapies*, pp. 161–176, Informa Healthcare USA, Inc., New York.
53. Dudley M.E., Wunderlich J.R., Yang J.C., *et al.* (2005). Adoptive cell transfer therapy following non-myeloablative but lymphodepleting chemotherapy for the treatment of patients with refractory metastatic melanoma. *J Clin Oncol* 23: 2346–2357.
54. Dudley M.E., Wunderlich J.R., Robbins P.F., *et al.* (2002). Cancer regression and autoimmunity in patients after clonal repopulation with antitumor lymphocytes. *Science* 298: 850–854.

55. Geiger J.D., Wagner P.D., Cameron M.J., *et al.* (1993). Generation of T-cells reactive to the poorly immunogenic B16-BL6 melanoma with efficacy in the treatment of spontaneous metastases. *J Immunother Emphasis Tumor Immunol* 13: 153–165.
56. Morgan R.A., Dudley M.E., Wunderlich J.R., *et al.* (2006) Cancer regression in patients after transfer of genetically engineered lymphocytes. *Science* 314: 126–129.
57. Feng H., Shuda M., Chang Y., Moore P.S. (2008). Clonal integration of a polyomavirus in human Merkel cell carcinoma. *Science* 319: 1096–1100.
58. Poulin D.L., DeCaprio J.A. (2006). Is there a role for SV40 in human cancer? *J Clin Oncol* 24: 4356–4365.
59. Viscidi R.P., Shah K.V. (2008). Cancer. A skin cancer virus? *Science* 319: 1049–1050.
60. Moens U., Johannessen M. (2008). Human polyomaviruses and cancer: expanding repertoire. *J Dtsch Dermatol Ges* 6: 704–708.
61. Mahdavi A., Monk B.J. (2005). Vaccines against human papillomavirus and cervical cancer: promises and challenges. *Oncologist* 10: 528–538.
62. Beaudenon S., Huibregtse J.M. (2008). HPV E6, E6AP and cervical cancer. *BMC Biochemistry* 9(Suppl 1): S4.
63. Shuda M., Feng H., Kwun H.J., *et al.* (2008). T antigen mutations are a human tumor-specific signature for Merkel cell polyomavirus. *Proc Natl Acad Sci USA* 105: 16272–16277.
64. Kim J., McNiff J.M. (2008). Nuclear expression of survivin portends a poor prognosis in Merkel cell carcinoma. *Mod Pathol* 21: 764–769.
65. Andersen M.H., Svane I.M., Becker J.C., thor Straten P. (2007). The universal character of the tumor-associated antigen survivin. *Clin Cancer Res* 13: 5991–5994.
66. Sorensen R.B., Svane I.M., thor Straten P., Andersen M.H. (2008). A survivin specific T-cell clone from a breast cancer patient display universal tumor cell lysis. *Cancer Biol Ther* 7: 1885–1887.
67. Schmidt S.M., Schag K., Muller M.R., *et al.* (2003). Survivin is a shared tumor-associated antigen expressed in a broad variety of malignancies and recognized by specific cytotoxic T cells. *Blood* 102: 571–576.
68. Andersen M.H., Pedersen L.O., Capeller B., *et al.* (2001). Spontaneous cytotoxic T-cell responses against survivin-derived MHC class I-restricted

T-cell epitopes in situ as well as ex vivo in cancer patients. *Cancer Res* 61: 5964–5968.

69. Coughlin C.M., Vance B.A., Grupp S.A., Vonderheide R.H. (2004). RNA-transfected CD40-activated B cells induce functional T-cell responses against viral and tumor antigen targets: implications for pediatric immunotherapy. *Blood* 103: 2046–2054.
70. Xiang R., Mizutani N., Luo Y., *et al.* (2005). A DNA vaccine targeting survivin combines apoptosis with suppression of angiogenesis in lung tumor eradication. *Cancer Res* 65: 553–561.
71. Wobser M., Keikavoussi P., Kunzmann V., *et al.* (2006). Complete remission of liver metastasis of pancreatic cancer under vaccination with a HLA-A2 restricted peptide derived from the universal tumor antigen survivin. *Cancer Immunol Immunother* 55: 1294–1298.
72. Rubinstein D.B., Karmely M., Pichinuk E., *et al.* (2009). The MUC1 oncoprotein as a functional target: immunotoxin binding to alpha/beta junction mediates cell killing. *Int J Cancer* 124: 46–54.
73. Kurzen H., Kaul S., Egner U., *et al.* (2003). Expression of MUC 1 and Ep-CAM in Merkel cell carcinomas: implications for immunotherapy. *Arch Dermatol Res* 295: 146–154.
74. Tang C.K., Katsara M., Apostolopoulos V. (2008). Strategies used for MUC1 immunotherapy: human clinical studies. *Expert Rev Vaccines* 7: 963–975.
75. Riethmuller G., Holz E., Schlimok G., *et al.* (1998). Monoclonal antibody therapy for resected Dukes' C colorectal cancer: seven-year outcome of a multicenter randomized trial. *J Clin Oncol* 16: 1788–1794.
76. Feinmesser M., Halpern M., Fenig E., *et al.* (1999). Expression of the apoptosis-related oncogenes bcl-2, bax, and p53 in Merkel cell carcinoma: can they predict treatment response and clinical outcome? *Hum Pathol* 30: 1367–1372.
77. Kennedy M.M., Blessing K., King G., Kerr K.M. (1996). Expression of bcl-2 and p53 in Merkel cell carcinoma. An immunohistochemical study. *Am J Dermatopathol* 18: 273–277.
78. Schlagbauer-Wadl H., Klosner G., Heere-Ress E., *et al.* (2000). Bcl-2 antisense oligonucleotides (G3139) inhibit Merkel cell carcinoma growth in SCID mice. *J Invest Dermatol* 114: 725–730.

79. Di Como C.J., Urist M.J., Babayan I., *et al.* (2002). p63 expression profiles in human normal and tumor tissues. *Clin Cancer Res* 8: 494–501.
80. Lo Muzio L., Santarelli A., Caltabiano R., *et al.* (2005). p63 overexpression associates with poor prognosis in head and neck squamous cell carcinoma. *Hum Pathol* 36: 187–194.
81. Au N.H., Gown A.M., Cheang M., *et al.* (2004). p63 expression in lung carcinoma: a tissue microarray study of 408 cases. *Appl Immunohistochem Mol Morphol* 12: 240–247.
82. Hu H., Xia S.H., Li A.D., *et al.* (2002). Elevated expression of p63 protein in human esophageal squamous cell carcinomas. *Int J Cancer* 102: 580–583.
83. Wang T.Y., Chen B.F., Yang Y.C., *et al.* (2001). Histologic and immunophenotypic classification of cervical carcinomas by expression of the p53 homologue p63: a study of 250 cases. *Hum Pathol* 32: 479–486.
84. Xu H., Bourne P.A., Spaulding B.O., Wang H.L. (2007). High-grade neuroendocrine carcinomas of the lung express K homology domain containing protein overexpressed in cancer but carcinoid tumors do not. *Hum Pathol* 38: 555–563.
85. Simon R., Bourne P.A., Yang Q., *et al.* (2007). Extrapulmonary small cell carcinomas express K homology domain containing protein overexpressed in cancer, but carcinoid tumors do not. *Hum Pathol* 38: 1178–1183.
86. Yantiss R.K., Woda B.A., Fanger G.R., *et al.* (2005). KOC (K homology domain containing protein overexpressed in cancer): a novel molecular marker that distinguishes between benign and malignant lesions of the pancreas. *Am J Surg Pathol* 29: 188–195.
87. Pryor J.G., Bourne P.A., Yang Q., *et al.* (2008). IMP-3 is a novel progression marker in malignant melanoma. *Mod Pathol* 21: 431–437.
88. Gu L., Shigemasa K., Ohama K. (2004). Increased expression of IGF II mRNA-binding protein 1 mRNA is associated with an advanced clinical stage and poor prognosis in patients with ovarian cancer. *Int J Oncol* 24: 671–678.
89. Pryor J.G., Simon R.A., Bourne P.A., *et al.* (2009). Merkel cell carcinoma expresses K homology domain-containing protein overexpressed in cancer similar to other high-grade neuroendocrine carcinomas. *Hum Pathol* 40: 238–243.
90. Wang T., Fan L., Watanabe Y., *et al.* (2003). L523S, an RNA-binding protein as a potential therapeutic target for lung cancer. *Br J Cancer* 88: 887–894.

91. Hammer N.A., Hansen T.O., Byskov A.G., *et al.* (2005). Expression of IGF-II mRNA-binding proteins (IMPs) in gonads and testicular cancer. *Reproduction* 130: 203–212.
92. Brunner M., Thurnher D., Pammer J., *et al.* (2008). Expression of VEGF-A/C, VEGF-R2, PDGF-alpha/beta, c-kit, EGFR, Her-2/Neu, Mcl-1 and Bmi-1 in Merkel cell carcinoma. *Mod Pathol* 21: 876–884.
93. Jager D. (2007). Potential target antigens for immunotherapy identified by serological expression cloning (SEREX). *Methods Mol Biol* 360: 319–326.
94. Li G., Miles A., Line A., Rees R.C. (2004). Identification of tumour antigens by serological analysis of cDNA expression cloning. *Cancer Immunol Immunother* 53: 139–143.
95. Hakim F.T., Flomerfelt F.A., Boyiadzis M., Gress R.E. (2004). Aging, immunity and cancer. *Curr Opin Immunol* 16: 151–156.
96. Van Gele M., Leonard J.H., Van Roy N., *et al.* (2002). Combined karyotyping, CGH and M-FISH analysis allows detailed characterization of unidentified chromosomal rearrangements in Merkel cell carcinoma. *Int J Cancer* 101: 137–145.
97. Becker J.C., Houben R., Ugurel S., *et al.* (2009). MC polyomavirus is frequently present in Merkel cell carcinoma of European patients. *J Invest Dermatol* 129: 248–250.
98. Garneski K.M., Warcola A.H., Feng Q., *et al.* (2009). Merkel cell polyomavirus is more frequently present in North American than Australian Merkel cell carcinoma tumors. *J Invest Dermatol* 129: 246–248.

Chapter 18

Establishing a Multidisciplinary Merkel Cell Carcinoma Clinic

Evans C. Bailey, Sandra L. Wong and Christopher K. Bichakjian

To date, treatment of Merkel cell carcinoma has suffered from a fragmented approach. Given the rarity of Merkel cell carcinoma and the lack of prospective clinical data, communication between clinicians of different specialties, a standardized treatment approach, coordination of clinical care, and patient awareness and education, are imperative for the delivery of optimal care. Current National Comprehensive Cancer Network (NCCN) treatment guidelines for Merkel cell carcinoma acknowledge the aggressive clinical behavior of this disease and the conflicting literature on the treatment and outcome of Merkel cell carcinoma.[1] The NCCN guidelines therefore specifically advocate multidisciplinary care for the management of patients with Merkel cell carcinoma. Creating a multidisciplinary clinic requires extensive coordination of care with multiple medical specialties. Once established, a multidisciplinary clinic provides a resource for institutions to provide the highest quality care to patients with Merkel cell carcinoma and their families. Prior to reviewing how a multidisciplinary clinic specific for Merkel cell carcinoma can be established, it is helpful to review some of the major advantages of such a clinic.

18.1 Benefits of Multidisciplinary Care

In an effort to improve the quality of medical care in the United States, The Institute of Medicine (IOM) proposed six aims for high quality care: care must be effective, safe, timely, efficient, equitable, and patient centered.[2] A national panel of cancer experts, convened by the National Cancer Institute (NCI), examined how these IOM goals can be specifically applied to caring for cancer patients.[3] In their report, the expert panel considered coordination of care among specialists to be an essential element of delivering high quality oncologic care.[3] Lack of coordination of care was considered to be a barrier that threatens every IOM aim for improving patient care. The integrated approach of a multidisciplinary clinic provides an avenue for fulfilling the IOM aims and allows institutions to consistently deliver high quality oncologic care.

A central aim identified by the IOM is that care must be effective, that is, based on the best clinical evidence.[3] It is rarely if ever possible for one clinician to be fully abreast of the latest developments in all areas of medical oncology, surgical oncology, radiation oncology, pathology, and mental health care that impact a cancer patient's care. This complexity of oncology, particularly in elderly patients with other medical comorbidities, often requires that patients be treated by multiple specialists. This is particularly true for Merkel cell carcinoma, in which patients are often seen by multiple specialties such as dermatology, surgical oncology, medical oncology, radiation oncology, otolaryngology, plastic surgery, dermatopathology, and psychiatry. Unlike other cutaneous malignancies such as melanoma, for which evidence-based treatment guidelines have been established, treatment of Merkel cell carcinoma requires determination of best-care guidelines from the existing, and at times conflicting, literature. Physicians from each specialty must critically review the literature and determine their role in a given patient's care. A multidisciplinary clinic can develop expert consensus guidelines that incorporate the best and most current data across multiple specialties, to provide the most effective care for each patient.[3,4]

The IOM report also determined that high quality medical care must be safe and equitable. Implementation of established treatment guidelines is an essential way in which multidisciplinary clinics achieve these goals. The NCI expert panel observed that cancer patients frequently receive inadequate care because cancer care is not delivered in a standardized fashion and established treatment guidelines are not followed.[3]

By ensuring that patients receive care that adheres to established best-care guidelines, and ensuring that all patients are offered this standard of care, multidisciplinary clinics deliver safe, high quality care in an equitable fashion to all patients. There are numerous reports demonstrating the beneficial impact on patient care made by multidisciplinary clinics.[5–7] In Europe, substantial variations from accepted melanoma practices are seen in patients treated outside an academic setting.[8] A multidisciplinary approach maximizes the chance that all patients are offered treatment that is consistent with the standard of care.

Another IOM goal for high quality medical care is that it must be efficient, and multidisciplinary clinics achieve this goal in several ways. It has been demonstrated for melanoma that multidisciplinary care at a large academic medical center that observes national guidelines can be more cost-efficient than a less organized traditional community-based approach.[9] When appropriately structured, the coordinated care provided by multidisciplinary academic clinics prevents duplication of tests, limits the number of physician visits, and delivers cost efficient, high quality care.

Beyond an immediate cost analysis, multidisciplinary care is also efficient as it uses its resources to deliver care while simultaneously striving to improve care. In providing a structured framework for treating patients, a multidisciplinary clinic provides a valuable opportunity to collect prospective data in an effort to continue to improve patient care and promote clinical and basic research. The number of patients needed to conduct any meaningful research for a disease as rare as Merkel cell carcinoma would be nearly impossible to obtain without a dedicated multidisciplinary clinic, which may serve as a regional, national, and international referral center. Such a clinic is an avenue for clinical trials, prospective documentation of patient demographics and clinical outcomes, and the establishment of a tumor tissue bank. The rarity of Merkel cell carcinoma is reflected in the scarcity of clinical data. Because of the severity of disease, there is a critical need for clinical and basic research to better characterize the biology of this disease, and determine optimal treatment modalities. A multidisciplinary clinic provides the resources to achieve these goals.

The fifth goal of the IOM is to ensure that care is provided in a patient centered fashion. An essential element of patient care is education, and multidisciplinary clinics provide an opportunity to educate patients and their families about their condition and available treatments. Lack of patient education has been specifically identified by the NCI as a major barrier to providing high quality oncologic care.[3] Through equipping patients and families with information on their condition and the treatments available, multidisciplinary clinics facilitate shared decision making. In a survey of cancer patients, over half of patients believed their physician did not provide them with sufficient information, illustrating the need for improvement in patient education.[10] A multidisciplinary clinic provides cancer patients with a centralized resource for information to help them understand their diagnosis and treatment options. A study examining an educational video designed for melanoma patients seen in a multidisciplinary clinic demonstrated an increase in knowledge and a decline in anxiety for patients who were provided this resource.[11] Such studies demonstrate the improvements in care that can be achieved by delivering patient centered care.

Finally, a sixth goal of the IOM and an essential component of quality care, is timely delivery of care. Even if all the abovementioned IOM goals are achieved, failure to provide timely care will prevent delivery of high quality care. Multidisciplinary clinics achieve the IOM goal of timely care by providing care in a coordinated, efficient fashion. Insufficient teamwork and communication among caregivers frequently results in treatment delays and prevents delivery of high quality care for cancer patients.[3] A multidisciplinary clinic provides a single clinical resource that facilitates information transfer among all members of the patient's care-team, coordinates the patients' appointments, and often allows patients to meet with multiple specialists on a single day. This coordinated care allows patients to receive their care in a timely, expedited fashion.

The care provided by multidisciplinary tumor clinics embodies the aims for high-quality care published by the IOM and overcomes known barriers to providing high-quality oncologic care. Patients with a rare and aggressive malignancy such as Merkel cell carcinoma greatly benefit from such an approach.

18.2 Developing a Multidisciplinary Merkel Cell Carcinoma Clinic

Numerous designs can be envisioned for the establishment of a multidisciplinary clinic. Each design, however, shares as a fundamental feature that all team members must be dedicated to the highest level of patient care. Dedication to patient care ensures an interdisciplinary team approach to managing each patient, and fosters cooperation among the various services. We describe a centralized intake hub model based on an established multidisciplinary melanoma and Merkel cell carcinoma clinic, designed to overcome the recognized barriers to the delivery of optimal oncologic care (Figure 1).[4,12]

18.2.1 *Intake*

The patient experience begins with a well trained nursing staff that serves as the centralized intake point for all patients. Patients with a biopsy proven diagnosis of Merkel cell carcinoma speak with a clinical coordinator who explains the process and gathers the required information. The clinical coordinator obtains demographic information, outside records, pathology slides, imaging studies and referring physician information. Pathology slides are reviewed by the dermatopathology team member prior to the patient's initial consultation to confirm the diagnosis of

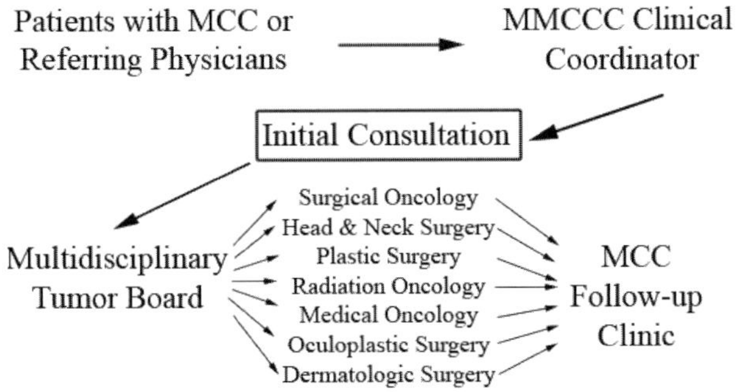

Figure 1. Centralized intake hub model for a multidisciplinary Merkel cell carcinoma clinic (MMCCC).

Merkel cell carcinoma. The pathology report and all of the patient's information are compiled in a report that is printed and distributed to all multidisciplinary team members prior to the patient's first clinic visit. An appointment is scheduled for an initial consultation in the multidisciplinary Merkel cell carcinoma clinic. Every attempt is made to see patients within one week of their referral. Because the diagnosis of Merkel cell carcinoma relies on the dermatopathologist, special attention is devoted to obtaining and reviewing the biopsy slides. The dermatopathology team member will review all slides immediately upon receiving them, often discussing the findings with team members prior to the patient's initial consultation. If all information is not received by the time of the patient's initial consultation, an addendum report is compiled and distributed to all team members after the supplemental information is received. Consultation with team members from various specialties, as well as preoperative visits, may be coordinated on the same day, if anticipated by the nurse coordinator.

18.2.2 *Consultation*

On the day of the initial consultation in the multidisciplinary Merkel cell carcinoma clinic, the patient is first seen by the dermatology team member specializing in cutaneous oncology. A comprehensive history is taken and complete skin and lymph node examinations are performed, with careful attention to the primary tumor site and draining lymphatics. During an hour-long consultation, the patient and their family members are extensively educated about Merkel cell carcinoma in general and as it relates to their particular circumstance. The patient is educated on how to perform, and the importance of performing, regular self skin and lymph node examinations. Patients are provided literature and guided to a variety of reliable Internet-based sources of information on cutaneous oncology in general and Merkel cell carcinoma in particular. Based on the history and the physical findings, the treatment options are discussed in detail. If additional tests are indicated (such as an imaging study or a fine needle aspirate of a palpable lymph node), these are discussed with the patient and performed the same day or scheduled at the earliest convenience. If the patient has additional appointments with other multidisciplinary team members, the pertinent information gathered from the initial consultation is relayed to the other team members. The patient is frequently able to meet other team members on the day of the initial consultation or shortly thereafter. Treatment is scheduled in a timely and appropriate fashion, typically within two to three weeks or sooner if medically indicated. Importantly, the patient and their family are provided the contact information for the physician from the initial consultation, who then serves as the contact point for managing their care and implementing the multidisciplinary plan. This provides a clear point of contact for patients when questions arise throughout their treatment. At the conclusion of this visit, a preliminary treatment plan is discussed with the patient and the case is then presented at the multidisciplinary tumor board meeting.

18.2.3 *Multidisciplinary tumor board meeting*

On a biweekly basis, the multidisciplinary tumor board meets to discuss all new patients seen since the last meeting and any follow-up issues concerning established patients with Merkel cell carcinoma. A preliminary plan of care is formulated and communicated to the patient and the family at the time of their first consultation. To expedite care, tumor board members communicate between tumor board meetings via email, allowing care plans to be formulated and surgeries to be scheduled in a timely manner. The final treatment plan for each patient is then reviewed and approved by the tumor board. A compilation containing all clinical and laboratory data on each patient to be discussed is provided to all tumor board members for review at the beginning of the meeting. The tumor board members discuss the recommendations for treatment, and formulate a final plan based on NCCN guidelines, treatment algorithms established by the tumor board from the best available evidence in the literature, and personal experiences of the individual members.[4,12] If indicated, additional tests are scheduled by the clinical coordinator.

18.2.4 *Treatment*

During this phase the patient may be treated by one or several team members from various specialties, such as surgical oncology, head and neck surgery, plastic surgery, oculoplastic surgery, radiation oncology, medical oncology, dermatology, and/or psychiatry (see Figure 1). If indicated throughout treatment, the patient may be re-presented at the multidisciplinary tumor board meeting to discuss relevant pathology results (such as a positive sentinel lymph node biopsy) or treatment response. Upon completion of the treatment plan as outlined by the tumor board, the patient is represented to determine an appropriate follow-up plan.

18.2.5 *Follow-up*

The last, but certainly not least, important role of a multidisciplinary clinic for a rare malignancy such as Merkel cell carcinoma is to establish appropriate follow-up care. Upon completion of therapy, follow-up is scheduled in the multidisciplinary Merkel cell carcinoma clinic with one of the dermatology team members, who will serve as a liaison to the other services involved in the care of the patient. At any time throughout the follow-up period, the patient can be represented to the multidisciplinary tumor board with any new findings that may require multidisciplinary input. This approach provides continuity of care and efficiency for the patient and ensures continuation of multidisciplinary care. It also results in significant efficiency for the clinic by eliminating clinic visits to multiple specialties for the same issues. Lastly, consistent follow-up provides an excellent opportunity to prospectively document outcomes in patients with a rare malignancy. On rare occasions, concerns specific to a certain specialty may require follow-up by more than one physician.

The described centralized intake hub model attempts to seamlessly integrate all the components of the complex care of patients with Merkel cell carcinoma involving multiple specialties into a single multidisciplinary clinic. This approach provides patients with the highest level of care, while providing multiple educational opportunities for those involved in delivering the care.

References

1. Miller S.J., Alam M., Andersen J., *et al.* (2009). Merkel cell carcinoma. *J Natl Compr Canc Netw* 7: 322–332.

2. An K.P., Ratner D. (2001). Merkel cell carcinoma in the setting of HIV infection. *J Am Acad Dermatol* 45: 309–312.
3. Aiello Bowles E.J., Tuzzio L., Wiese C.J., *et al.* (2008). Understanding high-quality cancer care: a summary of expert perspectives. *Cancer* 112: 934–942.
4. Bichakjian C.K., Lowe L., Lao C.D., *et al.* (2007). Merkel cell carcinoma: critical review with guidelines for multidisciplinary management. *Cancer* 110: 1–12.
5. Nesbitt C., Glendinnin R.J., Byrne C., *et al.* (2007). Factors that influence treatment strategies in advanced colorectal cancer. *Eur J Surg Oncol* 33(Suppl 2): S88–S94.
6. Newman E.A., Guest A.B., Helvie M.A., *et al.* (2006). Changes in surgical management resulting from case review at a breast cancer multidisciplinary tumor board. *Cancer* 107: 2346–2351.
7. Pawlik T.M., Laheru D., Hruban R.H., *et al.* (2008). Evaluating the impact of a single-day multidisciplinary clinic on the management of pancreatic cancer. *Ann Surg Oncol* 15: 2081–2088.
8. Grange F., Vitry F., Granel-Brocard F., *et al.* (2008). Variations in management of stage I to stage III cutaneous melanoma: a population-based study of clinical practices in France. *Arch Dermatol* 144: 629–636.
9. Fader D.J., Wise C.G., Normolle D.P., *et al.* (1998). The multidisciplinary melanoma clinic: a cost outcomes analysis of specialty care. *J Am Acad Dermatol* 38(5 Pt 1): 742–751.
10. Chen X., Siu L.L. (2001). Impact of the media and the internet on oncology: survey of cancer patients and oncologists in Canada. *J Clin Oncol* 19: 4291–4297.
11. Orringer J.S., Fendrick A.M., Trask P.C., *et al.* (2005). The effects of a professionally produced videotape on education and anxiety/distress levels for patients with newly diagnosed melanoma: a randomized, prospective clinical trial. *J Am Acad Dermatol* 53: 224–229.
12. Johnson T.M., Chang A., Redman B., *et al.* (2000). Management of melanoma with a multidisciplinary melanoma clinic model. *J Am Acad Dermatol* 42(5 Pt 1): 820–826.

Appendix I

Guidelines for Individualized Management and Opportunities for Further Research

Christopher A. Puleo, Jonathan S. Zager and Vernon K. Sondak

Introduction

These guidelines cover the main stages and presentations of Merkel cell carcinoma (localized, clinically nodal, distant disease), and are not intended to be comprehensive or cover every possible presentation of this disease. Special situations like in transit recurrence (Chapters 10 and 14) are covered in the textbook chapters themselves. The approach outlined here is based on the principles of management utilized by the Moffitt Cancer Center Cutaneous Oncology Program, as well as on guidelines developed by the National Comprehensive Cancer Network (NCCN) and other proposed guidelines (Bichakjian, *Cancer* 2007) for evaluation, management and follow-up. Like all guidelines, they are intended to inform decision-making, not mandate a standard of practice, and there could be many circumstances where specific details of an individual's case call for approaches different than those outlined herein. In the Moffitt Cutaneous Oncology Program, an emphasis is placed on individualized treatment, 'personalized cancer care,' rather than strict adherence to any algorithm. We have tried to highlight those areas where we routinely individualize decision-making with the term *individualize*. For example, rather than routinely use postoperative radiation therapy after all excisions of primary Merkel cell cancers, we individualize the use of radiation based on several clinical factors, most importantly the adequacy of the margins achieved around the primary tumor.

Furthermore, these guidelines try to identify specific areas where further research is needed to understand the role of an evaluation, management or follow-up strategy, using the tag *research*. In many cases, such as in the histopathologic assessment of the primary tumor to cite one prominent example, it is unclear how new information (like tumor thickness as an additional or alternative factor to assess primary tumors' risk of recurrence and metastasis) is to be used, but we believe it will be important to accumulate sufficient data to correlate this factor with outcomes. In other areas, such as the use of preoperative ultrasonography to evaluate regional lymph nodes prior to sentinel node biopsy, we can draw analogies to how this information is used in the management of melanoma, but research is needed to see if the results in Merkel cell carcinoma are similar or different before the approach is widely adopted.

As is stressed throughout this entire textbook, many important questions remain about the management of Merkel cell carcinoma, and few prospective studies have been conducted. Some of the approaches we use at Moffitt are different than those used at other high-volume centers; our approaches are not offered as 'definitive' but rather as 'representative' of an aggressive, multimodality approach. In particular, the use of radiation and chemotherapy in this disease varies widely worldwide. As we have assessed the literature, recent studies provide evidence that use of radiation should be individualized rather than routine, and that many patients can be treated without radiation with acceptable results. The literature also suggests strongly that the sentinel node negative basin can be safely observed without additional surgical therapy, whereas the sentinel node-positive basin should be treated with either radiation or completion node dissection, but only in specific situations with both. We have designated the decisions regarding radiation and completion node dissection as ones that should be 'individualized,' to reflect the strong support for different options and the evidence that there are identifiable factors that can be used to select among them. In contrast, for example, we have designated decisions regarding adjuvant chemotherapy as 'research' to reflect the strong differences of opinion in the literature and the lack of sufficient objective data to make a clear determination about its role. Please note that we are not indicating that adjuvant chemotherapy in this disease should be done only in a clinical trial setting, but rather that more research is needed before we can say for certain which patients, if any, most clearly benefit from its use. In fact, in our clinical practice and in other centers, adjuvant chemotherapy is frequently used, especially in younger patients and those with indications of very high risk for recurrence. The 'research' designation in this context should help clinicians discuss this option with their patients, and a balanced discussion should reflect that there is much we do not know about the optimum management of this disease.

Finally, follow-up guidelines represent our suggested approach, and we must acknowledge the limited or non-existent data to support any particular follow-up strategy. We call attention to the fact that in our guidelines, follow-up is extended compared to many guidelines that call for intensive surveillance only in the first two postoperative years, because recent studies document that many recurrences do occur after year 2, and with multimodality treatment delayed recurrences may become even more frequent in the future. In thinking about postoperative surveillance, we consider that recurrent and metastatic Merkel cell carcinoma is often more responsive to treatment than melanoma, but whether using imaging studies to identify recurrent or metastatic disease sooner results in better treatment outcomes or improves quality of life is completely unknown at present. Recently, we have come to rely more on PET-CT fusion imaging than on contrast-enhanced CT scans, but comparative data is very limited, and in fact we feel that the available data is insufficient to make any specific recommendation about postoperative imaging surveillance, even in clinically node-positive patients. We use it, but more research is clearly needed, and at present even among practitioners at our own center no consensus has emerged. We have not found any type of blood testing to be of value in the follow-up of Merkel cell carcinoma patients.

A. Clinically Localized Cutaneous Merkel Cell Carcinoma

1. *Clinically node negative (stage I and II)*

a) Pathology assessment of the primary tumor (see Chapter 5).

1. Tumor diameter.
2. Immunohistochemical staining to establish the diagnosis and rule out metastatic lung cancer (AE1/AE3 cytokeratins,

cytokeratin 20 and TTF-1); consider S-100 and/or leucocyte common antigen as needed to rule out melanoma or lymphoma.
3. *research* Tumor thickness.
4. *research* Presence or absence of angiolymphatic invasion.

b) Wide excision of the primary tumor (see Chapters 10 and 11).
1. *research* 1 vs. 2 cm margin of excision around the primary tumor or biopsy scar.
2. *individualize* Postoperative radiation to the primary tumor site (see Chapters 10 and 13).
   (a) Close or positive margins on final pathology.
   (b) *research* Tumor thickness, diameter or angiolymphatic invasion as indicators for postoperative radiation.

c) Assessment of the regional lymph nodes.
1. Preoperative lymphoscintigraphy with sentinel lymph node biopsy (see Chapters 10 and 11).
2. Immunohistochemical staining (AE1/AE3 cytokeratin) routinely used to evaluate the sentinel node.
3. *research* Preoperative lymph node ultrasonography with guided fine needle aspiration cytology of suspicious nodes, done either prior to or after lymphoscintigraphy but before sentinel lymph node biopsy (see Chapter 9).
4. If sentinel node positive on final pathology, go to **Microscopically node positive** (item 2 below).

d) Follow-up for the sentinel node negative patient.
1. Years 1 through 3: Physical examination every three to four months; dermatologist follow-up every six to 12 months as needed.
2. Years 4 and 5: Physical examination every six months; dermatologist follow-up every six to 12 months as needed.
3. Beyond year 5: Physical examination every 12 months; dermatologist follow-up every 12 months.

Routine laboratory determinations and imaging studies are not routinely indicated but should be used for evaluation of symptoms or physical examination findings.

2. ***Microscopically node positive (sentinel node biopsy positive, pathologic stage III)***

a) Postoperative management of the primary as discussed above (item A.1).
b) *individualize* Node dissection alone, radiation to the nodal basin alone or node dissection plus postoperative radiation is recommended based on whether or not the patient will undergo radiation to the primary site and the histologic findings at sentinel node biopsy (number of positive nodes, presence or absence of extracapsular extension in the sentinel node); if completion node dissection is done, post-dissection radiation is individualized based on the histologic findings in the non-sentinel nodes as well.
   a. **Radiation therapy to the nodal basin without node dissection:** for patients who are going to undergo radiation to the primary site, with "low volume" sentinel node metastasis without extracapsular extension.
   b. **Completion lymph node dissection without nodal irradiation:** for patients who are not going to undergo radiation to the primary site and who have no extracapsular extension in the sentinel or non-sentinel lymph nodes.
   c. **Complete lymph node dissection with postoperative radiation:** for patients with extracapsular extension in the sentinel or non-sentinel node, and/or for patients with multiple positive lymph nodes *individualize* based on the nodal basin site and the total number of positive nodes; the threshold number of positive nodes that signifies sufficiently high risk of regional recurrence to justify the morbidity of postoperative nodal irradiation is still undetermined, but it is recognized that the morbidity of postoperative radiation is greatest after inguinal node dissection.
c) Follow-up: as per A.1d above; *research* **the role of routine imaging studies in the follow-up of the microscopically node positive patient has not been established at this time**.

B. Clinically Node-Positive Cutaneous Merkel Cell Carcinoma Including Unknown Primary and Recurrence in a Regional Nodal Basin (Clinical Stage III)

1. Management of the primary, if present, as discussed above (item A.1).
2. Preoperative imaging with PET-CT scan or contrast-enhanced CT scan of the chest and abdomen (with pelvis for lower extremity and lower trunk primary sites or neck for head and neck primary sites).
3. Brain MRI only for evaluation of symptomatic patients.
4. Complete lymph node dissection with postoperative radiation.
5. *research* **Adjuvant postoperative chemotherapy has not been established to improve relapse-free or overall survival, but is widely used, particularly for younger patients** (see Chapter 15).
6. *individualize* 'Neoadjuvant' chemotherapy and/or radiation is considered for patients with unresectable nodal disease based on involvement of major vessels or nerves.
7. Follow-up: As per A.1d above except imaging studies are more commonly used in follow-up, but **the optimum modality and frequency of imaging for node-positive patients has not been established at this time**.

C. Metastatic Disease Beyond the Regional Nodal Basin (Stage IV)

1. Imaging with PET-CT scan or contrast-enhanced CT scan of the chest, abdomen and pelvis (see Chapter 9).
2. Brain MRI only for evaluation of symptomatic patients.
3. Radiation therapy for symptomatic lesions or asymptomatic bony metastases in critical or weight-bearing sites (see Chapter 13).
4. Systemic chemotherapy with platinum- or doxorubicin-based regimen (see Chapter 14).
5. *individualize* Consider surgery for isolated resectable metastases in patients with good functional status, with or without preoperative systemic or radiation therapy (see Chapter 10).

Appendix II

Merkel Cell Carcinoma: Information for Patients, Families and Caregivers Frequently Asked Questions

Mary H. Lien, Darcelle Welker, Stephanie Andrews and Paul Nghiem

1. **What is Merkel cell carcinoma?**
   Merkel cell carcinoma is a rare form of skin cancer that often grows rapidly and can be fatal in one-third or more of cases. It is believed to originate from Merkel cells, which are neuroendocrine cells that have nerve and hormone functions and also act as touch receptors.

2. **What does Merkel cell carcinoma look like?**
   Merkel cell carcinoma may look like an ordinary cyst or a flesh-colored, red or purple bump on or under the skin. It can occur anywhere on the body but is typically on sun-exposed skin such as the head, neck and arms. In most cases, the Merkel cell tumor is not painful or tender. There are no absolutely characteristic features to indicate when something is a Merkel cell tumor, and this makes diagnosis particularly difficult.

3. **Who gets Merkel cell carcinoma?**
   Patients who develop Merkel cell carcinoma typically are 65 years of age or older, fair-skinned individuals who have had significant past sun exposure. Some but not all patients who develop Merkel cell carcinoma have weakened immune systems, such as patients with organ transplants or HIV. There is no evidence that Merkel cell

carcinoma is passed on through families. The specific causes of Merkel cell carcinoma are not entirely known at this time, but there is increasing evidence that at least some cases of Merkel cell carcinoma may be associated with a virus called Merkel cell polyoma virus (MCPyV). It is not known exactly how many cases of Merkel cell carcinoma are linked to the virus or whether those cases behave better, worse or the same as those not related to the virus.

4. **Is Merkel cell carcinoma contagious?**
   Although Merkel cell carcinoma has been linked to a virus, it has never been shown to be transmitted from one person to another by contact with an affected individual. Therefore it is *not* considered contagious.

5. **How would I know if I have Merkel cell carcinoma?**
   Only a biopsy (removal of all or part of the tumor for analysis under the microscope by a pathologist) can tell for certain if a person has Merkel cell carcinoma. Often specialized testing is required in the pathology laboratory to determine that a tumor is Merkel cell carcinoma and not a different form of cancer arising from the skin or elsewhere in the body.

6. **What is the treatment for Merkel cell carcinoma?**
   After the biopsy, Merkel cell carcinoma is usually treated with a surgical procedure to remove any remaining tumor. Additionally, in many cases a sentinel lymph node biopsy is performed at the time of surgery to check the state of the lymph nodes. A sentinel lymph node biopsy is a procedure in which a radioactive tracer and a blue dye are injected into or around the tumor site, and any nearby lymph nodes which take up the dye are identified and surgically removed. The sentinel lymph node biopsy is a sensitive procedure that is utilized to detect any spread of the cancer at its earliest stage before the lymph nodes become enlarged and before it can be seen on scans. Imaging scans such as X-rays, CT scans, MRI, bone scans, and PET scans are utilized in certain circumstances to find out if Merkel cell carcinoma has spread to the lymph nodes and elsewhere in the body. In most

cases, a multidisciplinary team of surgical oncologists, dermatologists, medical oncologists, and radiation oncologists will be involved to determine the best course of management.

7. **What other treatment options are there besides surgery for Merkel cell carcinoma?**
In addition to surgery, radiation is another type of important treatment used to treat Merkel cell carcinoma. Radiation therapy is administered by radiation oncologists and it is used to treat the tumor site and/or any affected lymph nodes. Another method to treat Merkel cell carcinoma is chemotherapy, which uses drugs to treat the cancer by killing the tumor cells. Chemotherapy is often reserved for the later stages of Merkel cell carcinoma. For early Merkel cell carcinoma that has not metastasized (spread to other parts of the body), surgery and radiation therapy are the most commonly recommended treatments.

8. **What are the chances of survival with Merkel cell carcinoma?**
Like other forms of cancer, the outlook for survival depends on how advanced the Merkel cell carcinoma is at the time of diagnosis and what the response is to treatments that are administered. Merkel cell carcinoma is staged as local (in the skin), nodal (in the lymph nodes) or metastatic. When the Merkel cell carcinoma is metastatic, it may spread through the blood or lymphatic system to other organs, including the brain, lung, bone and liver, and lymph nodes throughout the body. The prognosis for survival correlates to the stage of Merkel cell carcinoma. The local stage has the highest cure rate, while the metastatic stage has the lowest survival. Merkel cell carcinoma will be fatal in approximately 30% of patients overall. The chance for survival is better if the cancer has not spread to the lymph nodes or beyond, and may also be better for patients with a normal immune system.

9. **What is the recommended follow-up?**
Follow-up recommendations, like treatment recommendations, vary from person to person based on the preferences of the treatment team and the stage of the cancer. Most recurrences of Merkel cell carcinoma occur in the first three to five years after diagnosis, so follow-up is the

most intensive during that period of time and may be less frequent thereafter. There are no specific blood tests or X-rays that can always detect recurrent Merkel cell carcinoma. For early stages of the disease, follow-up emphasizes skin and lymph node examinations and relies relatively less on X-rays and scans. Scans may be used more often in patients with later stages of disease. Regardless of the follow-up intervals and tests ordered, Merkel cell carcinoma patients noticing new lesions or other unexplained signs or symptoms that do not go away promptly should let their doctor know so that they can be evaluated if necessary prior to the next scheduled visit.

10. Could my children inherit Merkel cell carcinoma?

There have been no reports to date where Merkel cell carcinoma developed in the other family members of Merkel cell carcinoma patients. No genetic susceptibility to Merkel cell carcinoma has ever been identified.

11. Where can I find a patient support group for Merkel cell carcinoma?

An interactive support group for Merkel cell carcinoma can be located at http://groups.google.com/group/merkelcell to further discuss Merkel cell carcinoma with other patients, families and caregivers.

Appendix III

Internet Resources Relating to Merkel Cell Carcinoma for Providers, Patients, Family Members and Caregivers

Rosalind E. Atchison, Angie Paniagua and Jane L. Messina

Introduction

The Internet can be a valuable and powerful tool for researching medical information. However, for those who have no medical or technological background, 'surfing the web' can be challenging and a bit intimidating, especially when looking for factual data. Unfortunately, information (often called 'content') on the Internet does not have to be checked and validated before it is made public, and the quality of the information can range from very good to poor. Some helpful tips to remember:

1. **Consider the source.** Who has written the content? What are the author's qualifications? Do they give their contact information?
2. **Know your domain.** Different domains (the two or three letters after the period or 'dot' in the Internet address) contain different types of information.
   - **.gov**. U.S. government (non-military)
   - **.mil**. U.S. military
   - **.edu**. Educational site, often a college or university
   - **.com**. Commercial business

- **.net**. Networks and internet service providers
- **.org**. U.S. non-profit organizations

As a general rule, information found on **.gov**, **.mil**, and **.edu** sites are considered to be most accurate, but this is just a generalization and not a guarantee of accuracy.

3. **Check the date.** When researching medical information, it is important that the content be up to date. Check to see if the site has a 'last updated' date stamp, or any other indication of how often the information has been reviewed and updated.
4. **Check the level.** Is the information appropriate for your academic level? Is it easy to understand for a person with no medical background, or is it written for a healthcare professional?
5. **Support.** Is the website easy to navigate? Does it offer support/assistance? Does it give you gateways, which are links to other high-quality content?

Using the Internet as a research tool for medical information has given patients empowerment to gather information about their health conditions, so that they may take charge of themselves. In doing so, they can better prepare themselves for their doctor's appointments and ask pertinent questions regarding their healthcare. Because of the rarity of Merkel cell carcinoma, online information is still scarce. This Appendix reviews and evaluates the features of the major websites devoted to this subject. It is our intent that these resources will be advantageous in a patient's search for valuable information on this rare disease. Please recognize, however, that the information available on the Internet changes all the time — no one resource can ever keep up with all of the changes and information that is out there in 'cyberspace.'

Merkel Cell Carcinoma Websites

http://www.merkelcell.org/

This website was developed by the Fred Hutchinson Cancer Research Center/Seattle Cancer Care Alliance, a member of the National Comprehensive Cancer Network (NCCN). It is an excellent and concise resource created by Dr. Paul Nghiem and his team, with a grant from the

American Cancer Society and the Jerry Wachter Fund, to educate patients and their physicians about Merkel cell carcinoma. This site features frequently asked questions (FAQ's), a glossary of terminology, information about the disease itself, diagnosis, photographs, staging, prognosis, treatment, referral centers, news, and useful links. *English only.*

http://www.cancer.gov/cancertopics/pdg/treatment/merkelcell/patient/
(National Cancer Institute-PDQ) The National Cancer Institute's (NCI) cancer information database contains summaries on cancer care for both patients and health care professionals. Easy to understand information on the disease, including prevention, treatment and clinical trials, is available, and the site provides gateways to other helpful sites. There are toll-free telephone numbers for more information, which are also available for the deaf and hearing impaired. The summary on this website lends itself well to printing for patient handouts. *Also available in Spanish.*

http://www.cancer.gov/cancertopics/factsheet/Sites-Types/merkel-cell
(National Cancer Institute) This website provides information on prevention, genetics, causes and treatment of Merkel cell carcinoma. There is a guide that will assist in searching for cancer treatment and clinical trials. It also includes NCI-supported research, special reports and statistical information related to cancer incidence, mortality and survival. *Also available in Spanish.*

http://www.moffitt.org/EducationalLinks.aspx?spid=8BF2079F7A564ED0B2E2EA20439F8838
The H. Lee Moffitt Cancer Center and Research Institute, an NCCN member, created this educational link, which offers an overview of Merkel cell carcinoma covering description, stages and treatment options. You can also access the Moffitt Cutaneous Oncology Program website or go to 'Cancer Answers' and find a toll-free phone number or email a Moffitt physician or nurse with your cancer-related questions. *Also available in Spanish.*

http://www.dana-farber.org/can/cancer
The Dana Farber Cancer Institute, an NCCN member, sponsors this site. Most of the information on this website is available in two formats: one

written for patients, another written for medical professionals. The patient version uses easy to understand terminology. Sections include information on clinical trials (updated regularly), screening and detection, supportive care, symptom management, diagnostic tests, integrative therapies and further resources on the Web. *English only.*

http://www.massgeneral.org/conditions/condition.aspx?ID=302&type=conditions
The Massachusetts General Hospital Cancer Center, an NCCN member, sponsors this website which offers an overview on Merkel cell carcinoma with common questions asked regarding this disease. There is a link to 'connect with others' that offers a variety of ways to communicate with support groups, survivors and family members. *English only.*

http://www.mayoclinic.com/health/merkel-cell-carcinoma/DS00802
This accredited website, written by the Mayo Clinic staff, gives a comprehensive overview of Merkel cell carcinoma. It covers definitions, symptoms, causes, risk factors, complications, tests, treatment, and prevention. It is easy to understand and navigate for patients, family and health care professionals. A unique and helpful feature is the ability to contact the staff by e-mail with questions. *English only.*

http://www.emedicine.com/derm/topic262.htm
This website from WebMD, with contributions from leading physicians in dermatology and pathology, provides detailed information for both patient and healthcare providers. It includes pathophysiology and a multi-media file. *English only.*

http://www.nccn.org/professionals/physician_gls/PDF/mcc.pdf
The National Comprehensive Cancer Network (NCCN) website is run by a panel of physicians from 21 leading cancer institutions, who have worked together to develop clinical practice guidelines for a current approach in treating cancer. Guidelines address surgery, staging, chemotherapy, radiation, and clinical trials. The guidelines are updated yearly. This site is tailored for health care professionals. *Subscription required*

Support Groups

http://groups.google.com/group/merkelcell
This website was created by a group of patients with Merkel cell carcinoma for the use of patients, family members and other professionals to share their experience with this rare disease. There is a current membership of approximately 320 patients and family members.

References

Guadagnino C. (July 2000). 'Using Medical Information on the Internet.' <www.physiciansnews.com/spotlight/700.html>

Pearson Education Development Group (2005). 'Finding Information on the Internet.' <http://www.infoplease.com/homework/u4evalinfo.html>

Place E., Kendall M., Hiom D., Booth H., Ayres P., Manuel A., Smith P. (2006). 'Internet Detective: Wise Up to the Web.' 3rd Ed. Intute Virtual Training Suite <http://www.vts.intute.ac.uk/detective/>

Index